the truth about FOOD

The Good, the Bad and the Downright Dangerous

by Gillian Drake

SHANK PAINTER PUBLISHING

The Truth About Food

The Good, The Bad and The Downright Dangerous

The information provided in this book is intended to educate the reader, and nothing in this book should in any way be taken to constitute a medical diagnosis nor treatment for any disease or condition. Those people with a medical condition or disease are advised to seek the help of a health care provider.

BOOKS MAY BE ORDERED FROM:

GillianDrakeTruthAboutFood.com

OR:

SHANK PAINTER PUBLISHING
P. O. Box 720, North Eastham, MA 02651

PUBLISHED BY:

SHANK PAINTER PUBLISHING

ISBN:
978-1-888959-49-9

PRINTED IN USA

This book is dedicated to the

TRUTH

and to all who seek it

and to David Hawkins, MD, PhD

1927—2012

whose book *Power vs. Force*

shows how we can all learn to tell

Truth from Falsehood

Acknowledgements

I AM GRATEFUL TO THE FOLLOWING PEOPLE from whom I have learned so much over the years: Dr. David Leaf, Dr. Pamela Latimer, Dr. Paula Sperry, Dr. Kevin Lowey, Dr. Michael Singleton, Fred Allen, Kim Allen, PA, Lynne Delaney, and Dede Dunbar, all sane voices in what so often seemed like an insane world.

My deepest appreciation to: my dedicated editorial assistants, Anne Garton and Debi Boucher Stetson; Gail McMeekin and Berta Walker, whose support, advice and enthusiasm meant so much to me; all my friends who offered me encouragement, friendship and understanding during the production of this book: Lynne, Allison, Laura, Joyce, Kate, Kristina, Richard, Jim, Nick, Karen and Julian; and last but not least, my family—Ron, Tessa, Mick, Ewa, Leigh, Judith, and Clive.

Thanks are due to my local supermarket, the Stop & Shop in Orleans, MA, where I spent hours doing research for this book, and to my local food stores—the Orleans Whole Foods Store, Chatham Natural Market, Phoenix Fruit & Vegetables, and Friends Market—my life here on Cape Cod would be very different without you. Thanks also to the wonderful folk who run the Cape Cod Farmers' Markets and the local farmers who manage to raise delicious food in this sandy soil.

My deepest appreciation also to the following people who have inspired me over the years by sharing their stories and their wisdom in books, newsletters and lectures: Christopher Bird, Wayne Dyer, David Hawkins, Bruce Lipton, Joseph Mercola, Edgar Mitchell, Lynne McTaggart, Rupert Sheldrake, Brian Weiss, David Williams, and Marianne Williamson—they are the heroes of our time, exploring new frontiers and leading the way forward.

Table of Contents

"Illnesses do not come upon us out of the blue.
They are developed from small daily sins against Nature.
When enough sins have accumulated, illnesses will suddenly appear."

— HIPPOCRATES

Introduction

"A definitive review and close reading of medical peer-review journals and government health statistics shows that food frequently causes more harm than good. . . . [and] you will quickly come to the conclusion that food is the leading cause of death and injury in the United States."

— *From the Science-Based Medicine website*

THE TRUTH ABOUT FOOD IS THAT we are not told the truth about food—not by the medical profession, nor by the government, and certainly not by the food industry. The truth is that the nutritional level of food in the average supermarket is now so poor that we are literally poisoning ourselves and our children, condemning them to a life of ill health. According to a report in the *New England Journal of Medicine,* for the first time in 200 years, the current generation of children in America is expected to have shorter life expectancies than their parents.

This low-quality processed food is made from the cheapest ingredients and developed for a long shelf life, not for nutritional value. These foods realize huge profits for the food industry, profits that are being made at the expense of the U.S. population. This food is so bad for us that it has led to an epidemic of obesity and degenerative diseases which is causing untold suffering among the U.S. population, placing a huge financial burden on the country in the form of soaring health care and insurance costs and lost productivity.

The kinds of diseases caused by a poor diet are different from the type of illnesses or infections caused by a bacteria or virus which can be treated with an antibiotic or other drug. Degenerative diseases that are caused by diet are diseases that develop gradually over time, the result of a constant and continuous assault on the fine-tuned workings of the body, and cannot be cured with a simple drug. These are chronic conditions that start at the cellular level and, over time, lead to a breakdown in various functions and organs of the body. The most common are heart disease, cancer, diabetes, arthritis, osteoporosis, and dementia. Heart disease is the number one killer of American citizens, and cancer now affects one out of every three women, and one out of every two men. Nutritional experts have suggested that if we don't change our diets, in the next 40 years or so we will *all* lose our lives to cancer. Countless scientific studies have been performed trying to blame these diseases on various causes—it's the water we drink, the chemicals under our sink, pollution in the air. But the truth is, three or more times a day, day in and day out, most of us are unwittingly eating food that is really bad for us.

Most of us are confused about what we should eat to be healthy. We are constantly being bombarded with conflicting information: Cholesterol is bad! Eat vegetarian! Red meat causes cancer! Raw foods are best! Animal protein is good! Avoid eggs! Take vitamins! Drink pomegranate juice! How are we supposed to figure it all out? Much of the confusion comes from advice from well-meaning people who seem not to have studied the facts, or by those who have a vested interest in influencing what we eat, such as scientists developing blockbuster new drugs, vendors marketing highly-profitable processed foods, vitamins and supplements, or the latest exotic fruit juice that is guaranteed to cure all ills. How are we to find objective, factual, scientifically-driven information about which foods are healthy to eat and which are not?

This book answers that question by introducing a unique new way of determining the quality of food based not on a breakdown of its components—vitamins, minerals and so on—but on its *total nutritional value,* which includes its vitality, or life force energy—a crucial aspect of food that scientists have so far ignored.

We do in fact have an innate sense of which foods are healthy for us and which are not. At heart we know the difference, often we can actually *see* the difference—just compare a tomato fresh off the vine to the average supermarket variety, or a home-made pie compared to one from the frozen dessert section of a grocery store. It's the difference in water from a mountain stream compared to city water treated with chlorine, or a ripe peach plucked from a tree in summer compared to one from the local supermarket, hard as a bullet or mushy from being transported hundreds of miles. We can sense in them the life force energy that nourishes us as much as the air we breathe and the sun that shines upon us.

Up until now there's been no way of identifying exactly which foods are good for us and which aren't; that is, to identify the *quality* of a food—its intrinsic, aggregate nutritional value. And that's what this book is all about. We could say that the last thing the world needs is another book about diets, but this isn't just another diet book—it's a survival manual, a revolutionary new way of identifying which foods are good for us to eat and which are not, and the direct impact they have on our health.

Mass-produced food has not turned out to be the miracle it was intended. The corporate processed food industry has managed to push the bounds of ethics by using political influence to push through laws and subsidies that are in their best interests, not the consumer's.

The whole purpose of processing food is so it lasts longer on the shelf, which means that the most important part of food—its vitality, or life force energy—is removed in the interests of extended shelf-life. Thus the consumer is deprived of the most important nutrient of all while the food industry generates enormous profits at our expense. And let's not forget that cheap food is a political decision—when food is cheap and plentiful, there's money left over in the household budget for people to buy the latest electronic gadgets and new appliances. So in effect, the economy grows on the back of cheap food. But we do eventually pay the price—in poor health, soaring health care costs and lost productivity.

Most people trust the grocery stores where they buy their food—they are invariably bright and clean, filled with friendly staff, the shelves stocked with appealing looking products in a variety of seductive packages. But appearances lie, despite what the labels tell us. This food is far from healthy—in fact, in some cases it is deadly. Most people also trust the food industry ads, but slowly the truth is coming out and now we are realizing it's about making money, not providing us with healthy food. And it's even worse when it comes to food for children and pets.

Those magazine articles about how to make "delicious recipes" using processed supermarket food ("Just add a can of Campbell's mushroom soup to make this casserole a family favorite!") are mostly funded by advertising paid for by the corporate food industry, so of course they are going to be pushing their own money-making products. The media is largely owned by corporate America these days, so we can't expect to find honest information about the food we eat in magazines or on television. Even Public Television is now supported by grants from corporations.

It's interesting to look up the various definitions of "food." The one by Wikipedia says: "Food is any substance consumed to provide nutritional support for the body . . . to produce energy, maintain life, or stimulate growth." If this could be adopted as the legal definition of food by the U.S. government, then it might save a lot of lives and much suffering—highly processed food is not *food* in the acknowledged definition of the word since it does not nourish the body.

When I first read the book *Sugar Blues* by William Dufty many years ago, I was intrigued by his description of an encounter he had with Gloria Swanson, the Academy Award-winning actress, at a business meeting. As he was about to pop a sugar cube into his coffee, she hissed in his ear, "That stuff is poison. I won't have it in my house, let alone my body." Swanson, a legendary beauty, was known for following a healthy regime. She continued, "I used to get positively livid when I watched people eating poison, but I've learned that everyone has to find out for themselves—the hard way. Go ahead, eat your white sugar—kill yourself. See if I care." Swanson's advice changed Dufty's life, and was the inspiration for his book.

But I do care, and that's why I've written this book, so people can see and understand just what processed food is doing to us—to our health, to our children, to the future of this country.

After some serious health issues in 1990, I banished wheat and sugar from my diet and have remained wheat- and sugar-free since then. This new diet helped me regain my health, and the thrill of feeling really good and full of energy was incentive enough for me never to be tempted to revert to my former diet. But when people ask me how I remain so healthy and I tell them it's because I don't eat wheat or sugar, they immediately think it would impossible for them to do the same thing—which is just how I felt when I first realized I needed to change my diet to regain my health.

Changing our diet can be challenging because refined

carbohydrates have become dietary staples. And one particular combination—wheat and sugar—creates products that can be extremely addictive. A woman who works in a bakery said to me, "If I can't eat baked goods, my life would not be worth living." It might not be easy to give up these foods completely, but cutting way back might be good enough. And nowadays there are plenty of wheat-alternative products on the market, while cutting sugar out of your diet altogether just makes good sense. But it's good to know that we do have a choice, so we can look forward to years of good health rather than indulge in foods that will make us so ill we will become a burden on our family and on society.

I am distressed at what we as a nation are feeding ourselves and our families, assuming that the food we buy in the grocery store will nourish us and keep us healthy. This simply is not the case. I find it just heartbreaking that parents are doing their best to raise healthy kids, buying them everything they need, saving for college and planning a bright future, but feeding them inferior food. We CANNOT raise healthy kids on junk food like pizza and Pepsi—they need quality protein to build healthy flesh and bones. Pizza is just about one of the worst foods we can eat. I went to a birthday party recently where the adults had brought dishes of shrimp and chicken to share, but the three teenage boys present were provided with pizza and Coke—ironic, when they were the ones who really NEEDED the protein. This is being played out all over the country, and it is nothing short of a national tragedy.

My hope is that this book will raise awareness about how dangerous our food supply has become. America's future depends on raising healthy kids, our future citizens. We MUST feed our children healthy food—the consequences if we don't are too grim to think about.

For my part, I spend my money where I feel it makes the most difference, buying organic when possible, and choosing independent food producers and the "small guys" over the major food corporations. I buy eggs from a woman in the next town who raises chickens, and meat from a local farm. I go to Whole Foods Market and Trader Joe's when I can, frequent my local health food store and the independent shop that sells fresh fruit and vegetables, and visit my local farmer's market from May through November. Yes, it may cost more, but I rarely go to the doctor—I don't need to—and we all know how much money that saves.

As consumers, we need to take responsibility for our own health and wellbeing, and demand our basic rights for access to healthy food, clean air, pure water, and non-toxic treatment for diseases. But most of all we need a system that promotes the wellbeing of all Americans, not the wellbeing of the corporations. This is why "voting with our wallets"—buying only high-quality food—is an essential part of this game plan. And this book shows you how to do that by identifying the foods that are good for us, those that are bad, and those that are downright dangerous.

"He who has health has hope;
and he who has hope, has everything."
— THOMAS CARLYLE

CHAPTER 1

How to Read the Charts and What They Tell Us

WE LITERALLY ARE WHAT WE EAT, and our health is directly related to the nutritional level of the foods we consume. The intent of this book is to provide a way of making an informed choice about what kind of foods will keep us and our family healthy. The most important nutrient in our food is its vitality, or life force energy. Food is more than a breakdown of its parts—it is a living entity which nourishes our body at the cellular level. And it is the health of our cells that determines whether we are healthy or sick—healthy food creates healthy cells which create healthy people.

Science has shown us that all things in nature vibrate, including food and disease states, and these vibrational levels can be measured. These vibrational measurements are shown on the chart in two columns: **Comparative Vibrational Levels of Health and Disease States** in the left-hand hand column, and **Comparative Nutritional Levels of Various Food Groups** in the right-hand column. When a person consistently consumes low-grade food that vibrates at the level of disease, that disease will eventually occur in the body. There is a more extensive explanation of this vibrational energy in the chapter that follows.

In the center of each chart is an arrow showing the **Scale of Nutritional Value**: the top of the arrow represents the highest level—10,000—which is the level of perfect health equal to that of a healthy new-born baby, or primitive hunter-gatherer tribes who live on a diet free of processed foods. The scale gradually descends down to the level of the lowest vibrating foods that exist, those containing refined sugar, at 50. Death, represented by the level of 0, is at the very bottom of the scale.

These charts show the true nutritional levels of over 1,500 foods found in the average supermarket, presenting the information in a visual format. Each chart is accompanied by a narrative that provides a review of the major nutritional research for that particular food group. All this information shows quite clearly that it is the increased consumption of processed and refined foods in the average Western diet that has caused the epidemic of chronic degenerative diseases that we are seeing today.

A review of nutritional research over the past 100 years reveals that key aspects of this knowledge have been repressed or manipulated by the major corporations that profit from the deception that processed food is nutritious, such as the American Medical Association, the Food & Drug Administration, the USDA, the giant food corporations, and the political lobbyists who work for them. It points to an ongoing battle between the processed food industry's primary goal, which is to make a profit, and the consumer's need for access to healthy food and truthful information, and it is only education and a search for the truth that can turn this situation around, both on a personal and a political level.

These charts also show that the more processed a food is, the lower its nutritional value, and the more dangerous it is to our health. The life force energy of a food is a vital nutrient, and without it we cannot survive. The whole idea of processing foods—removing the vitality so they won't deteriorate—is in itself a flawed concept, as it removes the very thing that the body needs from it as nourishment. When you consider this fact, you can see the folly in it—by destroying the vitality of food so it lasts longer, the processed food industry is depriving consumers of this essential nutrition. They have created dead food, and it is slowly killing us.

Healthy people, nourished by whole, living foods, are energetic, productive individuals who take responsibility for their own health and are not a drain on their loved ones, nor on society. They do not have a succession of ailments and degenerative diseases brought on by a poor diet, nor do they take expensive and debilitating pharmaceutical drugs—instead, they have peace of mind because they do not live in fear that they may have some kind of deadly but silent disease lurking in their body, and can enjoy a better quality of life.

Comparative Vibrational Levels of Health and Disease States		How To Read the Charts & What They Tell Us
10,000 = Level of Optimal Health e.g. a healthy newborn baby / hunter/gatherer tribes	10,000	This is the level of the highest quality foods which confer the highest levels of health.
	9,500	
	9,000	
	8,500	
	8,000	
	7,500	
	7,000	
	6,500	Eating "above the line" means that you will be healthier than someone who eats "below the line."
AVERAGE LEVEL OF HEALTH IN USA Inflammation	6,000	This is the health level of average Americans. Inflammation signals the start of the disease process.
Arthritis starts to manifest	5,500	The more processed the food, the lower it calibrates, i.e. the more unhealthy it is for us to eat.
Heart Disease starts to manifest	5,000	Eating a steady diet of processed foods eventually leads to the diseases listed in the left column.
Cancer cells form: Breast, Prostate, Lung, Colon, Pancreas	4,500	Many familiar foods that we are told are healthy for us are in fact very unhealthy.
Diabetes • Osteoporosis	4,000	This is the true nutritional level of Kellogg's Rice Krispies and Raisin Bran, for instance.
Lymphoma • Leukemia • Dementia	3,500	
Congestive heart disease Brain cancer • Multiple sclerosis	3,000	This is the level of Wesson canola oil and Egg Beaters.
Breast cancer metastasizes	2,500	This is the level of parboiled, enriched white rice.
Prostate cancer metastasizes • Common cold/ flu	2,000	This is the level of bleached wheat flour products, such as a McDonald's hamburger bun.
Melanoma	1,500	This is the level of frying oils used by fast food restaurants.
Metastatic bone and lung cancer	1,000	This is the level of Bisquick Pancake Mix.
	500	This is the level of muffins, brownies, and Oreo cookies, and baked goods made with sugar.
	50	This is the level of sugar and most things made with it, including candy and jam.
Decay and Death	0	

BETTER HEALTH

WORSENING HEALTH

Measured in Bovis Units of Life Force Energy

CHAPTER 2

The Science Behind the Calibrations

"The farther you search, the greater you will realize the simplicity of all creation."
—*Paracelsus*

THE NEW WAY OF OBSERVING AND UNDERSTANDING our physical world, known as quantum theory, was pioneered in the early 20th century by German theoretical physicist Max Planck, who won a Nobel prize in Physics in 1918 for his work. His theory revolutionized human understanding of atomic and subatomic processes, but in the nearly one hundred years since then, the new ideas and theories that have subsequently developed have not been embraced by other branches of scientific investigation. The truth is, at the quantum level, standard physics—the kind we learned in high school—starts to fall apart, to be replaced by a set of phenomena and theories that are unsettling to those who firmly believe only in a four-dimensional world. Quantum physics has shown that there is more to life in this universe than what can be seen and measured by conventional means; when we dig deep enough, we discover atoms, particles and sub-particles, or quanta, which behave in strange ways, a discovery that has led many scientists to believe that there must be some kind of Intelligent Designer behind it all, even an Infinite Spirit. For one thing, quanta are not exactly *things*, they can be waves or vibrations of energy, or they can be particles—and sometimes both at the same time; it seems they may be able to change their form. This discovery suggests that there is no such thing as mass, only energy, an idea that is disconcerting to scientists who have been trained to believe otherwise. "Resistance was the way it had always been in science," writes Lynne McTaggart in her book *The Field*. "New ideas were always considered heretical."

But this new way of looking at the world is like Pandora's box—it's been opened and we can't go back. Rather like falling down a rabbit hole, we have been transported into a different world where things don't work the way we expect or the way we were told they would. We need to accept these new theories and move forward, but much of the scientific community, and especially the medical industry in the U.S., seem reluctant to do so. Energy medicine is the way of the future, yet much of modern medicine still lives in the world of chemical reactions, where drugs are used to alter a perceived chemical imbalance in the body, rather than using energy, or the knowledge that "new physics" has given us, to heal. This is also true of nutritional science, and in this chapter, I endeavor to explain how the new physics can help us look at ourselves, our world and our nourishment in a new way.

"At our most elemental, we are not a
chemical reaction, but an energetic charge."
—*Lynne McTaggart, from her book*
The Field: The Quest for the Secret Force of the Universe

The Reductionist Approach to Nutrition Has Failed Us

The question is, how do we determine what constitutes healthy food? Scientists can analyze food and break it down into its various parts, telling us what kinds of vitamins, minerals, enzymes and antioxidants and so on that it contains. But food is more than a breakdown of it parts—it contains vital nutrients beyond those which scientists have identified. You can take a machine apart and put it back together again, but you can't do that with a living thing—the parts of a living thing form a synergistic balance of perfection that man can't possibly hope to match.

From the reductionist point of view, the objective of science is to reconstruct reality by its parts. In the mid 20th century, nutritional scientists were thrilled to discover by analysis that food consisted of various components, namely vitamins and minerals, which they believed would be the cure for many diseases. The fact that they "cured" diseases that were caused by the depletion of nutrients in processed foods in the first place seemed to have escaped them, and in their exuberance they ridiculed the traditional way scientists and the community at large had regarded nutrition since the time of Hippocrates.

Hippocrates, who lived more than 2,300 years ago, believed and taught that all foods served the same purpose, that they all contained a basic nourishment which he called the "universal aliment." All these years later, it seems that Hippocrates was right all along, that he had identified the most important element of food—its vitality, or life force energy, an essential nutrient that is present in all fresh foods. We are coming full circle, returning to this simple but profound ancient belief, but it is an idea that the reductionist approach to nutrition has missed altogether.

In her paper, "Transcending Reductionism in Nutrition Research," scientist Ingrid Hoffmann points out that the reductionist approach has traditionally been and continues to be the dominant approach in nutrition research. But this brings up the question about whether the parts add up to the whole. She writes, "With the recognition about the whole being more than the sum of its parts, the limitations on the applicability of the reductionist approach, and the growing knowledge about parts of diet . . . new research strategies are needed to reveal more about the relationship between diet and health. This implies that a system as a whole has features not found in any one of the parts."

Here is an example from the LiveStrong website where a reader wrote in asking which of two breakfast dishes from McDonald's—the Egg McMuffin and the Big Breakfast with Hot Cakes—would be the healthiest to eat. Please note that this is not intended to be a criticism of the LiveStrong website, it is merely a demonstration of the difficulties in identifying healthy food using conventional methods:

"McDonald's offers both healthy and unhealthy breakfast options. The popular Egg McMuffin contains 300 calories, 12 g of fat, 260 mg of cholesterol, 820 g of sodium, 30 g of total carbohydrate and 18 g of protein. It also provides 10 percent of the recommended daily value of vitamin A, 30 percent of the daily value of calcium and 20 percent of the daily value of iron, based on a 2,000-calorie diet. On the other end of the spectrum, the large-sized Big Breakfast with Hotcakes contains a whopping 1150 calories, 60 g of fat, 575 mg of cholesterol, 2260 g of sodium, 116 g of total carbohydrate and 36 g of protein. It also contains 15 percent of the daily value of vitamin A, 2 percent of the daily value of vitamin C, 30 percent of the daily value of calcium and 40 percent of the daily value of iron."

The article on the website concludes that the former is healthier than the latter. But in fact, if a calibration is made of the *quality* of the food, the Egg McMuffin clocks in at a very low 3,000 Bovis units of life force energy, while the Big Breakfast with Hotcakes comes in at 2,000, not that much different. Hold the syrup on the pancakes and they are dead even; so both breakfasts are really bad for you. Obviously, this method of evaluating food is not providing us with information that is accurate and useful.

So if food contains more than the sum of its parts, what do we call the part that hasn't yet been officially identified by scientists? We can call it radiance, vitality, cosmic energy, or life force energy.

The Life Force Energy Content of Food is an Essential Nutrient

"Living things emit a weak radiation . . . through scientific experiment [scientists have] demonstrated that there may be such a thing as a life force flowing through the universe."

— *Lynne McTaggart, author of*

The Field: The Quest for the Secret Force of the Universe

Science has proven that all things radiate; this radiation emanates from all substances and beings here on earth and throughout the universe. Nobel-prize-winning physicist Louis-Victor de Broglie (1892-1987) established that every particle, down to a photon of light, is associated with a specific wavelength. These vibrational wavelengths, or radiation, are what we might call life force energy, for they represent life itself. Without this kind of energy flowing through our bodies, we cease to function. In Chinese medicine this life force is called chi; in ayurvedic Indian tradition it is called prana; in the Polynesian culture it is called mana; in Europe, Rudolf Steiner referred to it as "cosmic etheric forces." Edward Bach based his system of Bach Flower Remedies on the premise that every living thing radiates energy, and homeopathy stems from this same truth.

Healthy plants, and the animals that eat them, radiate this energy. And if we eat food that contains high levels of life force energy, that energy will cause us to be vibrant and healthy too. The higher the vibrations of the food we eat, the healthier we will be, and the more we will show a certain radiance—some people would say we "glow with good health."

We also receive life force energy from other sources, such as from the water we drink, the air we breathe, the planet that we live on, and the sun that gives us light and life. So, in order to be healthy, we need high-energy food, clean water, unpolluted air, a direct connection to the earth, and exposure to sunlight. If any of these are missing, it affects the healthy functioning or our body, and if all are missing, we'll sicken and die.

Incidentally, some nutritional consultants advocate a raw food diet because they believe that raw foods contain more life force energy than cooked foods. I have not found this to be true—in fact, many of the foods we eat, such as potatoes and other root vegetables, are actually more nutritious when cooked.

The Life Force Energy of Food has been Found to Consist of Biophotons

Biology is a quantum process, and quantum mechanics governs all living systems. The cosmic energy, or life force energy, that is in the food we eat—in plants and the animals which eat them—has been identified by scientists as biophotons. Biophotons are weak light emissions that radiate from the cells of all living beings and are an expression of the functional state of a living organism. This energy is absorbed by the body from the food we eat and creates an atmosphere of coherence at the cellular level.

Many scientists working independently, among them Stuart Hameroff, M.D., physicist Herbert Frohlich, scientific scholar Marco Bischof, and German biophysicist Fritz-Albert Popp, Ph.D., discovered that all the living cells of our body transmit photons, or molecules of light. Quantum coherence is a state where the cells of the body are healthy and working in accord, also called "global coherence," or "super-radiance."

Popp found that in healthy people, these photons showed an exquisite coherence at the quantum level, but in cancer patients, the lines of internal communication were scrambled and the photons lost their coherence. Popp began to realize that this light in the body held the key to health and to illness. In one experiment, he compared the light emitted from free-range eggs to those produced by caged hens. The photons in the eggs produced by the free-range chickens were far more coherent than those in the other eggs. He went on to use biophoton emissions as a tool for measuring the quality of food. *The healthiest food had the most coherent intensity of light.* Health was a state of perfect subatomic communication, he discovered, and ill health was a state where communication breaks down. We are ill when our waves are out of synch. He believed that biophoton emissions orchestrate all bodily processes, and that biophoton vibrations cause molecules to vibrate and create their own signature frequency, which acts as its unique driving force and also its means of communication. Water in the body was essential for these healthy vibrations, he realized, and he found that water can "hold" or "remember" a signature electromagnetic frequency.

Lynne McTaggart explains this process elegantly in her book, *The Field:* "When we eat plant foods . . . we take up the photons and store them. This energy becomes the driving force for all the molecules in our body. Photons switch on the body's processes like a conductor launching each individual instrument into the collective sound. At different frequencies they perform different functions . . . these biophotons provide a perfect communication system to transfer information to many cells across the organism."

Parallel research was also carried out by Dr. Kikuo Chishima, a professor at the Nagoya Commercial University in Japan, who theorized that the energetic information contained in food is even more important than the nutrients scientists have so far identified. He believed that the vibrations of the food we eat raises the vibrations of the body's tissues, and that food laden with pesticides and chemicals and contaminated with antibiotics and growth hormones has a chaotic vibratory oscillation that derails the coherence of our nutritional energy needs. Our food has to vibrate at the highest level, he said, so it can be absorbed into our cells in the form of biophoton energy. Like Popp, he also discovered that a healthy cell radiates coherent light, while a diseased cell radiates chaotic light. So when we are healthy, we are actually radiating light. In essence, we are beings of light.

The discovery of biophoton emission also lends scientific support to methods of healing based on concepts of homeostasis, or self-regulation of the organism, such as homeopathy and acupuncture, and various somatic therapies which integrate the body's mental, emotional, spiritual and physical aspects.

It has also been found that consciousness is a global phenomenon that occurs everywhere in the body and that consciousness at its most basic is coherent light. "The universe is a vast dynamic cobweb of energy exchange," writes Lynne McTaggart in *The Field.* Our food and the effect it has on our bodies and our consciousness is part of this energy exchange. That's why our food has to be *live* food—it feeds a living body. "Illness is a disturbance in the quantum fluctuations of an individual," she writes. So, dead food creates a dead body, eventually.

Healing, as Popp's work suggests, might be a matter of reprogramming individual quantum fluctuations to operate more coherently. This can be done in several ways—by eating high quality food, drinking fresh water, being connected to the earth, and breathing in fresh, unpolluted air. In fact, we are nourished by the four elements that have been celebrated throughout human history: fire (sun), water, earth and air—all are essential nutrients for the body, and provide us with radiance and information that is essential for our wellbeing. We can also increase the vibrational level of the cells in our body by using vibrational remedies such as homeopathy, sound vibrations, crystals, and essential oils. These all raise the level of life force energy in the body and are therefore equally important. But in this book we will focus on just one of these sources—the food we eat.

"The physical universe is an aggregate of frequencies."
—*Buckminster Fuller*

Where Science and Metaphysics Collide

There is much talk these days about "the end of science," with a book of that title by John Horgan becoming a best seller. But this idea was not born from the sense that there is nothing left to discover, but rather that we lack the instruments with which to measure the phenomena that quantum mechanics are revealing to us. Quite simply, we need a new way of investigating and measuring things—or "new research strategies," as scientist Ingrid Hoffmann put it. Nobel-prize-winning physicist Louis-Victor de Broglie agreed, saying: "It is premature to want to assess vital processes according to the very insufficient physio-chemical concepts of the 20th century."

We have lived in a left-brained world for the past 200 years or so, and now it seems that the analytical influence of the left brain has taken us as far as we can go in scientific investigation. It may be time for the mainstream to recognize the value of the right-brained way of experiencing the world we live in; however, the right brain cannot be activated by logic—we can access information through the right side of our brain only by what are variously termed intuition, meditation, hypnosis, dream states, emotions, hunches or gut feelings, and "second sight."

So in fact, the "new research strategies" that Hoffmann alluded to might well include intuition and divination. The word "divination" is derived from the Latin noun *divinus*, meaning "one inspired by the gods." The English dowsing expert Malcolm Rae is quoted in the book *The Divining Hand* by Christopher Bird as saying, "Physics is approaching very closely the limits of observation achievable with non-living instruments." He believed that living detectors may be required to measure patterns of energy emanating from or influencing life and that the dowsing faculty may become an important probe for penetrating the unknown in search of understanding and wisdom.

History tell us that scientists have long depended on their intuitive side. Albert Einstein once said, "All great achievements of science must start from intuitive knowledge. I believe in intuition and inspiration . . . At times I feel certain I am right while not knowing the reason." He intuited his theory of relativity and then spent the rest of his life proving it mathematically. Isaac Newton and Archimedes both credited intuition for their earth-shattering theories while in reverie or in a dream. This is when we get those bursts of insight—when the brain is allowed to relax enough to make associations that are the flash of genius. This is how a generalist rather than a specialist can come up with new thoughts and ideas—they can make intuitive leaps that take them outside the conventional box constructed by scientific conventions.

The importance of being able to use the right side of the brain is that it gives us access to our subconscious mind and to the vast store of information in the collective unconscious, also called the Zero Point Field, which represents the larger unseen world that our rational brain imagines does not exist. The Zero Point Field has been investigated at length by Lynne McTaggart in her extraordinary book, *The Field.* She describes it as "an ocean of microscopic vibrations in the space between things." This field has also been termed the Akashic Records and the "Mind of God," and has been described as a "universal supercomputer" which contains all knowledge of human experience and the history of the cosmos. This is where all the thoughts and memories of the universe are stored for those who have the ability and intention to access them; it is where the truth lies, and where new ideas come from. We all have equal opportunity access to this information, it's just a question of allowing and training our minds to access this great storehouse of thought, idea, and information. Many scientists feel that this is the new frontier.

There is much about the mysteries of nature that we still don't know. In fact, as advances in quantum mechanics have shown us, it seems to be a case of the more we know, the more we realize we don't know. The mysteries of nature only seem more mystical and extraordinary the more we delve into them. We still don't know what matter really is, nor what a proton or an electron is made of, nor what type of energy gravity represents. French scientist Louis Kervran said that physicists are mistaken in claiming that physical laws are the same for the living as for inanimate matter, and it is becoming evident that many new theories and discoveries at the quantum level are in direct conflict with "known" facts and principles about the physical world.

"We cannot deny the existence of something just because we don't know about it," said Kervran. The secret of life is still that, a huge secret.

> "If a person does not feel shocked when he
> first encounters quantum theory,
> he has not understood a word of it."
>
> —*Niels Bohr, winner of the Nobel Prize in Physics in 1922*

Who Are the New Scientists?

Well, that could include you and me, according to British physicist Rupert Sheldrake, whom Deepak Chopra calls "one of the most innovative and visionary scientists of our times," regarding him on the same level as Newton and Darwin. Many professionals have taken potshots at the "authority of science," at the idea that you have to be a career scientist to even participate in the exploration of our physical and metaphysical worlds. And Sheldrake agrees, saying: "In the past, some of the most innovative scientific research was carried out by amateurs. Charles Darwin, for example, never held an institutional post. He worked independently at his home . . . just one of the many independent researchers who, not reliant on grants or constrained by the conservative pressures of anonymous peer review, did highly original work." That kind of freedom is almost nonexistent today, he says, and he believes that science has become increasingly professionalized to the point where there are only a handful of independent scientists working today.

Modern computing power and access to a vast amount of information on the Internet has changed the scientific landscape forever. Science can once again be nourished from the grass roots up, Sheldrake believes, and research can grow from a personal interest in the nature of nature, even in those who are not professional scientists.

Sheldrake says that science has always been elitist and undemocratic, but believes that in fact it can be as unlimited as the human imagination. "Science needs democratization," he declares. He doubts that all the phenomena of life can ever be explained entirely mechanistically, and it now appears that the new frontier of science beckons us inward, into the realm of the mystical and the imagination. And this is a place where many scientists and their instruments are unable, or unwilling, to go.

How We Can Learn to Determine the Truth About Anything

"Genuine truths exude a beauty, a rightness, a self-evident quality that gives them the power of revelation."

—*John Horgan, author of* The End of Science

You can only write a book called *The Truth About Food* if you have a means to identify the truth. And due to the ground-breaking work of Dr. David Hawkins, as described in his book *Power vs. Force: The Hidden Determinants of Human Behavior,* we can all now learn how to determine the truth about anything. In theory anyway; in practice, probably about one person in 50 will be able to learn and effectively use the method he describes in his book. But even so, having one person in 50 among us who can identify the truth is better than none.

Dr. Hawkins proved beyond doubt that his method works, having performed millions of calibrations on thousands of test subjects of all ages and personality types, from all walks of life, over a 20 year period. He found that in all cases, without exception, the results were identical and entirely reproducible, fulfilling the fundamental requirement of the scientific method: perfect experimental replicability.

And this is true of my calibrations of the food products in this book: allowing for small variations in some foods due to differences in batches, growing conditions, or production techniques, the results are reproducible again and again.

The basis of this method, Applied Kinesiology, is a well-established science based on the testing of muscle response stimulus that was originated in 1964 by chiropractor George J. Goodheart. Correlating muscles with acupuncture meridians and energy flows, Dr. Goodheart developed Applied Kinesiology through his research and from the study of medical, osteopathic and chiropractic journals and books. He began teaching this method to other chiropractors, and now about 40 percent of chiropractors in the U.S. use it, whether their patients are aware of it or not. Psychiatrist John Diamond was intrigued by Applied Kinesiology and adopted it in his practice, becoming the first qualified medical member of the International College of Applied Kinesiology in the 1970s. He found that a patient thinking an anxious thought "weakened" a previously strong muscle, and that he could reach the core of emotional problems for people far faster than by using orthodox counseling. This changed his entire practice.

As Dr. Hawkins says in his book: "Applied kinesiology reflects the human organism's capacity to differentiate not only positive from negative stimuli, but also anabolic (life-threatening) from catabolic (life-consuming), and most dramatically, truth from falsity."

Measuring the Vitality and Vibrational Content of Food

"Everything in the universe constantly gives off an energy pattern of a specific frequency that remains for all time and can be read by those who know how."

—*Dr. David Hawkins, author of* Power vs. Force

I first learned to calibrate the vibrational level of foods years ago when my chiropractor showed me how to use Applied Kinesiology to test for foods I might be allergic or sensitive to. I became very adept with this method, going around food markets testing foods to find those that would be best for me to eat. So it came naturally to me to expand my ability using this method to test foods for their levels of quality and vitality when I learned about the work of Andre Bovis.

Bovis was a French scientist working in Paris during WWI who discovered that he could measure the intrinsic vitality and relative freshness of different foods from the power of their radiations. He believed that plant foods are filled with solar radiation and that their radiance rises slowly to a peak while ripening, decreasing to zero at putrefaction. He developed a machine he called a *biometre*, or the Bovis meter, to measure these vibrations based on a measurement range from 1 to 10,000 angstroms.

Another scientist, Andre Simoneton, had used Bovis's technique just after WWI when he was stricken by tuberculosis and was able to test for the healthiest foods to eat to aid in his recovery. At the time, he was working with physicist Louis de Broglie, the scientist who would establish that every particle, down to a photon of light, is associated with a specific wavelength. With this background and experience, Simoneton realized the importance of Bovis's work, and by using the system developed by Bovis, he was able to establish empirically that one could measure specific wavelengths from foods that indicated vitality and freshness.

It is a combination of the knowledge explained in this chapter along with the methods of calibration developed by Andre Bovis and Dr. David Hawkins that I use in measuring the life force energy, or total nutritional content, of the foods listed in the charts in this book. In order to honor Andre Bovis for his work, I decided to adopt the scale that he had developed nearly one hundred years ago to demonstrate the levels of functioning nutrition of various food items and the difference between healthy and unhealthy food—even though modern science has shown us that the radiance, or vitality, being measured is actually an indicator of the biophoton coherence in the food being calibrated. All systems of measurement are conventional, they are merely devised as a convenient system of comparing one thing to another. What is important is being able to make the comparison, not the scale of measurement used.

How a Diet of Processed Foods Causes Degenerative Diseases

Ill health starts at the cellular level, caused by years of eating inferior foods which fail to nourish the body at the most profound level. When this happens, the cells, and eventually the whole body, starts to vibrate at a progressively lower level. Microbes, viruses, and diseases also vibrate at a low level, but these disease-causing organisms can only affect a human body when its vitality has been lowered to a point where cells resonate at a corresponding wavelength. A healthy body, on the other hand, radiating with vitality and good health, remains immune to attack by microbes and disease. If this fact were not true, then we all would come down with a contagious illness during an epidemic. But we don't. Not everyone gets sick, only those with lowered immunity—lowered vibrations—catch the flu or plague or whatever is the current infection or epidemic.

Processed foods, which vibrate at a much lower level than healthy foods, eventually cause disease because the body absorbs the lower energy of the food. If a person consistently eats a diet of low quality food, then the cells of their body will also begin to consistently vibrate at a lower level, leading to systemic ill-health and disease.

A chronic condition of low vibration in the body causes a low level of general health which can lead to more serious ailments than catching a cold. Ill health at this level affects all the cells in the body, leading to systemic problems and chronic degenerative diseases such as circulatory diseases, diabetes and cancer. Fritz-Albert Popp found that the radiation given off by cancer patients calibrates at a lower rate than a healthy person, equal with the vibration of the disease itself, and Marco Bischof found that cancer cells and healthy cells of the same type can be identified by differences in their biophoton emissions.

However, a body can be generally healthy but can be stressed by a temporary negative emotion or situation, giving an opportunistic microbe the chance to strike. Most of us know that when we get a cold or the flu, we can usually trace the moment of infection back to feeling stressed or tired or overworked, or to an evening out when maybe we overdid it a bit. Refined sugar is the biggest culprit here, it lowers our immunity dramatically and calibrates at the lowest level of all the products we eat, just above the vibrational level of anti-freeze and weed-killer.

A Good Diet Leads to Good Health

With this knowledge and these charts, we now have important tools to help us to be as healthy as possible by knowing which foods promote good health and which we need to avoid or minimize. We all share a common goal—the wish for a long life with good health so we can explore all that life has to offer without having to worry about getting some deadly disease or the idea that our hard-earned inheritance will go to a nursing home, not to our children. Life is challenging enough without having to worry about these things, and we all deserve to be able to live a life where our focus can be on productive things, rather than on fear of disease and its financial burden.

CHAPTER 3

The Standard American Diet (SAD)

"Humans today suffer more chronic and debilitating diseases than ever before. And there can be little doubt that our food choices play a major role in this development."

—Dr. Joseph Mercola, founder of the world's most popular natural health website www.mercola.com

NEVER WAS AN ACRONYM SO APT, for the SAD diet is just that, sad—because it's slowly killing us. The Standard American Diet is largely based on processed foods, food items that are manufactured from the cheapest ingredients to ensure the greatest profits, supported by government farm subsidies and huge advertising budgets, and with little regard to the effect they are having on our health. These foods are cheap, addictive, and readily available, and they are the reason that Americans are now overfed, overweight and undernourished.

In the charts on the following pages, we can see that the highest level of health is given a value of 10,000—that of a newborn baby, or primitive hunter-gatherer tribes who eat a traditional diet. But the same charts show that the average diet of Americans now stands at 6,000, the level where inflammation sets the stage for degenerative diseases. Up until 1920, the average level of health in America was at the optimum level. Back then, many Americans lived in rural areas and had ready access to raw milk and fresh farm produce. But as more people moved to urban areas and as processed foods became more available, the average level of health of Americans has fallen to the dangerous level it is today.

An article in *Time* magazine in October 2011 showed that the amount of money spent on food in America has decreased in the same proportion that spending on health care has increased. In 1950, 22 percent of the average household budget was spent on food, while in 2010, it was only 7 percent, and during the same period, health care costs rose from 3 percent to 16 percent of household budget. It is not hard to draw a direct correlation between the reduction in the cost, and presumably quality, of the food we consumed over those years and the rising costs of sickness care. We really have to ask ourselves, what have we gained by having access to cheaper food? It's only made us sicker. America is now one of the sickest developed nations in the world—the World Health Organization placed the U.S. at the bottom of a list of 37 industrialized nations in levels of general health, even though the U.S. spends more than any other nation on health care.

Eric Schossler, author of *Fast Food Nation*, states in his book that about 90 percent of the money that Americans now spend on food goes to buy processed food. In the average supermarket, about 98 percent of the food on sale is processed food, which leaves only two percent of high nutritional quality. If we choose to shop at Whole Foods Market, we'll find that 90 percent of the food is high quality, with Trader Joe's coming in at about 60 percent. But most people shop at their local supermarket, where the quality of food is poor, the shelves and freezers laden with packaged food products.

The cumulative effect of a steady diet of processed food has a devastating effect on our health. The body struggles to maintain a stable blood sugar level and the liver does its best to filter out the toxins, but eventually they reach overload. This used to happen around middle age, but now doctors are reporting cases of non-alcoholic fatty liver disease and type 2 diabetes in young children. In most countries, malnutrition is the result of poverty, but in America, it's the result of ignorance, self-indulgence, and a rushed lifestyle where people don't have enough time to plan healthy meals.

The main problem with refined foods is that essential nutrients are lost in the refining process. Once food has been processed and deprived of its life force energy, which represents the aggregate of all its goodness—its vitality, vitamins, minerals, antioxidants, phytonutrients, all that scientists have so far been able to detect in our food and more—it cannot be introduced back in, no matter how many vitamins and minerals the food processors might add. The food is essentially dead. So most people are spending good money on dead food. No need to guess where that leads.

Comparative Vibrational Levels of Health and Disease States	Bovis Units	Comparative Nutritional Levels of **Foods in the Standard American Diet**
10,000 = Level of Optimal Health e.g. a healthy newborn baby / hunter/gatherer tribes	10,000	Organic vegetables, fruits, grains & nuts • Wild and organic/naturally-raised poultry, meat, fish & eggs Organic lard • Sea salt • Raw honey/maple syrup • Unprocessed dairy products • Extra-virgin olive oil
	9,500	Starkist tuna fish • Kerry Gold butter • Supermarket onions, grapefruit, tangerines
BETTER	9,000	Most supermarket vegetables and fruits • Quaker oatmeal cereal
	8,500	Supermarket red grapes, Kiwi fruit, plums, oranges, lettuce • Bird's Eye frozen peas
	8,000	Lard (from corn-fed cattle) • Supermarket apples, bananas • Cream of Wheat
HEALTH	7,500	Supermarket green peppers, red peppers, celery, pears • Ben & Jerry's vanilla ice cream
	7,000	Supermarket strawberries • Budweiser Beer
	6,500	Average supermarket steak • Arnold's rye bread • Morton's salt • Starbuck's coffee, black
AVERAGE LEVEL OF HEALTH IN USA Inflammation	6,000	Purdue chicken • Farmed shrimp • Mott's apple juice • Arnold's whole-grain bread
WORSENING Arthritis starts to manifest	5,500	Supermarket eggs • Land O' Lakes butter • Oscar Meyer/Plumrose bacon • Philadelphia cream cheese
Heart Disease starts to manifest	5,000	Generic supermarket milk and cheese • Average supermarket ground beef, bacon, sausages
Cancer cells form: Breast, Prostate, Lung, Colon, Pancreas	4,500	Kellogg's Cornflakes • McDonald's hamburger, no bun • Yoplait yogurt
Diabetes • Osteoporosis	4,000	Kellogg's Rice Krispies & Cheerios • Oscar Meyer hot dogs • Minute Maid apple juice • Wonder Bread
HEALTH Lymphoma • Leukemia • Dementia	3,500	Peanut oil • Haagen Dazs Chocolate Chip ice cream • Jiffy-Pop popcorn • Pepsi • Egg Beaters • Pita bread
Congestive heart disease Brain cancer • Multiple sclerosis	3,000	McDonald's Hamburger & Egg McMuffin • Swanson's frozen dinners • Wesson corn and canola oil • Campbell's tomato soup • Starbuck's coffee w/sugar & cream • Dunkin' Donuts bagel • Average pizza
Breast cancer metastasizes	2,500	Sara Lee cheesecake • McDonald's Big Mac & Fries • Goldfish Crackers • KFC chicken wings
Prostate cancer metastasizes • Common cold/ flu	2,000	Coca-Cola • Sara Lee Pound Cake • Goya white rice • Crisco • Cottonseed oil • Hellmann's mayonnaise
Melanoma	1,500	Planter's Cocktail Peanuts • Wheat Thins Crackers • Miracle Whip • Campbell's Baked Beans • Kellogg's Frosted Flakes • Campbell's Cream of Mushroom Soup • Hostess Coffee Cake
Metastatic bone and lung cancer	1,000	Diet Coke • Heinz Tomato Ketchup • Donuts • Saltines • Campbell's Cream of Chicken Soup
	500	Oreo cookies • Starbucks Danish • Coffee cake • Brownies • Pop Tarts • Fruit Loops • Cheetos • Mrs. Smith's fruit pies • Costco hot dog • Pancakes & waffles with imitation "maple" syrup
	50	Sugar • HF Corn Syrup • Twinkies • Chocolate • Candy • Sorbet/sherbert • Aspartame/Splenda • MSG
Decay and Death	0	These calibrate at 5 Bovis Units: Anti-freeze • Roundup Weed Killer • Pesticides

Measured in Bovis Units of Life Force Energy

The Real Cost of Cheap Food

There's no such thing as cheap food when you include the health care costs to treat the diseases it causes. Poor quality food causes disease while good quality food makes us healthy, so there is a direct correlation between the quality of a person's diet and the level of their health.

In the days before the advent of processed foods, when the average food in a market or restaurant was likely to have been grown on a local farm and naturally raised, eating without thinking much about it wasn't a dangerous enterprise. But now that processed foods, made with highly refined ingredients, much of them genetically-modified, make up such a large percentage of our food supply, eating has reached a whole new level of danger. And that's where we are today—at the danger level, with rates of diabetes, cancer and heart disease at all time highs.

Currently, the U.S. spends about $2.6 trillion every year on medical care, ten times what was spent in 1980. But medical care in the U.S. has not always been so expensive. In 1950, five years before the first McDonald's opened, Americans spent $8.4 billion on medical care, or $70 billion in today's dollars. We now spend as much on health care every 10 days as we did in the entire year of 1950. If other costs had risen this dramatically, we'd be paying $55 for a dozen eggs, $48 for a gallon of milk, and $134 for a dozen oranges. The most scandalous fact is that this increase in spending hasn't made us any healthier—in fact quite the opposite, and today, we are experiencing an epidemic of largely preventable diseases which are being "treated" with expensive drugs, but are not being cured nor prevented.

The TV program "60 Minutes," which aired on CNBC in February, 2012, stated, "The one thing that could bankrupt America is uncontrolled medical care costs." You would think that with the spectre of bankruptcy and universal sickness looming in our future, the government might be concerned. But they seem oblivious, not even managing to legislate a functioning national health care program. The U.S. is the only industrialized nation without one, and the ever-rising cost of health care is taking a devastating toll on just about everyone. The annual health insurance premium paid by the average American family now exceeds the gross yearly income of a full-time minimum wage worker, and every single day people are filing for bankruptcy due to the overwhelming costs of health care. It even impacts businesses: Starbucks spends more on the health insurance of its workers than it does on coffee.

Many researchers have exposed the current government policy of farming subsidies as immensely flawed. Subsidizing mass-produced food leads to cheap ingredients which leads to substandard food. It also leads to cheap animal feed, which produces an inferior product, since grains are not a natural food for cattle and swine. And there is no escape from genetically-modified corn and soy—they are in just about every food we eat, unless it's home-grown or labeled organic. They are also fed to most confined feedlot animals—and when we eat the animals, we are eating the feed too.

When we consider that the government, i.e. the taxpayer, is covering a large part of the costs of treating the resulting diseases, to the tune of $846 billion a year for Medicare and Medicaid programs alone, we can see what a self-defeating plan this is. And when we include the cost of farm subsidies, the real cost is astronomical.

The idea of growing cheap food ingredients to provide low-cost food to the masses is not sound policy—it creates an unhealthy and unproductive workforce, causes diseases that cost a fortune to treat, causes countless suffering to domesticated animals, and thanks to pesticides, herbicides and GMOs, destroys the environment.

Which brings us to the question, why is the U.S. government allowing this threat of personal and national bankruptcy to threaten the future of this country?

The Truth About the Health Care Industry

One reason is the strangle-hold the medical and pharmaceutical industries have on healing. They have systematically defeated and eliminated any challenge to their supremacy as the ONLY approved method of treatment, so if you have health insurance, you can only go one route—conventional care. If you prefer an alternative treatment, or vitamins and supplements, they are not covered so you have to pay for them yourself. Which means that many people are having to pay for health insurance on top of their chosen forms of treatment.

The underlying issue here is the basic concept of a for-profit health care system. A profit-making system is not interested in healing patients at the lowest cost, as a state-run system would seek to do; they are interested in making the largest profit possible. A for-profit health care system has serious conflicts between providing affordable, quality care to patients and making a profit for investors.

The health-care stocks that are soaring on the stock market these days are the ones that make drugs for diabetes. You can see the analysts on the TV money shows wringing their hands in joy at the anticipation of the many millions more people who will contract diabetes in the future. Imagine! Each one on a lifetime of expensive drugs, and with no "cure" in sight. No wonder they don't want doctors to tell their patients that type 2 diabetes can be cured by diet.

If anyone should be telling us how to eat a healthy diet, it should be the American Dietetic Association. But they actually

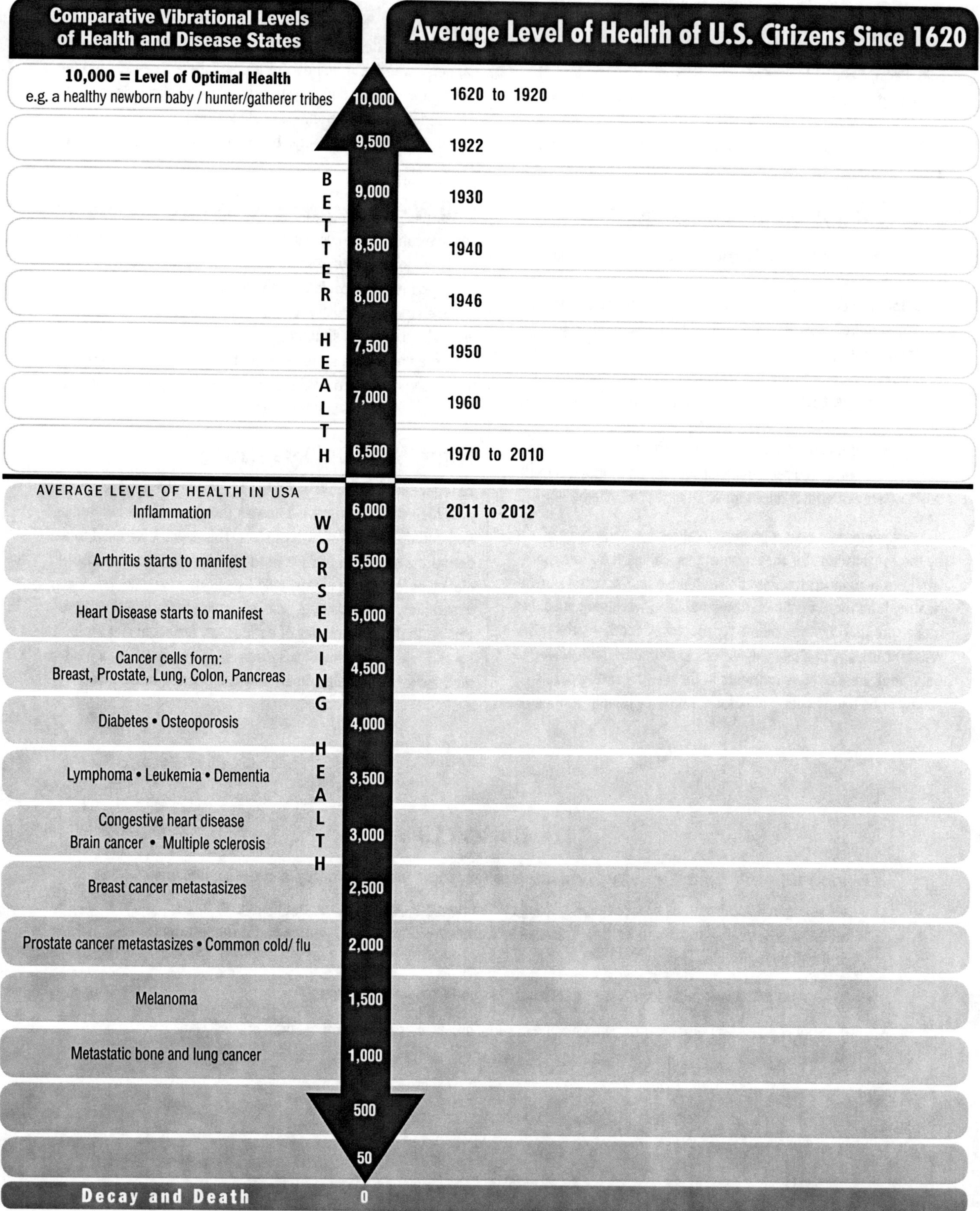
Comparative Vibrational Levels of Health and Disease States
Average Level of Health of U.S. Citizens Since 1620
10,000 = Level of Optimal Health
e.g. a healthy newborn baby / hunter/gatherer tribes
10,000
1620 to 1920
9,500
1922
BETTER HEALTH
9,000
1930
8,500
1940
8,000
1946
7,500
1950
7,000
1960
6,500
1970 to 2010
AVERAGE LEVEL OF HEALTH IN USA
Inflammation
6,000
2011 to 2012
WORSENING HEALTH
Arthritis starts to manifest
5,500
Heart Disease starts to manifest
5,000
Cancer cells form:
Breast, Prostate, Lung, Colon, Pancreas
4,500
Diabetes • Osteoporosis
4,000
Lymphoma • Leukemia • Dementia
3,500
Congestive heart disease
Brain cancer • Multiple sclerosis
3,000
Breast cancer metastasizes
2,500
Prostate cancer metastasizes • Common cold/ flu
2,000
Melanoma
1,500
Metastatic bone and lung cancer
1,000
500
50
Decay and Death
0
Measured in Bovis Units of Life Force Energy

receive payments from processed food producers such as Coca-Cola, Pepsi, General Mills, Kellogg's, Hershey, Unilever, and Abbott Nutrition, a division of pharmaceutical giant Abbott Laboratories, so don't expect them to suggest that we can improve our health by eliminating sugar and refined carbohydrates from our diets.

How is the Government Helping?

Well, not much, actually. In fact, it's obvious that our government has failed us by:

1. Not protecting us from unsafe farming practices, substandard food ingredients, and the predatory marketing practices of the food industry.
2. Caving in to the American Medical Association which has systematically restricted the art of healing to the medical profession.
3. Allowing these gigantic for-profit entities to influence the political system with direct financial support and lobbyists to the point where our vote is impotent to change the system.

The government seems content to allow our country to be run by the corporations for the corporations, calling it a "free market." But how much freedom do we have when we can't purchase healthy food for our children? Meanwhile, government subsidies make sure that the ingredients for processed foods—primarily wheat, corn, soy and sugar—are cheap and abundant. Never mind that there are few nutrients in them—the voting public seems to be happy eating junk food, and they blindly assume that the medical system will take care of them when the inevitable happens, whether it be heart disease, diabetes, cancer, and the rest of the litany of degenerative disease. But these diseases represent profound systemic imbalances in the body caused by malnutrition, and the "magic bullet" of a pill just doesn't work in these cases.

Can We Do Anything to Change the System?

Yes, we can! We can vote with our wallets. If every penny we spent on groceries were spent on quality food, locally produced when possible, we could curb the food giants, regain our health, and the sickness industry would see their business dwindle. This would be a win/win situation.

We can also vote, state by state, to mandate labelling of GM foods, and demand that our local food stores label the foods they sell, otherwise we won't buy them.

What We Should be Eating

To regain our health, we need to eat "above the line" as much as possible—that is, above the line on the chart where inflammation and disease are shown to start. This is what we used to eat before the advent of processed food, when our diets consisted mainly of free-range meats, wild fish, eggs, raw dairy products, vegetables, fruit, and nuts. Many people are finding that by reverting to this simpler way of eating they are regaining their vitality and reversing many of the diseases associated with a modern diet, including diabetes, heart disease, obesity, and cancer.

The Bottom Line

- Avoid all foods that contain refined products, especially sugar, wheat, corn, soy, and GM ingredients
- Eat organic and naturally or locally raised foods when possible. It costs more, but it's worth it. The alternative—treatment for cancer, heart disease or diabetes—is expensive, traumatic, time-consuming, and mostly ineffective
- Demand that supermarkets provide us with healthy food from known sources
- Support your local grocery store, butcher, local suppliers, farmers, and farmers' markets

Comparative Vibrational Levels of Health and Disease States	Bovis Units	Average Level of Health of Selected Countries Showing the U.S. to be the Unhealthiest Country in the World
10,000 = Level of Optimal Health e.g. a healthy newborn baby / hunter/gatherer tribes	10,000	Primitive hunter/gatherer tribes: Masai, Aborigine, Maori, Bushmen, Inuit, etc.
	9,500	Average level of health in Argentina, Bolivia, Chile, Finland, Greenland
	9,000	Average level of health in New Zealand, Mongolia, Norway, Poland, Russia, Sweden, Thailand
	8,500	Average level of health in Denmark, India, Italy, Kenya, Mexico, South Africa, Turkey
	8,000	Average Level of Health in Brazil, Greece, Japan, Morocco, Tanzania
	7,500	Average Level of Health in Egypt, France, Germany, Iran, Nigeria, Spain
	7,000	Average Level of Health in Australia, China, Iraq, Mexico
	6,500	Average Level of Health in Canada, England, Ireland, Scotland, Wales
AVERAGE LEVEL OF HEALTH IN USA Inflammation	6,000	**Average Level of Health in USA**
Arthritis starts to manifest	5,500	
Heart Disease starts to manifest	5,000	
Cancer cells form: Breast, Prostate, Lung, Colon, Pancreas	4,500	
Diabetes • Osteoporosis	4,000	
Lymphoma • Leukemia • Dementia	3,500	
Congestive heart disease Brain cancer • Multiple sclerosis	3,000	
Breast cancer metastasizes	2,500	
Prostate cancer metastasizes • Common cold/ flu	2,000	
Melanoma	1,500	
Metastatic bone and lung cancer	1,000	
	500	
	50	
Decay and Death	0	

BETTER HEALTH ↑ / WORSENING HEALTH ↓

Measured in Bovis Units of Life Force Energy

CHAPTER 4

Diet-Related Diseases

"Serious diseases that are linked to what we eat kill an estimated three out of four Americans each year. These diseases include heart disease, high blood pressure, stroke, some types of cancer, and diabetes."
— *National Cancer Institute*

CHRONIC PREVENTABLE ILLNESSES THAT RESULT FROM "lifestyle choices," meaning any combination of a poor diet, drinking alcohol to excess, smoking, drug use, and lack of exercise, now account for seven out of every ten deaths in the U.S. and 75 percent of the $2.6 trillion that the U.S. spends annually on health care. We only have to look at the chart on page 21 to see how the average level of health of Americans has dropped over the course of the past 100 years or so.

The most serious of the diseases which are thought to be caused in the most part by inadequate nutrition are diabetes, heart disease, cancer, arthritis, dementia, and stroke, but diet also plays a part in the development of other conditions such as allergies, auto-immune diseases, osteoporosis, and candidiasis. All of these are briefly described in the following pages of this chapter.

In all these conditions, inflammation is believed to be the underlying cause. Research has shown that health problems caused by inflammation don't just happen overnight, but can build up over years. Inflammation is the body's natural immune response to illness, injury, or infection, and in a healthy person, when healing is complete, the process is normally turned off. But this process can be affected by other factors such as an unhealthy diet, stress, and lack of sleep, and this kind of inflammation can't be so easily controlled.

Some obvious symptoms of inflammation include aching joints, muscle tenderness and swelling, but other symptoms can be internal, silent and deadly, such as inflamed blood vessels which leads to heart disease. Arthritis is a disease that is most commonly linked to chronic inflammation, but inflammation can also affect internal organs—inflammation of the heart (myocarditis) can cause shortness of breath or swelling of the legs, inflammation of the bronchial tubes in the lungs can lead to an asthma attack, and inflammation of the kidneys can lead to high blood pressure and eventual kidney failure.

A poor diet combined with antibiotics that destroy gut flora are primary factors in rising disease rates due to inflammation, and recent research suggests that intestinal inflammation may play a role in the development of certain cancers. Refined grains, sugar, and processed foods all contribute to the destruction of gut flora, and also create an acidic state in the body which leads to inflammation and disease. Another cause is the imbalance in our diets of omega-6 and omega-3 essential fatty acids. This may come as a surprise to many people who have been led to believe that vegetable oils are healthy to eat, but they contain omega-6 fatty acids that can be inflammatory when consumed in abundance. Eating a healthy diet with a correct omega-6 to omega-3 EFA balance, quitting smoking, cutting down on alcohol consumption, exercising more, and controlling stress can all help reverse an inflammatory condition in the body.

The good news is, when diseases and chronic conditions are caused by an unhealthy diet, then a healthy diet can be the cure. The medical and pharmaceutical industries make their profits by diagnosing and treating these diseases with expensive drugs and medical tests, but the truth is, *virtually all these diseases can be prevented, ameliorated or cured by a healthy diet of whole foods devoid of refined and processed products.*

"Diet can have a more profound effect on your health than any other known modality of medical treatment."
—*Dr. Joseph Mercola, founder of the world's most popular natural health website www.mercola.com*

Obesity

The most obvious result of a poor diet is obesity. According to the American Obesity Association, obesity is now epidemic in the U.S. as well as in other developed countries. The number of overweight and obese Americans continues to rise and now about 127 million people are categorized as being overweight, and of these, 60 million are estimated to be obese. It is estimated that obesity causes at least 300,000 premature deaths in the U.S. each year, with healthcare costs of approximately $100 billion. A study published in the *American Journal of Preventive Medicine* predicts that close to 50 percent of Americans will be obese by 2030, and 11 percent of the population will be severely obese—or roughly 100 pounds overweight.

The cause of obesity is simply poor dietary choices that eventually interfere with the body's metabolism. A diet high in sugar, fructose and refined grains causes weight gain and malnourishment which in turn leads to a number of diseases including heart problems and diabetes.

The cost of obesity among full-time workers in the U.S. is thought to be $73 billion per year, the equivalent of hiring 1.8 million new workers at an annual salary of $42,000. Obesity's hidden costs, say researchers, stem from the fact that obese people tend to be less productive than normal-weight people while at work. The Rand Corporation, a research and analysis organization, released a study that found links between the increase in obesity and reported disabilities. Their study found a 39.4 percent increase in the number of people between the ages of 30 and 49 years who were unable to care for themselves due to obesity. Muscle-skeletal problems such as chronic back pain, which are linked to obesity, are one of the nation's leading causes of disability. The Office of the Surgeon General reports that obese people also have a higher risk of arthritis, asthma, sleep apnea, incontinence, gallbladder disease and reproductive difficulties.

Heart Disease and Blood Vessel Disease

Coronary heart disease currently affects about 14 million men and women in the U.S., and causes around 600,000 deaths every year. New studies show that atherosclerosis, the major precursor of cardiovascular disease—a hardening or "furring" of the arteries—can begin in childhood, with unhealthy changes appearing in the blood vessels of children as young as seven years old. There are many different causes and contributing factors to heart disease including an unhealthy diet, stress, obesity, diabetes, high blood pressure, and smoking. For many years, a high fat diet was considered a major cause of heart disease, but research has shown that the real culprit is a diet heavy in refined and processed foods, and especially foods sweetened with fructose.

Arterial disease is systemic, in other words, it affects the arteries and veins in the entire body, which includes the coronary arteries within the brain, leading to dementia and stroke.

Peripheral arterial and vascular diseases are diseases of the blood vessels outside the heart. The arteries are blood vessels that supply blood, oxygen and nutrients to the body from the heart. Narrow, hardened arteries make it more difficult for blood to flow through and reach body tissue, resulting in an inadequate blood supply to the extremities. Signs of peripheral vascular disease include varicose veins, spider veins, and intermittent cramping pain in the leg muscles on exertion, and complications can include sores that do not heal, ulcers, gangrene, and infections in the extremities. In rare cases, amputation may be necessary. About five percent of people over the age of 50 in the U.S. are believed to suffer from peripheral artery disease.

Renal artery disease is a form of peripheral artery disease that reduces blood flow through the renal arteries, which supply blood to the kidneys. Renal artery disease affects one in every 18 women aged 65 and older. Blood flow to the kidneys is reduced or cut off, which may cause high blood pressure and potentially permanent damage to the kidneys.

Stroke, which is cerebrovascular disease, or a disease of the blood vessels in the brain, claims 128,842 lives per year.

Cancer

Cancer is epidemic in modern society and now affects one of out every three women and one out of every two men in the U.S. A report by the American Cancer Society entitled *Cancer Statistics 2012* says that a total of 1,638,910 new cancer cases and 577,190 deaths from cancer are expected to occur in the U.S. in 2012. "This rise [in cancer cases] may be linked to the increasing prevalence of obesity," says the report.

It's well documented that eating a poor diet high in processed foods is a major contributor of obesity, and of cancer. Cancer is a complex disease with no known single cause; causes range from emotional issues to toxin overload to stress to poor diet. The multi-billion-dollar cancer industry still likes to assert that red meat, animal protein and fats cause cancer, but in fact, cancer tumors grow by feeding on sugar, and especially fructose, in the bloodstream. Refined carbohydrates provide plenty of this sugar, most often from refined grains, such as white flour, pizza, and pasta, and from sugar and HFCS and foods that contain them—candy, bakery products, alcohol, refined fruit juice, soda and sweetened drinks. Unhealthy fats, such as hydrogenated and trans-fats, also promote the growth of cancer cells by contributing to poor cell membrane permeability, which leads to malnourished cells and malfunctioning organs in the body.

Arthritis

Arthritis is a general term which actually means inflammation of a joint. Arthritis can affect people of all ages, but becomes more prevalent as people age, and over the years it can cause permanent destruction. Government surveys show that approximately 33 percent of adults in the U.S. currently suffer from some type of troublesome arthritis, and approximately half of all people over 65 years report having arthritis. Though arthritis can be caused by injury, the vast majority of cases are caused by an unhealthy diet, especially a diet high in grains and sugars. Many cases of all types of arthritis, including rheumatoid arthritis, have been helped by removing wheat and sugar from the diet, and others have been cured by removing a food allergy, such as milk. In other words, most cases of arthritis can be cured or greatly ameliorated when the diatetic cause is identified and removed. Significantly, arthritis is comparatively rare in African and Asian countries where processed foods do not make up the bulk of the daily diet.

Type 2 Diabetes

Type 2 diabetes is a disorder in which the blood contains more glucose than the body can process. In this type of diabetes, the pancreas does produce insulin, but the insulin produced is ineffective due to insulin resistance. A diet too high in refined carbohydrates—baked goods and sugary foods—is the main culprit. A constant intake of high carbohydrate foods causes the body to produce more and more insulin but eventually, the cells become insulin resistant when the "doors" to the cells, called cell receptors, close up. The body then produces even more insulin to try to get glucose into the cells. But the body is now producing too much insulin, to the point where the cells don't respond to the insulin any more. This results in even more insulin being pumped into the blood stream, which in turn creates more insulin resistance.

Nearly 70,000 people in the U.S. die from diabetes every year, and the results of long-term diabetes can be devastating, including blindness, kidney failure, and problems with circulation to the extremities, often resulting in amputation. Type 2 diabetes can be controlled, and even cured, some doctors have shown, by eating a healthy diet of whole organic foods.

Candidiasis

Candidiasis is a systemic yeast infection caused by an overgrowth of a naturally-occurring organism in the gut called *Candida albicans.* It can cause a wide range of symptoms in the body, including fatigue, migraine, fibromyalgia, food sensitivities, "brain fog," bowel disturbances including bloating, gas and severe constipation, and just plain "feeling bad all over." Candidiasis is caused by a combination of taking antibiotics, which kill off the "good" flora in the gut, combined with a high carbohydrate diet which feeds the *Candida albicans* its favorite food—sugar, just like any yeast. It can take just one course of antibiotics to create an imbalance between good and bad bacteria in the gut. The resulting yeast overgrowth can also disturb the intestinal tract lining, allowing allergens and toxins to "leak" through the gut into the blood circulation, resulting in a weakening of the immune system. Unfortunately, candidiasis is a condition that flies under the radar screen of most medical professionals and is not often diganosed.

Someone with a candida overgrowth will often crave the foods that feed it, especially sugary foods and refined wheat, such as bread and pasta. Now that sugar and HFCS are found in virtually all processed foods, including savory ones such as breads, soups, crackers, and peanut butter, avoiding sweeteners can be difficult. Candida can be diagnosed with a blood test, and can be treated by drastically reducing the amount of sugar and refined carbohydrates in the diet, and by taking antifungal supplements, such as garlic, along with acidophilus to repopulate the gut with beneficial flora. There is more information at the website yeastconnection.com.

Dementia and Alzheimer's Disease

Alzheimer's is the sixth-leading cause of death in the country, claiming 79,000 lives per year. During the period 2000-2008, deaths from Alzheimer's disease rose 66 percent, and health care professionals now consider Alzheimer's to be at the level of an epidemic. An estimated 5.4 million Americans are now living with the disease, according to the Alzheimer's Association's *2011 Disease Facts and Figures*, and the cost for care in 2012 is estimated to be $200 billion. It is projected that in the next 20 years, Alzheimer's will affect one in four elderly Americans, and if things continue at this rate, the care costs of Alzheimer's and other dementias will soar to a projected $1.1 trillion (in today's dollars) by 2050.

Alzheimer's disease is associated with inflammation in the body. Research conducted at the Mayo Clinic shows that people on a high calorie diet have twice the risk of mild cognitive impairment compared with a low calorie diet. A study from Columbia University in New York shows that those least likely to develop Alzheimer's disease eat a diet rich in foods such as nuts, fish, tomatoes, olive oil, poultry, broccoli and other cruciferous vegetables, fruits, and dark green leafy vegetables.

Strict vegetarian and vegan diets, which can be low in omega-3 and other fats, have been shown to increase the risk of Alzheimer's, whereas diets high in omega-3 fatty acids have a lower risk. "Trans fats have been shown to replace omega-3 fats in the cell membranes, and are associated with systemic inflammation, cardiovascular disease, and endothelial dysfunction. All those processes have an impact on memory, brain structure, and cognition," says the study.

Most of the information available about treating Alzheimer's stresses the importance of a healthy diet free from processed foods, sweetened foods, and "bad" fats—which leads us to believe that these may be the things that cause dementia in the first place. In fact, some doctors are calling Alzheimer's "diabetes of the brain" or "type 3 diabetes."

An article by George Monbiot in the U.K. newspaper *The Guardian* says, "A large body of evidence now suggests that Alzheimer's is primarily a metabolic disease. Some scientists have gone so far as to rename it type 3 diabetes . . . and believe it is caused largely by the brain's impaired response to insulin."

Prevention is the key here: eliminate or reduce refined and processed foods from your diet so you can avoid dementia and live a long life with your brain cells firing on all cylinders.

Osteoporosis

Osteoporosis, meaning "porous bones," is a bone weakness due to reduced mineral density that leads to an increased risk of fracture. Bones become weak and brittle when the creation of new bone doesn't keep up with the body's normal removal of old bone cells. About half of all women and one in five men in the U.S. over the age of 50 are estimated to have a fracture of the hip, wrist, or vertebra during their lifetime, and many become disabled from weakened bones. Hip fracture is one of the main reasons people are admitted to nursing homes. An Australian study has found that people over 60 years old who have had a fracture because of osteoporosis face a higher risk of death over the next 5 to 10 years compared to the general population. Causes of osteoporosis include malnutrition, mainly a high-carbohydrate acidic diet which leaches minerals from bones, and most especially the excessive consumption of alcohol, caffeinated drinks, and soda drinks, which contain phosphoric acid. Osteoporosis can be prevented, and reversed to a degree, by eating a healthy diet of whole foods and by participating in weight-bearing exercise.

Allergies & Immune System Problems

Autoimmune disorders stem from a dysfunctional immune system that attacks the body's own cells, tissues, and organs. There are more than 80 known autoimmune disorders which range from asthma, hay-fever, and eczema to lupus, multiple sclerosis, rheumatoid arthritis, and type 1 diabetes, as well as autoimmune related diseases like fibromyalgia and chronic fatigue syndrome. Experts estimate that the incidence of these diseases has doubled, tripled or in some cases even quadrupled over the past 20 years, and some studies now indicate that more than half of all Americans have at least one allergy. In her book *The Autoimmune Epidemic*, Donna Jackson Nakazawa states that 75 percent of autoimmune sufferers are women, and that the average American woman is eight times more likely to have an autoimmune disease than breast cancer.

These types of diseases occur when the immune system is overwhelmed by a combination of factors, including a poor diet, obesity, stress, lack of physical activity, air pollution, and toxic chemicals. All these diseases have inflammation at their base, and an anti-inflammatory diet can often help, and especially the Paleo diet, which at its most basic consists of meat, fats and cooked vegetables, preferably organic since average supermarket vegetables and meat are raised with the use of pesticides, herbicides, antibiotics, and hormones.

"After 30 years of practicing medicine, I have learned that for any chronic illness or ailment, treating underlying imbalances and dysfunctions is more important than making a diagnosis and naming the disease."

—*Dr. Frank Lipman, Huffington Post*

CHAPTER 5

Genetically-Modified Foods

A Threat to our Health, Our Food Supply, and the Environment

"It is estimated that about 75 percent of processed foods sold in the U.S. contain at least some genetically modified food ingredients. Unlike many other countries, there is no law in the U.S. requiring the labeling of foods that contain GM ingredients."

— *Health Freedom Alliance*

MOST DEVELOPED NATIONS DO NOT CONSIDER GENETICALLY-MODIFIED (GM) CROPS TO BE SAFE—in many countries around the world, including Australia, Japan, and the European Union, there are restrictions or bans on the production and sale of genetically-modified organisms (GMOs). India recently became the 50th nation in the world to require labels on GM foods. But in the U.S., the government has bowed to pressure from the biotech industry and so far has refused to legislate restricting or labelling GM products, and has approved GMOs based on studies conducted by the same corporations that created them.

A growing amount of evidence is connecting GM food crops with health problems and environmental damage. Other issues that have created a huge controversy all over the world include the violation of farmers' and consumers' rights, the effect on GM crops on natural ecosystems, gene flow into non GM crops, and corporate control of the food supply.

The American Academy of Environmental Medicine (AAEM) has stated that several animal studies indicate there are serious health risks associated with ingesting GM food, including infertility, immune problems, accelerated aging, insulin regulation, and changes in major organs and the gastrointestinal system. The AAEM has called on physicians to educate their patients, the medical community, and the public to avoid GM foods when possible and provide educational materials concerning GM foods and health risks. They have called for a moratorium on GM foods, and have requested that long-term independent studies be started. They also suggest labeling for GM foods. They conclude, "There is more than a casual association between GM foods and adverse health effects. There is causation as defined by recognized scientific criteria. The strength of association and consistency between GM foods and disease is confirmed in several animal studies."

Many pressure groups opposed to GM crops argue that governments should use independent studies rather than industry studies to assess crop safety, and have called for the EPA to require that independent researchers have free access to GM products for testing. But the truth about the effect of GM food crops on humans and the ecosystem is hard if not impossible to scientifically assess due to restrictive end-user agreements, so researchers are forbidden by law from publishing independent research in peer-reviewed journals without the approval of the agritech companies. Cornell University's Elson Shields, the spokesperson for a group of scientists who oppose this practice, submitted a statement to the Environmental Protection Agency (EPA) arguing that "as a result of restrictive access, no truly independent research can be legally conducted on many critical questions regarding [GM] technology." And the magazine *Scientific American* reported that several studies were blocked from being published when scientists found results that were "unflattering" to the industry, even though they were initially approved by agritech companies.

Meanwhile, grass-roots movements such as Food and Water Watch, the Organic Consumers Association, and Millions Against Monsanto are fighting corporate interests in the attempt to control the spread of GM crops and to legislate labeling of GM foods. We have a right to know what we are eating and what we are feeding to our children, and how these foods will affect us in the long-term.

Despite Promises, No Benefits Seen from GM Foods

Despite all the assurances, none of the GM products currently on the market seem to offer the benefits initially promised by the biotech industry, such as increased yield, drought tolerance, or enhanced nutrition. In fact, GM crops have been found to be more susceptible to disease than normal plants, and some crops have been shown to need twice as much water as non-GM crops.

GM crops are not more productive, according to data collected by the Union of Concerned Scientists in a report called "Failure to Yield." Corn, soy, cotton, canola, alfalfa, and sugar beets have all been modified with engineered DNA that either resist an herbicide or produce an insecticide. But insects and weeds quickly take up the altered DNA from the GM crops through the soil and develop herbicide and pesticide resistance themselves. These superweeds and Bt-resistant insects (Bt is a toxin made by the bacteria *Bacillus thuringiensis*) have become a chronic problem for farmers who grow GM crops. Over the past 16 years, it's estimated that more than a quarter of a million Indian farmers have committed suicide after being convinced to plant Monsanto's GM seeds, especially Bt cotton, then having their crops fail, leaving them in financial ruin.

Widespread adoption of GM crops would not help feed the world as their promoters claim, according to ActionAid. In fact, they believe that the dangers from GM crops will actually worsen the plight of the 800 million hungry people in the world, and that there should be a moratorium until more research is done. Only one percent of GM research is aimed at crops used by poor farmers in poor countries: "It is not the interests of poor farmers but the profits of the agrochemical industry that have been the driving force behind the emergence of GM agriculture. Four multinationals—Monsanto, Syngenta, Bayer CropScience, and Dupont—now control most of the GM seed market. About 91 percent of all GM crops grown in the world are from Monsanto seeds."

Monsanto's Herbicide Roundup and the Environmental Problems it Causes

Monsanto's Roundup Ready GM crops are engineered to be able to withstand heavy applications of Roundup, a broad-spectrum herbicide whose active ingredient is the isopropylamine salt of glyphosate. One of the results of heavy use of Roundup is that glyphosate resistance in weeds is on the rise. These super-hardy weeds are nearly impossible to get rid of—it is estimated that more than 130 types of weeds in 40 states in the U.S. are now herbicide-resistant, and farmers are applying ever increasing amounts of toxic herbicides to their crops in the attempt to control them.

Monsanto's scientists apparently did not believe that weeds could become resistant to glyphosate. When requesting government approval for the herbicide in 1993, Monsanto claimed that "glyphosate is considered to be an herbicide with low risk for weed resistance," and support for this viewpoint was given by several university scientists who agreed that "it is highly unlikely that weed resistance to glyphosate will become a problem."

In 2009, a French court found Monsanto guilty of falsely advertising its herbicide as "biodegradable," "environmentally friendly" and claiming it "left the soil clean." Even Monsanto's own tests showed that only two percent of the herbicide broke down after 28 days. Glyphosate has been found in the air and in rain samples that were collected in Mississippi and Iowa, according to a study published in the journal *Environmental Toxicology and Chemistry* in March 2011. Glyphosate was detected in 60 to 100 percent of all air and rain samples, which is further evidence that Roundup does not readily break down in the environment.

"The truth is, GM crops are designed to do nothing more than sell herbicides," explains Alexis Baden-Mayer, political director of the Organic Consumers Association. "That they've done successfully; Monsanto's RoundUp Ready GM crops have made Monsanto's RoundUp the number one herbicide."

Roundup Affects Fertility in Humans

There is considerable evidence that glyphosate is dangerous to humans, affecting the endocrine and reproductive systems and altering fertility by throwing off the delicate hormonal balance that governs the reproductive cycle. It has been shown to interfere with aromatase, which produces estrogen, and is highly toxic to the placenta in pregnant women. In a 2009 French study, scientists discovered that glyphosate can kill the cells in the outer layer of the human placenta which in turn can kill the placenta. Only 1/500th of the amount needed to kill weeds was able to kill these cells, an amount so small, according to the study's authors, that the "residual levels to be expected, especially in food and feed derived from Roundup formulation-treated crops, could be enough to cause cell damage and even [cell] death." Glyphosate has also been shown to inhibit other plant enzymes, and to affect animal enzymes. In April 2010, researchers at Russia's Institute of Ecology and Evolution of the Russian Academy of Sciences and the National Association for Gene Security found that after feeding hamsters GM soy for two years over three generations, most lost the ability to produce young by the third generation.

A group of international scientists has released a report detailing health and environmental hazards from the cultivation of GM Roundup-ready soy and the use of glyphosate. The report, "GM Soy: Sustainable? Responsible?," highlights new research by Argentine government scientist Professor Andrés

Carrasco who found that glyphosate causes malformations in frog and chicken embryos at doses far lower than those used in agricultural spraying. "The findings in the lab are compatible with malformations observed in humans exposed to glyphosate during pregnancy," said Carrasco. The report is released with testimonies of Argentine villagers whose lives have been radically disrupted by the cultivation of GM soy. In Argentina and Paraguay, doctors and residents living in GM soy producing areas have reported serious health effects from glyphosate spraying, and studies confirm links between exposure to glyphosate and premature births, miscarriages, cancer, and damage to DNA and reproductive organ cells. Carrasco said people living in soy-producing areas of Argentina began reporting problems in 2002, two years after the first big harvests of GM Roundup-ready soy. He said, "I suspect the toxicity classification of glyphosate is too low . . . in some cases this can be a powerful poison."

Children are Most Vulnerable to GM Foods

"Swapping genes between organisms can produce unknown toxic effects and allergies that are most likely to affect children."

—Dr. Vyvyan Howard, President of the International Society of Doctors for the Environment

GM organisms are now found in more than 75 percent of processed foods on sale in the U.S. A report released in October 2012 by the Environmental Working Group showed that Americans are eating their weight and more in genetically engineered food every year—an average of 193 pounds of GM foods annually. It is estimated that a child in the U.S. who eats processed foods on a regular basis consumes at least 10 percent GM ingredients, though the actual percentage may be far higher than that.

"What's shocking is that Americans are eating so much genetically engineered food, yet there have been zero long-term studies done by the federal government or industry to determine if its consumption could pose a risk health," said Renee Sharp, lead author of the report and the director of Environmental Working Group's California office. "If you were planning on eating your body weight of anything in a year or feeding that much food to your family, wouldn't you first want to know if long-term government studies and monitoring have shown it is safe?"

Glyphosate has been shown to build up in the body so its toxic effects are accumulative. This may become a serious concern for the next generation as most young children growing up today are eating a large amount of processed foods containing GM ingredients whether their parents are aware of it or not.

"There is no need for, or value in testing the safety of GM foods in humans."

—from the website of Monsanto Inc.

The GM Foods in our Food Supply and Supermarkets are Unlabeled

How do we know which foods contain GMOs? Unfortunately, we don't. The United States is one of the few countries in the developed world that doesn't require labeling of GM food, even though polls consistently show that a significant majority of Americans want to know if their food contains GMOs—a recent poll released by ABC News found that 93 percent of the American public wants the federal government to require mandatory labeling of genetically engineered foods. ABC News stated, "Such near-unanimity in public opinion is rare."

Although 50 countries around the world require labelling of GM foods, Monsanto continues to fight it. With an annual income of over $11 billion, the company has the money and power to push its agenda of controlling seed and food production around the world by influencing politicians and legislators. A ballot initiative was held in November of 2012 in California, the eight largest economy in the world, to mandate labeling of GM foods and food ingredients, but Monsanto and other food and pesticide producers including PepsiCo, Coca-Cola, Kellogg, General Mills, DuPont, and Bayer spent a sum believed to be in excess of $45 million to defeat the initiative. Vermont legislators, despite overwhelming public support, dragged their feet on a proposed GMO labeling bill because Monsanto threatened to sue the state if the bill passed.

According to OpenSecrets.org, "Monsanto basically lives at the doorsteps of legislators in Washington" where it spent $5.3 million in 2011 lobbying the nation's lawmakers. The power of Monsanto can be seen through its influence in Washington, including making contributions to Rep. Frank D. Lucas, chairman of the House Agriculture Committee, through which every farm-related piece of legislation must pass.

But this begs the question, if GM foods are not dangerous to our health, why is Monsanto so resistant to labeling them? Other more enlightened and ethical food companies, however, are volunteering to label their food as safe to eat, such as Green Mountain Gringo whose Tortilla Strips are made from GMO-free corn, which is clearly marked on the packet and on their website.

In the meantime, until our politicians come to their senses, the simplest way to avoid GM foods is to buy organic foods. By definition, growers of foods that are certified organic must never intentionally use GM ingredients, and the food must be produced without artificial pesticides and fertilizers and from animals reared without the routine use of antibiotics, growth promoters, or other drugs. Additionally, grass-fed beef will not have been fed GM corn feed.

CHAPTER 6

Nutritional Equivalents of Naturally-Produced Foods Compared to Processed Foods

AS PROCESSED FOODS HAVE BECOME MORE and more a major part of the American diet, our health has progressively deteriorated, so it makes absolute sense to eat the most nutritionally-dense foods we can get. People complain that organic food is expensive, but in fact, the actual cost of eating cheap food is enormous, it's just that people rarely think about it. When you add in the cost of medical treatment and other side effects, cheap food is no longer cheap.

The SAD diet is heavy in carbohydrate foods, which are a poor source of nutrition, and the truth is, the poorer the food in our diets, the more of it we will need to eat to reach our nutritional needs. This leads to overeating and weight gain, because if the body is fed inferior food it will keep on eating, trying to derive some nutritional value from the food being consumed. In this way, we consume excess calories, not to mention undesirable food additives, in this attempt to reach our body's nutritional goals, which leads to overeating, weight gain, and ill health.

There is no greater investment you can make in yourself and your family than eating the best food available. If you do, you will be in perfect health. This is the natural state for the body—we are born in perfect health, and if we feed our body the right foods, we will stay that way. We are not designed nor destined to get sick. Our body has extraordinary healing capacities, and when we feed it nutritious food, we are giving it the tools it needs to stay healthy.

One of the biggest advantages of being in optimal health is not having to worry about getting sick. Imagine not having to worry about whether we'll get cancer or heart disease, not having to take time off work for expensive and uncomfortable medical tests, and not being depressed about being overweight and out of shape. And most importantly, knowing we can look forward to many vibrant years as a senior citizen, allowing us to say NO to long-term care insurance, because we KNOW we will remain healthy in our later years.

Why Our Bodies Need Nutritious Food

The function of food is not to satisfy any deep psychological needs we might have, or titillate our taste buds, or relieve us from boredom. We need food because it is fuel for the body and provides the building blocks that the body needs in order to create new cells and tissues and repair itself.

Food cravings are often caused by imbalances in our nutritional intake. The body is an intelligent multi-celled organism that knows what it needs to be healthy, and if properly nourished, it will not generate food cravings. Most diet advice focuses on calories, but nutrition is not just about calories, which is simply a measurement of the energy a food produces when it is burned in the body. Yes, the body needs energy foods, but not getting enough energy foods is the least of our concerns as they are overabundant in the average diet. Most importantly we need building foods, elements in our diet that provide our body with the raw materials necessary to build and repair itself, such as high-quality proteins and fats. If it were all about the energy, we could eat two pounds of sugar a day and we'd be off and running like the Energizer Bunny. But we all know that's not the case.

On his website, nutritional expert Dr. Joseph Mercola writes, "What most people don't know is that you don't actually need carbohydrates—they are not essential for survival and the RDA for carbs is actually zero. If you ate no carbohydrates, like many traditional Eskimos do, you would survive as long as you had enough high-quality protein, fat, water and minerals."

Many of the ingredients added to our foods, as well as some of the ways our food is produced and grown, actually count as "anti-nutrition." For instance, sugar added to a food reduces its nutritional value dramatically—one cup of unsweetened applesauce calibrates at an optimum level of nutrition, while that same cup of applesauce sweetened with one teaspoon of sugar calibrates at the level close to poison. Due to "negative nutrition," you would have to eat four cups of sweetened apple sauce to gain the nutritional equivalent of one cup of unsweetened apple sauce, and you'd be consuming four teaspoons of unnecessary refined sugar.

A list of more comparisons between natural foods and processed foods is shown in the table on the opposite page. Remember that a healthy food consists of a combination of ALL the nutrients that are present in its original, natural state—including, but not limited to, vitamins, minerals, enzymes, antioxidants, phytonutrients, and energy from the sun, or life force energy. Processed foods, deprived of some or all of these components, are deficient foods and are the main reason why the average American is now overweight and undernourished.

Comparison of Organic vs. Supermarket Foods

True Nutritional Equivalents and Costs of a Sample Breakfast, Taking into Account Negative Nutrition

As we can see from these equivalents, we have to eat a much larger amount of processed foods compared to whole organic foods to reach our body's nutritional requirements. And the unhealthy food in this example would actually cost four times more than buying the equivalent nutritional value of a healthy breakfast of organic food.

All Organic/Naturally-Raised	*COST*		*Generic supermarket food:*	*COST*
1 organic orange	$1.50	=	32 oz. Tropicana orange juice	$2.20
2 oz. Applegate Farm organic bacon	1.75	=	1 lb. Oscar Meyer bacon	6.99
2 organic eggs	1.00	=	6 supermarket eggs	1.00
1 slice organic whole wheat bread	.55	=	1 loaf Pepperidge Farm Soft Wheat Bread	3.99
2 oz. organic oatmeal, milk & honey	.60	=	2 lbs. Cheerios (average price $3.79/18 oz.)	7.00
TOTAL COST	**$5.40**		**TOTAL COST**	**$21.18**

Nutritional Equivalent of Certain Foods

Comparison of Functional Nutritional Values

Organic/Naturally-Raised Food		Standard Supermarket Food
4 oz. grass-raised beef	equals	1 lb. corn-fed beef
4 oz. naturally-raised chicken	equals	10 oz. Purdue chicken or 16 oz. White Gem chicken
2 oz. naturally-raised bacon	equals	1 lb. Oscar Meyer bacon
1 egg from free-range chickens	equals	4 eggs from battery-raised chickens
4 oz. organic raw milk	equals	20 oz. of Hood low-fat milk, pasteurized and homogenized
4 oz. baked organic potato	equals	5 lbs. Cape Cod russet potato chips
4 oz. fresh organic corn kernels	equals	4 lbs. Lays corn chips
4 oz. fresh organic corn kernels	equals	2 1/2 lbs. Kellogg's corn flakes
2 oz. organic milled oats	equals	2 lbs. of Cheerios
1 slice of organic whole wheat bread	equals	2 loaves of Wonder Bread
1 slice of organic whole wheat bread	equals	1 loaf of Pepperidge Farm whole wheat bread
1 oz. Kerry Gold Irish Butter	equals	8 oz. Land O'Lakes butter or 2 oz. Horizon organic butter
1 oz. organic cream cheese	equals	6 oz. of Philadelphia cream cheese
1 medium-sized organic orange	equals	4 eight-ounce glasses of Tropicana orange juice
1 medium-sized organic apple	equals	2 eight-ounce glasses of Mott's apple juice
1 large organic apple	equals	3 whole Mrs. Smith's apple pies
1 medium-sized tomato	equals	20 oz. bottle of Heinz tomato ketchup
1 oz. organic mayonnaise (olive oil)	equals	20 oz. Hellmann's Mayonnaise (soy-bean oil)
1 oz. extra-virgin olive oil	equals	16 oz. refined canola, soy bean or sunflower seed oil
1 oz. extra-virgin olive oil	equals	20 oz. refined corn oil
1 oz. of raw walnuts	equals	6 oz. of candied walnuts
1 oz. of raw organic peanuts	equals	12 oz. of Beer Nuts
1 oz. of raw organic peanuts	equals	4 lbs. of chocolate-covered peanut M&Ms
1 oz. of raw organic peanuts	equals	12 oz. jar of Skippy peanut butter
1 oz. of raw organic peanuts	equals	16.3 oz. jar of Skippy Roasted Honey Nut Super Chunk
1 oz. of unsweetened raw chocolate	equals	12 oz. of Hershey's milk chocolate

CHAPTER 7

Grains

"There's no human requirement for grains. [We are not] hard-wired as a species to eat grains. You can get by just fine and meet every single nutrient requirement that humans have without eating grains. And grains are poor sources of vitamins and minerals compared to fruits and vegetables and meat and fish."

— *Dr. Loren Cordain, an expert on Paleolithic lifestyles at Colorado State University*

THE MAIN SOURCE OF CARBOHYDRATE IN THE U.S. DIET TODAY is grains, mainly wheat, corn, and rice. Grains have been part of the human diet since the early days of agriculture some 10,000 years ago, when people began cultivating plants that had previously grown wild. But before that time, grains were not part of the human diet, and many nutritional experts believe that grains are not a natural food for mammals to eat (and yes, that includes us). They argue that, biologically, our digestive systems are not adapted to eating grains, as we cannot digest raw grains in the stomach—they must be sprouted or cooked first.

Grains are problematic for the human digestive system because they contain naturally-occurring toxins made by the plants as protection against predators. Dr. Loren Cordain, a professor at Colorado State University and an expert on Paleolithic lifestyles, explains why: "Grains are the seeds of a plant. They're its reproductive material, and plants don't make their reproductive material to give away for free to other animals. If they did they'd become extinct, and so the evolutionary strategy that many plants, particularly cereal grains, have taken to prevent predation is to evolve toxic compounds so that the predator of the seeds can't eat them, so that they can put their seeds in the soil where they're meant to be to grow a new plant and not in the gut of an animal to feed it." Cattle, whose natural food is grass, have to be given antibiotics when fed corn otherwise they'd get sick from eating it. Birds, however, are able to digest grains—they have a special organ, the gizzard, which can grind up the grains along with grit and small stones.

The appeal of grains as a food source is that they can be mass-produced, providing food for huge numbers of people and animals, and, when refined, can be stored and sold on the open market as a commodity. The total annual yield of wheat and corn in the U.S. is valued at over 20 billion dollars, and much of that is sold oversees, making it an important export. Because of farming subsidies, grains provide a very low-cost ingredient for many processed foods. And politicians like to keep the cost of food down because the less money we spend on food, the more is left over to buy such things as cars and consumer electronics that boost economic growth.

We have been given the message for so long that grains are an important part of our diet that we now believe this to be true. The Government USDA Food Pyramid recommends 6 to 11 servings of carbohydrates—bread, cereal, pasta, rice—per day. But we have to ask ourselves how the USDA, a government body set up to promote agriculture and sell agricultural commodities, can be trusted to make dietary recommendations. There seems to be a conflict of interest in helping farmers sell more wheat, corn, and soy, and at the same time trying to convince people to consume healthier food.

There are other issues associated with the consumption of grains in the modern diet, including allergies, weight gain, chemical toxins, and genetically-modified strains. Consuming grains in excess increases the incidence of diabetes, and also makes the body more acidic. This causes the body to draw calcium and other alkaline minerals from the bones and teeth to buffer the acidic condition in the blood and leads to such diseases as arthritis, osteoporosis, and dental decay, as well as hardened arteries and high blood pressure. Some people have an allergy to gluten, a component of wheat and other grains such as rye, barley and to some degree oats, which causes severe digestive problems.

The High Carbohydrate Diet is a Scourge of Modern Civilization

"What you begin to review the evidence stacked up against whole grains, it becomes self-evident that our reliance on wheat and other grains may be one of the primary culprits for the poor health of so many."
—*Dr. Joseph Mercola, founder of the World's No. 1 Natural Health Website www.mercola.com*

A diet high in refined carbohydrates, such as white bread, pizza, pasta, cakes, cookies, pastries, and candy, causes nutritional deficiencies which lead to many of the modern degenerative diseases that are epidemic today. But grains are not, in fact, an essential part of our diet and most people would be much better off never eating them.

Grains have become a problem in our diets because of their ubiquitous nature. If we eat cereal or bread for breakfast, a sandwich for lunch, pizza or pasta for dinner, and snack on chips, pretzels and cookies between meals, we are eating grains throughout the day, every day. This dependence upon one food item, particularly wheat, results in allergies and sensitivities—or even addiction in susceptible individuals.

Grains originally found their way into our diet as a substitute for more expensive (but more nutritious) animal proteins. It is ironic that the traditional diet of poor Italian peasants, *la cucina povera*, has been adopted by the richest country in the world as a healthy alternative to eating meat. Pizza and pasta have become accepted in our culture as suitable fare for a hearty meal, replacing the "meat and two veg" that was for so long considered a perfect dinner.

But eating grains in excess causes weight gain—bear in mind that beef cattle are fattened on corn because their natural food, grass, keeps them lean. Over the past 40 years or so, the medical profession has encouraged us to increase our intake of carbohydrates and reduce our fat intake because it was thought this would lower the risk of heart disease, but during this period of time the rate of heart disease, diabetes and cancer actually rose to almost epidemic levels, leading nutritional experts to seriously question this advice.

Today, a high-carbohydrate diet is known to be the primary culprit in virtually all of today's common degenerative diseases—diabetes, heart disease, cancer, arthritis, osteoporosis and Alzheimer's. Study after study shows that a diet high in quality animal protein protects against these diseases, while a diet high in refined sugar and starch causes them.

Carbohydrates are a source of energy that is metabolized by the body more quickly than proteins or fats. A diet too high in carbohydrates can upset the delicate balance of the body's blood sugar level, resulting in fluctuations in energy and mood that can leave a person feeling irritated and tired, inducing them to consume even more carbohydrate for a "quick lift." And too many carbohydrates causes insulin resistance, eventually leading to diabetes. It's estimated that 68 percent of Americans are now obese, and cases of diabetes in the U.S. have risen from 1.6 million in 1958 to 25.8 million in 2011. Even more shocking is that scientists estimate that one in every three children born this year in the U.S. will develop diabetes in their lifetime.

Grains Are Not a Complete Protein

A complete protein contains all the essential amino acids in quantities sufficient for growth and repair of body tissue. Most proteins from animal sources contain all the essential amino acids and are therefore considered to be complete proteins. However, plant proteins, including grains, lack the full range of essential amino acids. For example, corn lacks tryptophan, rice lacks threonine, soybeans lack methionine, and lysine is missing from corn, rice, and wheat. Vegetarians and vegans who consume no animal proteins in their diets are at risk of malnutrition as they may be deficient in one or more essential amino acids. However, consuming grains in combination with certain protein-rich plant foods, such as beans with rice, can result in a complete protein.

Grains Can Be Addictive

"Addiction is characterized by compulsive behavior, cravings, seeking, and use that persists even in the face of negative consequences."
— From "Drug Abuse and Addiction: Signs, Symptoms, and Effects"

Allergies and/or addictions to grain carbohydrates are linked to a variety of illnesses and conditions including chronic fatigue, lack of energy, chronic pain, brain fog, fibromyalgia, arthritis, bone loss and osteoporosis, metabolic diseases including weight gain, obesity, pre-diabetes, diabetes, autoimmune diseases, fertility problems and many more.

New scientific studies are showing a link between carbohydrate consumption and its effects on the brain. Research has confirmed what has been long suspected: food makes us feel good. It is believed that carbohydrate addiction may affect as many as one out of every two people worldwide. Craving an extra slice of toast or pizza is a strong indicator that you have become addicted to grain carbohydrates. And strangely, we crave what we may be allergic to.

Grains have significant effects on glucose levels in the blood and can also trigger the release of neurological chemicals such as tryptophan and serotonin that can cause addictive eating patterns. Tryptophan is a naturally occurring tranquilizer, basically an opioid chemical, with a direct relationship to serotonin levels in the brain, similar to pharmaceutical drugs like Valium. It affects the brain much like an addiction to opium. Researchers at the University of Wisconsin have demonstrated the effect of opiates on rats in several areas of the brain, and have recently shown that opioids affect the prefrontal cortex, where impulse control and cognition is located. Just as drugs and alcohol have a direct effect on these areas of the brain, the study shows that food creates neurological and biological pathways that foster physical and psychological addiction.

When people are driven by addictive food cravings, just as with drugs or caffeine, they are more likely to overindulge. This is one reason why diets so often fail—they attempt to limit the amount of food a person eats, but not the *type* of foods. Women seem to be especially prone to experiencing the negative effects from consuming excessive amounts of carbohydrates, which include weight gain, fibromyalgia, osteoporosis, infertility issues, heavy and painful menses, and polycystic ovary syndrome. Acne and other skin and autoimmune diseases, including lupus and rosacea, may also be linked to grain carbohydrates acting as toxins—in these cases, the only solution is to remove grains entirely from the diet.

Corn and Corn Products

IN MOST COUNTRIES AROUND THE WORLD, CORN, sometimes called Indian corn, or maize, is considered to be animal feed and not fit for human consumption. With a protein content of only 3 grams per 100 grams of corn compared to wheat germ at 23 grams per 100 grams, corn lags way behind other grains in nutritional content. But in the U.S., corn has become a staple ingredient in snack foods and processed foods, such as pop-corn, corn flakes, and corn chips, and is the base for high fructose corn syrup (HFCS), which is widely used as a sweetener for soft drinks and other products. HFCS is produced by milling corn to produce corn starch, then processing that starch to yield corn syrup, which is almost entirely glucose. Enzymes are then added that change some of the glucose into fructose.

The corn that is so familiar to us today was first cultivated and developed by early humans about 7,000 years ago, most probably in the area that is now central Mexico. It is a plant that does not exist naturally in the wild and can only survive if planted and protected by humans. Corn is thought to have evolved from a wild grass called teosinte, which looked very different from the corn that is grown today, with much smaller kernels. Indians throughout North and South America eventually came to depend upon this crop for much of their food, but it was unknown in other parts of the world until Columbus and his fellow explorers visited America's shores and took such items as corn, potatoes and tobacco back to Europe with them. Corn is recorded as being grown in Spain as early as 1498 and cultivation of corn quickly spread throughout Europe, and later to Africa and India. While natural corn varieties can grow to nearly 40 ft. tall, most commercially grown varieties have been bred for a standardized height of around 8 ft. Sweet corn, a genetic variant that contains more sugar and less starch, is usually shorter than field corn varieties. In England, the word "corn" can be used to describe any cereal crop, but most usually wheat, which can be a bit confusing.

Corn is the most widely grown grain crop in the world, with an annual harvest of 817 million tons. The U.S. is the largest producer of corn in the world with 332 million tons grown annually on over 400,000 farms. Nearly 80 million acres of land in the U.S. are planted with corn every year, and hybridization has meant that the yield from one acre of farmland has increased from 20 bushels of corn in 1900 to 138 in the 1990s. According to the National Corn Growers Association, about 80 percent of all U.S. corn is consumed by livestock and poultry and used in fish production, both in the US and abroad. About 12 percent of the U.S. corn crop is used for human food and the balance is used for corn ethanol, an oxygenate in auto fuels.

The Environmental Working Group shows that corn subsidies in the United States totaled $81.7 billion from 1995 to 2011. Corn has become a popular animal feed because it's cheap—it costs about $2.25 for a bushel of corn, which is 56 pounds, or about four cents a pound. Because of the subsidies, it actually costs less to buy corn than it costs to grow, but, since the U.S. Government pays the farmer to grow the corn, there is in fact a hidden cost to this supposedly cheap feed.

When ground into flour, corn yields more flour with less bran than wheat does, but it lacks the protein gluten of wheat and therefore does not make satisfactory baked goods. However, it can be used to make such dishes as corn bread, hominy, grits, hushpuppies, and Indian pudding, as well as polenta, which is a traditional food in parts of Northern Italy. Corn may not be a particularly nutritious food for humans, but the biggest danger is that the vast majority of corn used for animal feed and human food is genetically modified (GM), and unlabeled as such.

Comparative Vibrational Levels of Health and Disease States	Measured in Bovis Units of Life Force Energy	Comparative Nutritional Levels of **Corn & Corn Products**
10,000 = Level of Optimal Health e.g. a healthy newborn baby / hunter/gatherer tribes	10,000	Organically-grown corn • Organic popcorn • Corn bread and corn muffins made with organic ingredients and honey or maple syrup as a sweetener (not sugar)
	9,500	Quaker corn meal • Colavita polenta • Indian Head stone-ground corn meal
BETTER HEALTH	9,000	Bird's Eye frozen corn
	8,500	
	8,000	Green Giant Niblets frozen corn • Green Giant canned corn • Allen's Golden Hominy, canned
	7,500	
	7,000	Del Monte canned corn
	6,500	Generic supermarket popcorn
AVERAGE LEVEL OF HEALTH IN USA Inflammation	6,000	Generic corn-on-the-cob, corn meal and polenta • Orville Redenbacker's Gourmet Popping Corn
WORSENING HEALTH Arthritis starts to manifest	5,500	Green Mountain Gringo Tortilla Chips (non GM)
Heart Disease starts to manifest	5,000	Microwavable popcorn in bag with artificial "butter"
Cancer cells form: Breast, Prostate, Lung, Colon, Pancreas	4,500	Kellogg's Cornflakes
Diabetes • Osteoporosis	4,000	Jiffy-Pop Butter-flavored Corn • Orville Redenbacker's Gourmet Popcorn w/Movie Theater Butter
Lymphoma • Leukemia • Dementia	3,500	Mazola corn oil
Congestive heart disease Brain cancer • Multiple sclerosis	3,000	Wesson corn oil
Breast cancer metastasizes	2,500	
Prostate cancer metastasizes • Common cold/ flu	2,000	Pepperidge Farm corn bread stuffing • Goya corn meal • Kenyon's corn meal • Corn Sun Chips
Melanoma	1,500	Arnold's corn bread stuffing mix • Kellogg's Frosted Flakes
Metastatic bone and lung cancer	1,000	GV corn muffin mix • Jiffy corn muffin mix • Betty Crocker cornbread mix • Grande tortilla chips
	500	Thomas' Corn Toast R Cakes • Tostito's white corn chips • Santitas tortilla triangles • Argo corn starch
	50	Wise Cheez Doodles • Frito's corn chips • Dorito's nachos • Wise popcorn • Smartfood popcorn
Decay and Death	0	At 30: Cheetos Puffs, Twisted Puffs, and Crunch Puffs

Genetically Modified Corn

Many people still don't realize just how much of our food supply has been genetically modified (GM). Currently, about 88 percent of corn grown in the U.S. is genetically engineered, mostly seed from Monsanto that is "Roundup Ready." When you consider that 94 percent of U.S. sugar beets are also GM, it means that just about every processed food on sale in supermarkets that is not labeled "100 Percent USDA Organic" is likely to contain at least one GM component. This is a serious problem, as GM corn and soy have been shown to reduce fertility in animals, and glyphosate, the active ingredient in Monsanto's weed killer Roundup (glyphosate), which is heavily used on GM crops, has been shown to affect humans in a variety of ways, including altering fertility and killing kidney cells.

Monsanto continues to deny allegations that GM foods are harmful to humans and to the environment, and is fighting to prevent labelling of GM foods. With an annual income of over $11 billion, Monsanto has the money and power to push its agenda of controlling seed and food production around the world by influencing politicians and legislators.

Another sign that GM foods and the heavy application of the herbicide Roundup to our crops are causing environmental problems was reported by National Public Radio who revealed that the corn rootworm has developed resistance to one of the genes inserted in GM corn that is designed to kill them. Top experts on corn pests are urging the EPA to take action to halt the use of such GM crops. According to NPR: "The researchers are calling on farmers in some parts of the country to stop planting corn with anti-rootworm genes altogether, or to plant such corn only intermittently . . . If the recommendations in this letter were, in fact, put into practice, it would compel wrenching changes in the way that major seed companies like Monsanto and DuPont breed and market their corn seed."

Corn as a Protein Food

Corn is deficient in certain amino acids and B vitamins which has led to nutritional diseases such as pellagra and kwashiorkor in some parts of the world where the population was ignorant about the traditional method of preparing corn by soaking it in an alkaline solution.

Corn lacks readily accessible niacin, so corn was traditionally cooked with an alkali, a process known as nixtamalization. The ancient Aztec and Mayan civilizations developed this method using lime (calcium hydroxide, not the citrus fruit of the same name) and ash (potassium hydroxide) to create alkaline solutions. The Hopi used the ashes of various native plants and trees, while some contemporary Maya use the ashes of burnt mussel shells. The corn is treated by boiling it in water to which several tablespoons of lime have been added. The mixture is left to stand for a few hours, and the corn is then washed well with fresh water. The hulls are removed and the kernels are dried and ground. This is called *masa harina,* or instant masa flour.

The term hominy may refer to whole, coarsely ground, or finely ground nixtamal, or to a cooked porridge prepared from any of these. Corn cooked with lime in this way provides niacin in the diet, and when corn is eaten with another form of plant protein, such as beans, the full complement of amino acids is achieved.

In the United States, European settlers did not always adopt the nixtamalization process, except in the case of hominy grits, though corn became a staple among the poor of the southern states; unfortunately, the reliance on corn as a staple food caused outbreaks of pellagra in the American South during the early 1900s.

Corn and Toxins

Corn is especially vulnerable to aflatoxins, which are naturally occurring molds, or mycotoxins, that are produced by many species of Aspergillus, a fungus. Aflatoxins are among the most carcinogenic substances known. They are very common and can colonize and contaminate grain before harvest or during storage, especially during times of high-humidity or drought conditions. Aflatoxins are found in soil, decaying vegetation, hay, and grains, and can also be found in the milk of animals that are fed contaminated feed. High-level aflatoxin exposure can lead to cirrhosis and/or carcinoma of the liver. It is thought that most of the peanut butter sold in the U.S. contains minute quantities of aflatoxin but it is usually far below the FDA's recommended safe level.

All animal species are susceptible to the acute toxic effects

Retail behemoth Walmart says it will soon be selling a new variety of genetically modified sweet corn developed by Monsanto. This is the same corn that other big names like Whole Foods and General Mills have already rejected. "After closely looking at both sides of the debate and collaborating with a number of respected food safety experts, we see no scientifically validated safety reasons to implement restrictions on this product," *a Walmart rep explained to the* **Chicago Tribune.**

of aflatoxins, including humans. Adults have a high tolerance for aflatoxin exposure and rarely succumb to acute aflatoxicosis, but children are particularly affected by aflatoxin exposure, which can lead to stunted growth and delayed development, and chronic exposure has been shown to be a factor in developing liver cancer. Medical research has shown that a diet rich in vegetables like carrots, parsnips, celery and parsley reduces the carcinogenic effects of aflatoxin.

Other environmental toxins that plague corn are fumonisins. They are produced by *Fusarium* molds that grow in the field or develop during storage, and have been found worldwide. More than ten types of fumonisins have been isolated and characterized. Studies have not yet shown definite associations between fumonisins and human cancer, but human health risks are possible. The nixtamalization process significantly reduces the mycotoxins produced by *Fusarium verticillioides* and *Fusarium proliferatum*, molds that commonly infect corn.

Allergies to Corn

Allergies to corn are quite rare when compared to wheat allergies, but the dangers are very real and can range in severity from mild to potentially fatal. Some people must consume corn to see a reaction, while others may show signs of an allergic reaction if they are within close proximity to it. Learning how to avoid corn protein is the biggest challenge for people with corn allergies as corn is in just about everything, from foods to hair care products, surgical gloves and adhesives.

Corn

The Bottom Line

THE GOOD: Organically-grown sweet corn • organically-grown masa corn flour and products

THE BAD: Corn oil (non-GM)

THE DOWNRIGHT DANGEROUS: Conventionally-grown GM corn and corn products such as high fructose corn syrup, corn flakes breakfast cereal, corn chips, taco shells, corn flour, pop-corn, and corn oil

Rice and Rice Products

RICE IS THE THIRD MOST-PRODUCED CEREAL CROP in the world after wheat and corn, and is the most important grain with regard to human nutrition, providing more than one fifth of the calories consumed worldwide by the human species.

There are many varieties of rice and preferences tend to vary regionally, for instance, in the Far East there is a preference for softer, stickier varieties. Because of its importance as a staple food, rice has considerable cultural importance, and is often directly associated with prosperity and fertility, evidenced by the custom of throwing rice at weddings. The nutritional value of rice varies and is based on a number of factors including the strain of the rice, the nutrient quality of the soil it is grown in, and if and how it is processed and enriched. Since rice is lacking in the amino acids lysine and threonine, it needs to be combined with other sources of vegetable protein such as nuts, seeds, beans, lentils, or peanuts to form a complete protein.

Rice cannot be digested in its raw state and needs to be prepared for human consumption. The seeds of the rice plant are milled to remove the chaff, the outer husk of the grain, and the result is brown rice, complete with the germ and bran. To produce white rice, the milling and refining process is continued and the bran and germ are discarded. However, this processing removes much of the nutrients, and it has been found that a diet high in white rice can cause beriberi, a nervous system ailment caused by a thiamine (vitamin B1) deficiency. Brown rice is much more nutritious since it represents the whole grain, and beriberi is not seen in communities where people eat a diet high in brown rice.

White rice has a longer shelf life but is lacking in nutrients, so is often enriched by manufacturers by adding vitamins that have been lost during the milling process. The cheapest method of enriching rice involves adding a powdered blend of nutrients to the grains, but this easily washes off, and in the U.S. rice enriched by this method requires a label warning against rinsing. Another method of enriching rice involves coating the grains with a substance insoluble to water which is resistant to washing off. White rice may also be polished by buffing with glucose, starch or talc powder to improve its appearance. Despite the hypothetical health risks of consuming talc, such as stomach cancer, talc-coated rice remains popular in some countries, but has been banned in others. It is no longer widely used in the U.S.

In many parts of the world, especially the Far East, parboiled rice is popular. Parboiled rice is made by partially boiling rice in the husk by a special process that requires soaking, steaming, and then drying. This method causes nutrients from the outer husk, especially thiamine, to be drawn into the grain to boost its vitamin content. This method also increases the formation of type 3-resistant starch which can act as a prebiotic, a great benefit to the health of the intestines. Most parboiled rice is then milled in the same way as white rice. Parboiling rice turns the starch in the grains translucent and gelatinous, and the rice takes less time to cook and is firmer and less sticky. In North America, parboiled rice is either partially or fully precooked before sale.

Rice is the seed of the monocot plants *Oryza sativa* (Asian rice) and *Oryza glaberrima* (African rice). The term "wild rice" is usually reserved for species of the grass genus *Zizania*, both wild and domesticated. Rice bran, called *nuka* in Japan, is a moist, oily inner layer of the rice grain and is a valuable commodity in Asia. It can be used in many ways, including being heated to produce oil, and as a pickling bed in making rice bran pickles and *takuan,* a popular traditional pickle made from daikon radish.

Rice is comprised of long chains of glucose and has virtually no fructose, which is a benefit, since fructose is far too abundant in many diets and is now known to be a primary cause of obesity. Rice is also gluten free, making it safe for people with celiac disease and gluten sensitivities.

Comparative Vibrational Levels of Health and Disease States		Comparative Nutritional Levels of **Rice & Rice Products**
10,000 = Level of Optimal Health e.g. a healthy newborn baby / hunter/gatherer tribes	10,000	Organically-grown whole brown rice, steamed or boiled • Rice Dream organic rice milk
	9,500	Canadian Lake wild rice
BETTER HEALTH	9,000	Conventionally-grown brown rice • Carolina whole-grain brown rice • River brown rice • Sesmark Rice Thins • Rice Dream rice milk (not organic)
	8,500	
	8,000	Ka-me Rice Crackers
	7,500	Blue Diamond Nut Thins nut & rice crackers
	7,000	
	6,500	Sesmark Cheddar Rice Thins
AVERAGE LEVEL OF HEALTH IN USA Inflammation	6,000	
Arthritis starts to manifest	5,500	
Heart Disease starts to manifest	5,000	
Cancer cells form: Breast, Prostate, Lung, Colon, Pancreas	4,500	
Diabetes • Osteoporosis	4,000	Kellogg's Rice Krispies
Lymphoma • Leukemia • Dementia	3,500	
Congestive heart disease Brain cancer • Multiple sclerosis	3,000	Organic white rice
Breast cancer metastasizes	2,500	Conventionally-grown parboiled enriched white rice
Prostate cancer metastasizes • Common cold/ flu	2,000	Conventionally-grown enriched white rice by Goya, River etc. • Carolina Basmati White Rice
Melanoma	1,500	Quaker Rice Cakes
Metastatic bone and lung cancer	1,000	Quaker Rice Snacks
	500	Rice Krispies "Treats"
	50	Rice pudding made from average supermarket ingredients (white rice, milk and sugar) • Quaker Rice Snacks: Caramel Corn, Apple Cinnamon
Decay and Death	0	

WORSENING HEALTH

Measured in Bovis Units of Life Force Energy

Toxins in Rice

The moist, nutrient-rich environment of brown rice can serve as a breeding ground for a variety of molds, bacteria and fungi.

There are many molds, bacteria and fungi that can grow on brown rice, but Aspergillus section flavi is among the most dangerous. This fungus, known as an aflatoxin, has the potential to cause cancer if consumed. The risk of aflatoxin poisoning is relatively low, but proper preparation and storage of rice can help avoid many of the dangers associated with eating contaminated brown rice. It is important to properly prepare rice and consume it as soon as possible after cooking to eliminate the risk of consuming aflatoxins. Tryptophan, an amino acid present in brown rice, can be converted by some of these microorganisms to a compound called alpha-picolinic acid. If consumed, alpha-picolinic acid can cause rice hypersensitivity and apoptosis, a condition involving accelerated cell death and tissue damage.

When storing cooked rice for future use, rapid cooling is advised since cooked rice can produce an emetic toxin called *bacillus cereus* when left unrefrigerated. This disease has been associated with fried rice that has been cooked and then held at warm temperatures for several hours, such as at Chinese restaurants. One of the enterotoxins produced by *bacillus cereus* is heat-resistant; reheating contaminated rice kills the bacteria, but does not destroy the toxin already present. Cooked rice should be stored in the refrigerator for no more than four to seven days.

As for naturally-occurring toxins, white rice is virtually toxin-free, and has far fewer toxins than brown rice. The vast majority of toxins in white rice are destroyed by cooking and it is known to be a good choice for people with a high level of food allergies.

Arsenic in Rice

According to scientific reports, rice contains potentially dangerous levels of arsenic if consumed in large quantities over time. Rice can become contaminated with arsenic because of previous pesticide use in the soil where it is grown, and when metals and toxins produced by heavy industry find their way into the soil. Arsenic, a powerful poison, can cause tissue damage, organ failure and death in humans, and is also associated with the development of certain cancers. Rice is a plant that is efficient at absorbing arsenic from the soil, regardless of whether the resulting products are considered organic. Brown rice seems to have the highest concentrations of arsenic, particularly rice that is produced in the U.S.

According to a study published in the journal *Environmental Health Perspectives,* Dartmouth environmental chemist Brian Jackson and his colleagues reported elevated arsenic levels in some cereal bars and energy bars sweetened with brown rice syrup. These toxins are also ending up in top-selling baby foods, but manufacturers insist the levels are so low they do not pose a health risk. However, scientists and food campaigners are calling for efforts to eliminate the chemicals from mass-produced products that are eaten by millions of youngsters.

A new study has also found high arsenic levels in pregnant women who eat rice and experts are concerned because arsenic is able to cross the placenta and may harm a developing baby. Studies have linked high arsenic levels to an increased risk of miscarriage, and exposure to arsenic in the womb has been associated with lower birth weights in children and an increased risk of infant mortality. Two years ago, Britain's Food Standards Agency issued an official warning that young children should not drink rice milk because of arsenic contamination.

"Rice, which I think a lot of people would think of as very healthy, may be a real source of exposure to inorganic arsenic," says Michael S. Bloom, PhD, an assistant professor at the University at Albany in New York. Bloom is studying the health effects of chronic arsenic exposure and believes that the average person may be receiving an additional daily dose by eating rice. Researchers calculated that women who ate just a half cup of cooked rice each day—the average amount eaten in the study—would be getting just as much arsenic as if they drank a liter of tap water at EPA's maximum allowable limit for arsenic.

Allergy to Rice

Any food eaten frequently enough can trigger a food allergy, and the truth is that there is no universally "safe" food. A person with allergic tendencies can become allergic to anything. In China, for instance, where rice is the most commonly eaten grain, more people are allergic to rice than to wheat. Rice allergy symptoms can include bloating, intestinal problems, skin rashes, and acne.

In the West, a rice allergy is thought to be quite rare as rice is considered to be fairly non-allergenic, but more cases of it seem to be occurring. An allergy to rice can be triggered by many things—the proteins in the rice, a particular amino acid such as lysine, a particular mineral or vitamin in the grain such as vitamin B, or even chemicals used in the growing and processing of the rice. With thousands of toxins involved in modern food production, it is no wonder that so many people are developing allergies.

Refined Rice as a Cause of Diabetes

Approximately 85 percent of the calories in rice come from carbohydrates, and white rice is classified as a simple carbohydrate. Researchers at Harvard School of Public Health in Boston have found that there is a much higher incidence of diabetes among South Asian, African and African-Caribbean communities due to their consumption of white rice. Type 2 diabetes is up to six times more common in South Asian communities than in Western countries as a whole, and three times more common among people of African and African-Caribbean descent. Other experts have warned that further studies are needed to determine a conclusive link, even though another study, the Chennai Urban Rural Epidemiology Study (CURES) in India, which evaluated the association of refined grains consumption with diabetes in an urban south Indian population, showed that higher intake of refined grains was associated with insulin resistance and metabolic syndrome, which lead to diabetes.

Rice

The Bottom Line

THE GOOD: Organically-grown brown rice

THE NOT-SO-GOOD: Conventionally-grown brown rice

THE BAD: White rice, even when organic

THE DOWNRIGHT DANGEROUS: Rice cakes • White rice combined with sugar, as in rice pudding • Sweetened breakfast cereals made with rice, such as Rice Chex, Barbara's Honey Rice Puffins, and Kellogg's Rice Krispies, and "treats" made with them

CHAPTER 8

Bread and Wheat Products

"Modern technology has transformed bread, once the staff of life, into a mere broken reed, contributing to widespread vitamin and mineral deficiencies. To get the conveniences of high-tech food processing, mass-production, mass-marketing, long shelf life, uniformity of final product, even coloration, and soft texture, we create nutritional deficiencies. The food processing industry deceptively markets its products as more convenient versions of what grandmother once did in her kitchen. That is far from the truth!"

— Elmer M. Cranton, M.D., former Chief-of-Staff at a U.S. Public Health Service Hospital, and former Editor-in-Chief of *Journal for Advancement in Medicine* and *Journal of Holistic Medicine*

AH, THE SMELL OF FRESHLY BAKED BREAD! Manna from heaven, the "staff of life," our proverbial daily bread. For millennia this humble food, made from flour, yeast and water, has been a staple for a large sector of the world's population, wheat being second only to rice as the main human food crop. But how does the "staff of life" fare today? Not so well. The process of extending the shelf-life of wheat, a quality so desirable to food producers and distributors, has resulted in a refined and degraded product that offers virtually zero nutritional value to consumers, and is dangerous to our health.

Wheat grain has a high protein and vitamin content, but it is found mainly in the germ, but it is this nutritious germ that is removed in the flour-making processes. A grain of wheat, or berry, consists of three layers: the inner layer, or germ; the endosperm, which consists of starch and gluten; and the outer layer, which consists of fiber, or bran. Freshly ground whole wheat, which includes the germ, is a power-house of nutrients. But modern flour, grown from hybridized grains treated with pesticides, divested of the wheat germ, then refined and bleached, is a ghostly and toxic substance compared to the robust whole ground wheat of days gone by.

It was the invention of high-speed milling machines in the late 19th century that led to the widespread use of refined and bleached flour in the diets of industrialized nations. But bleached white flour was at one time outlawed in parts of the U.S. Back in the early 1900s, flour mill executives agreed that flour bleaching was unnecessary and harmful to those eating the flour and was deceitful to the public buying it, and in 1910, bleached white flour was declared unfit as human food by the Federal Western District Court of Missouri. But, according to H. W. Wiley, first chief of the FDA, in his book *The History of a Crime Against the Pure Food Law,* the enforcement of this law was "halted through the political influence of the flour millers." Sounds like one of the first instances of political lobbying.

But the lack of nutrients in refined flour did not go unnoticed. Due to nutritional deficiencies seen in U.S. military recruits at the start of World War II, including pellagra and beriberi (deficiencies of niacin and thiamine, respectively), in 1941 the U.S. government mandated the fortification of white flour-based products with thiamin, riboflavin, niacin, and iron. Folic acid was added to this list in 1998 because of its important role in preventing birth defects. Since that date, the rate of neural tube defects has decreased by approximately one-third in the U.S.

World trade in wheat is greater than for all other crops combined. Wheat is an important commercial product because of its high starch content, and, when mixed with warm water, creates a paste that can be used as a thickening, stiffening or gluing agent. It is used as an adhesive in the paper making process and is the basis for wallpaper paste. When eaten by humans, refined flour, virtually a pure starch and totally lacking in fiber, forms a kind of "glue" in the intestines and is a leading cause of constipation and other bowel problems, especially for those with a sensitivity to gluten.

This chapter on wheat is long, but it's important information to cover because bread and wheat products, the mainstays of our diet, have been turned into a poison, and it's essential we understand how this has happened and what the effects are on our health.

Comparative Vibrational Levels of Health and Disease States		Comparative Nutritional Levels of **Bread & Wheat Products**
10,000 = Level of Optimal Health e.g. a healthy newborn baby / hunter/gatherer tribes	10,000	Organic whole-wheat grain and most products made from it • Packaged organic bread, such as Vermont Bread
	9,500	
	9,000	
	8,500	
	8,000	
	7,500	
	7,000	
	6,500	Conventionally-grown whole-wheat grain and spelt grain • Arnold's rye bread • Panera whole-wheat bread • Stop & Shop "Fresh Bakery" whole-wheat bread
AVERAGE LEVEL OF HEALTH IN USA Inflammation	6,000	Most whole-wheat breads: Pepperidge Farm whole-wheat, Nature's Pride multi-grain, Vermont Bread whole-wheat, Arnold's 100% whole grain, Arnold's Health Nut, Arnold's 12 Grain
Arthritis starts to manifest	5,500	Pepperidge Farm Soft Honey Oat • Nature's Pride 100% whole-wheat • Vermont English muffins & oat bread • Freihofer's 12 Grain, Double Fiber, whole wheat • Home Pride wheat • J.J. Nissen wheat
Heart Disease starts to manifest	5,000	Pepperidge Farm oatmeal bread • Nature's Promise Oats & Honey
Cancer cells form: Breast, Prostate, Lung, Colon, Pancreas	4,500	Most white breads: Wonder 100% Wheat • Nature's Pride Country White & Honey Wheat • Vermont Bread Cinnamon Raisin • Thomas's Whole Grain English muffins
Diabetes • Osteoporosis	4,000	Wonder Bread Classic White • Sunbeam White Sandwich Loaf • Thomas's English Muffins and Toaster Cakes
Lymphoma • Leukemia • Dementia	3,500	Pepperidge Farm Cinnamon Raisin Swirl • Arnold's Sandwich Thins and Whole Grain Rolls • Weight Watchers Multi-grain • Joseph's Pita bread
Congestive heart disease Brain cancer • Multiple sclerosis	3,000	Pepperidge Farm Hot Dog and Hamburger Buns • Dunkin' Donuts bagels
Breast cancer metastasizes	2,500	Generic supermarket English Muffins and Wheat Sandwich bread
Prostate cancer metastasizes • Common cold/ flu	2,000	McDonald's & Burger King hamburger buns • Generic supermarket hot dog & hamburger buns
Melanoma	1,500	Pillsbury refrigerated dough: Biscuits, Bread Sticks, Dinner Rolls, Country French Loaf, Country Italian • Thomas' Sahara White Pita Pockets, Tortilla Wraps, and Whole Wheat Breakfast Thins
Metastatic bone and lung cancer	1,000	
	500	
	50	
Decay and Death	0	

BETTER HEALTH

WORSENING HEALTH

Measured in Bovis Units of Life Force Energy

The Development of Refined Wheat Products

By looking at the charts on the opposite pages, it's clear that commercially-produced wheat products are not good for us. But why are they so dangerous for our health? The answer lies in the amount of insecticides applied to the growing wheat, and in the refining and bleaching process which strips the grains of virtually all their nutrients. But there are also issues with the new forms of hybridized wheat that are now being grown.

Domestic strains of wheat were developed over millennia by the cultivation and repeated harvesting and sowing of the seeds of wild grasses. Stone-ground wheat, with all its nutrients intact, is a highly nutritious food. Before the invention of high-speed milling machines, whole wheat berries were ground between large stones to turn them into flour, and all the nutrients from the original grain remained in the finished product—vitamins, minerals, micro-nutrients, wheat germ, and bran. But wheat-germ oil quickly becomes rancid, at about the same rate that milk becomes sour, so refrigeration of whole grain flours was necessary. Modern food processors learned that by discarding the wheat germ and adding preservatives, the flour could last for weeks without going stale. But the resulting product, containing only a fraction of the nutrients of the original grain, has proved to be disastrous for our health.

In his book, *Nutrition and Physical Degeneration,* Dr. Weston A. Price describes just how much "life force energy" is eliminated from whole grain by the refining process: "Modern white flour has had approximately four-fifths of the phosphorus and nearly all of the vitamins removed by processing in order to produce a flour that can be shipped without becoming infested with insect life. I have been advised by millers that they could not ship flour if the minerals and vitamins were not removed. At once, we have an important measure of the value of a food, namely, the quality of insect life that it can support. The more valuable the product for human food, the more insect life it will support . . . highly refined white flour will support almost no insect life."

He recounts how he took a piece of coarse homemade rye bread from a rustic home in the Swiss Alps back to his laboratory to examine it, but just a short while later all that remained of the bread was a pile of bran left by the insects that had eaten it.

To contrast Dr. Price's experience, Roger Bennatti, a teacher at George Stevens Academy in Blue Hill, Maine, tried an experiment for his students to demonstrate the effects of additives and preservatives on food. He placed an unwrapped Twinkie (a kind of small, chocolate cake roll) on his blackboard where it remained for 30 years. A Fig Newton lasted for 15 years, and is believed to be still standing, untouched by time or predators.

In what might be considered an encouraging sign of the times, Hostess, the maker of the Twinkie, filed for bankruptcy protection in January 2012, citing debt of $860 million. According to Associated Press, changing eating habits have caused a decline in sales and profits: "Health-conscious Americans favor yogurt and energy bars over the dessert cakes and white bread they devoured 30 years ago. Last year, 36 percent of Americans ate white bread in their homes, down from 54 percent in 2000, according to NPD Group."

The Reality of Modern Wheat Production

New hybrid strains of wheat, developed after World War II, may deliver higher yields but they need the application of greater quantities of nitrogen, herbicides and pesticides. Many pesticides may legally be used in commercial wheat production, including herbicides, insecticides, fungicides, vertebrate poisons, and vertebrate repellents, and strychnine can legally be sprayed on wheat as a poison for birds, deer, and rodents.

Wheat seeds are treated even before they start to grow. Pesticides are applied to the seed prior to planting, in the form of a seed treatment, or coating, to protect against soil-borne risks to the plant. These coatings can also provide supplemental chemicals and nutrients designed to encourage growth. Young wheat plants are also sprayed with hormone-like substances such as Cycocel which act as plant growth regulators, and which are toxic to humans, domestic animals and wildlife. More pesticides are added in the field as the growing season progresses, and after harvesting, the wheat grain is stored in bins which have been coated with insecticides. The grain is then fumigated to kill any insects that normally live in the grain.

Comparative Protein Content of Commonly Eaten Grains & Starches:

	Wheat Germ	Wheat Grain	Rice	Corn	Potato	Cassava
Protein component of raw grain/starch per 100g	23 g	12.6 g	7 g	3 g	1.7 g	1.4 g

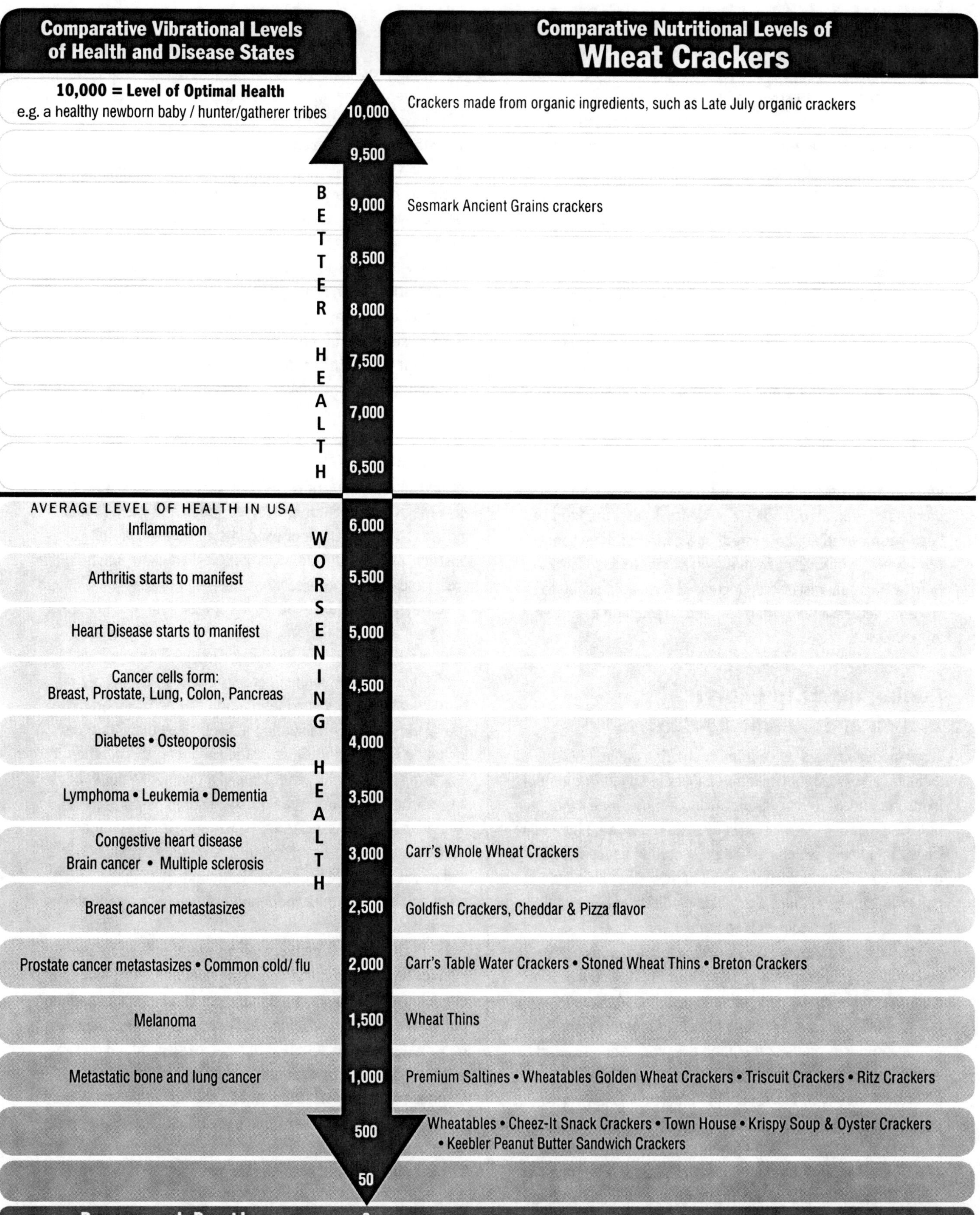

Comparative Vibrational Levels of Health and Disease States
Comparative Nutritional Levels of
Wheat Crackers
10,000 = Level of Optimal Health
e.g. a healthy newborn baby / hunter/gatherer tribes
10,000
Crackers made from organic ingredients, such as Late July organic crackers
9,500
BETTER HEALTH
9,000
Sesmark Ancient Grains crackers
8,500
8,000
7,500
7,000
6,500
AVERAGE LEVEL OF HEALTH IN USA
Inflammation
6,000
WORSENING HEALTH
Arthritis starts to manifest
5,500
Heart Disease starts to manifest
5,000
Cancer cells form:
Breast, Prostate, Lung, Colon, Pancreas
4,500
Diabetes • Osteoporosis
4,000
Lymphoma • Leukemia • Dementia
3,500
Congestive heart disease
Brain cancer • Multiple sclerosis
3,000
Carr's Whole Wheat Crackers
Breast cancer metastasizes
2,500
Goldfish Crackers, Cheddar & Pizza flavor
Prostate cancer metastasizes • Common cold/ flu
2,000
Carr's Table Water Crackers • Stoned Wheat Thins • Breton Crackers
Melanoma
1,500
Wheat Thins
Metastatic bone and lung cancer
1,000
Premium Saltines • Wheatables Golden Wheat Crackers • Triscuit Crackers • Ritz Crackers
500
Wheatables • Cheez-It Snack Crackers • Town House • Krispy Soup & Oyster Crackers
• Keebler Peanut Butter Sandwich Crackers
50
Decay and Death
0
Measured in Bovis Units
of Life Force Energy

The flour is then stripped of its natural nutrients, contained in the germ and the bran, and fortified with chemical vitamins and minerals while the germ and the bran are packaged and sold separately. Hippocrates, a physician who lived in ancient Greece and is considered to be the "father of modern medicine," recommended stone-ground flour for its beneficial effect on the digestive tract. But today, more than three-quarters of the dietary fiber (bran) is removed from commercial flour.

Irradiated Wheat

Wheat and wheat flour were some of the first foods the FDA approved for irradiation. A 1963 ruling approved the irradiation of imported grains, and in 1968, the FDA approved irradiation for U.S. wheat berries and flour to control insects. Irradiation is the practice of using either high-speed electron beams or high-energy radiation to break chemical bonds and ionize molecules that lie in their path. This is done to eradicate the pests in grain and prevent mold growth—all supposedly without health consequences. But research has shown that the dangers of irradiated foods are evident whether the food has been freshly irradiated or stored for a period of time. Long-term health implications from eating irradiated foods include lowered immune resistance, decreased fertility, damage to kidneys, depressed growth rates, and a reduction in certain vitamin levels.

Adding Insult to Injury: Bleach and Chemical Additives

Flour manufacturers use a form of chlorine gas to bleach and artificially "age" flour. The chlorine gas reacts with the flour, oxidizing and whitening it, producing a pure white product, but the process leaves residues of toxic chlorinated hydrocarbons and dioxins which have been shown to cause nervousness and seizures in animals. The EPA identifies chlorine gas as a flour-bleaching, aging and oxidizing agent that is a powerful irritant, dangerous to inhale, and lethal.

This might be thought bad enough, but an unintended by-product of this process is that it converts a dough additive called xanthine into a toxic substance called alloxan. Alloxan is a glucose analogue which has been shown to destroy insulin-producing cells in the pancreas when administered to rodents and other animals, causing diabetes with characteristics similar to type 1 diabetes in humans. Alloxan's harmful effects on the pancreas are so severe that the *Textbook of Natural Medicine* calls the chemical "a potent beta-cell toxin." Even though the toxic effect of alloxan is common scientific knowledge and has proven to be toxic to the liver and the kidneys in high doses, the FDA still allows companies to use it in processing foods for human consumption.

The International Medical Veritas Association believes that alloxan promotes the development of diabetes: "Studies show that alloxan, the chemical that makes white flour look 'clean and beautiful,' destroys the beta cells of the pancreas. Scientists have known of the alloxan-diabetes connection for years yet there seems to be a conspiracy that defends the integrity of the FDA, which allows dangerous chemicals that can cause diabetes to be used in drugs and food."

Interestingly, it has been found that we can reverse the effects of alloxan by supplementing our diet with vitamin E—precisely the nutrient that is removed from the flour when the wheat germ is discarded! According to Dr. Gary Null's *Clinicians' Handbook of Natural Healing*, vitamin E effectively protected lab rats from the harmful effects of alloxan.

Bleaching agents have been banned for use in bread flour in Germany since 1958 and in the UK since the late 1990s. In the United States, however, bleached flour continues to be a major ingredient in processed foods and the fast-food industry. Most of the flour used in supermarket bread, cakes, pastries, pies, muffins, donuts, cookies, crackers, pasta, pizza crust, and breakfast cereals has been bleached.

Another controversial additive is potassium bromate, used as a flour improver that strengthens dough and prevents it from falling when handled between proofing and baking, yielding higher volume bread. Potassium bromate has been classified as a carcinogen, and has been banned by the World Health Organization as well as by many nations, including Canada and those of the European Union. Though not banned in the U.S., the Center for Science in the Public Interest has petitioned the FDA to do so. In response, the American Bakers Association, which opposes such a ban, published a statement saying that potassium bromate is converted to harmless potassium bromide during the baking process. Flours that are bromated are labeled as such on the packaging.

More than 30 different chemicals are approved by the FDA for addition to bread to extend shelf life, including ethylated mono- and triglycerides, potassium iodide, sodium propionate, calcium propionate, benzoyl peroxide, tricalcium phosphate, calcium sulfate, sulphur dioxide, sodium metabisulphite, cysteine hydrochloride, ammonium chloride, and magnesium carbonate. But, usually only up to eight are used at any one time. The use of these preservatives allows bread to be shipped long distances and to remain on the shelf for a longer period of time without refrigeration.

Comparative Vibrational Levels of Health and Disease States	Bovis	Comparative Nutritional Levels of **Pizza & Pasta**
10,000 = Level of Optimal Health e.g. a healthy newborn baby / hunter/gatherer tribes	10,000	Pizza crust & pasta made from organic ingredients • Amy's Frozen Pizza: Vegetable & Soy Cheese
	9,500	
	9,000	Hodgson Mill Organic Penne
	8,500	Annie's Homegrown Macaroni & Cheese, made with organic pasta
	8,000	Annie's Homegrown Penne Pasta Alfredo, made with organic pasta
	7,500	
	7,000	
	6,500	
AVERAGE LEVEL OF HEALTH IN USA Inflammation	6,000	Newman's Own Frozen Pizza, Margherita
Arthritis starts to manifest	5,500	
Heart Disease starts to manifest	5,000	
Cancer cells form: Breast, Prostate, Lung, Colon, Pancreas	4,500	Celeste Pizza for One: Original Flavor (frozen)
Diabetes • Osteoporosis	4,000	Domino's cheese pizza • Pizza Hut pizza • Celeste Pizza for One: pepperoni, vegetables, sausage
Lymphoma • Leukemia • Dementia	3,500	Frozen Pizza: DiGiorno Supreme, Freschetta, California Pizza Kitchen • Stouffer's French bread pizza
Congestive heart disease Brain cancer • Multiple sclerosis	3,000	DaVinci whole wheat fettucine • Ronzoni Healthy Harvest whole grain pasta • Stouffer's lasagna
Breast cancer metastasizes	2,500	California Pizza Kitchen, Thin Crust: BBQ Chicken, Hawaiian • Dried pasta: Colavita, Racconto
Prostate cancer metastasizes • Common cold/ flu	2,000	Dried pasta: Barilla, Rienzi, Ronzoni, Prince, Pastene • Couscous
Melanoma	1,500	Kraft Easy Mac • Campbell's Chicken-Noodle soup • Nissin Cup Noodles, chicken flavor
Metastatic bone and lung cancer	1,000	Wacky Mac Veggie Bows, canned • Pennsylvania Dutch egg noodles • Campbell's Spaghetti Os
	500	Chef Boyardee Beef Ravioli, Beefaroni, Spaghetti & Meatballs, Lasagna • Kraft Mac & Cheese
	50	Chef Boyardee Macaroni & Cheese • Knorr Teriyaki Noodles
Decay and Death	0	

BETTER HEALTH ↑ / WORSENING HEALTH ↓

Measured in Bovis Units of Life Force Energy

Why is Eating Wheat Such a Problem for So Many People?

One of the reasons is that the type of wheat now grown in the U.S. has been highly hybridized and a large number of people are exhibiting sensitivities to its various components.

After World War II, in order to increase yield, modern agricultural scientists created two hybrid strains of wheat, and now more than 90 percent of the wheat grown worldwide comes from those two hybrid strains. These hybrid wheat strains show only 95 percent of the same proteins as the parent wheat strains, and the remaining five percent is an entirely unique protein. Many nutritional experts believe that this unique protein is responsible for wheat sensitivities in many people. Every day more evidence is coming to light about the perils of consuming foods containing unnatural substances that were created in a lab, and many scientists believe that just about everyone is allergic or sensitive to modern wheat in some way.

There is much evidence to show that wheat sabotages digestive function and can even affect IQ levels. Dr. Paul Jaminet, author of *The Perfect Health Diet,* recommends a high-fat diet, also known as the Paleolithic, Paleo or Caveman diet, with 20 to 30 percent of daily calories in the form of rice or potatoes, which he terms "safe starches." The only grain he recommends is rice.

"One of the strengths of the Paleo diet is that it's very low in toxicity," Dr. Jaminet says. "The toxins in wheat can actually have a large health impact." He cites a recent study from Japan that shows that children who eat wheat every day are almost four IQ points lower than children who eat rice. "The nice thing about rice is that the toxins are destroyed in cooking. Cooked white rice is very low in toxins. That gives us a measure of how much wheat may be impacting health. It could be just the difference between eating wheat and rice."

Wheat is Inflammatory

Wheat and other grains are high in pro-inflammatory omega-6 fatty acids, so eating grains will worsen any condition that has chronic inflammation at its root. One of these conditions is arthritis, an inflammatory life-style disease with malnutrition as its cause. About one in five adults, or nearly 50 million Americans, have been diagnosed with arthritis, the most common form of which is osteoarthritis. If action is not taken to reverse the loss of cartilage in the joints, arthritis can become progressively worse until a person is not able to carry out normal daily activities.

Another issue is that hybrid wheat flour consists of 33 percent glutamic acid, an inflammatory amino acid, and has a high level of aspartic acid, making wheat potentially excitotoxic. Excitotoxicity is a pathological process where glutamic and aspartic acid cause an over-activation of nerve cell receptors, which can lead to calcium-induced nerve and brain injury. These two amino acids may contribute to neurodegenerative conditions such as multiple sclerosis, Alzheimer's, Huntington's disease, and other nervous system disorders such as epilepsy, ADD/ADHD and migraines.

Wheat Affects Blood Sugar Levels

The consumption of wheat products plays havoc with blood sugar levels and is a major contributing factor to the development of diabetes and of metabolic syndrome, a combination of medical disorders that increases the risk of developing cardiovascular disease and diabetes. Metabolic syndrome affects one in five people in the United States, though some studies have shown the prevalence might actually be as high as one in four.

Wheat is high on the Glycemic Index, which measures how long it takes the glucose from food to enter the blood stream after consumption. Studies have linked the consumption of foods high on the GI index to a risk of obesity, diabetes, heart disease, and cancer. The highest level is pure glucose at 100, and wheat bread, astonishingly, measures at between 90 and 100, close to the level of glucose.

Having a chronically elevated insulin level is now the number one medical problem seen by doctors in the U.S. When a person consumes any form of sugar or carbohydrate, their body pumps out insulin to absorb the glucose into the body and stabilize blood glucose levels. Blood glucose levels have to stay within a very narrow range otherwise the body would die, so the body is constantly trying to balance this level. The more sugar a person eats, the more insulin the body pumps out, and if this persists, the pancreas keeps on producing even more insulin, until eventually the cells become resistant to insulin and the pancreas wears out. When this happens, the results is

---

"Eating wheat may not be beneficial to your health . . . each grain contains about one microgram of Wheat Germ Agglutinin (WGA). Even in small quantities, WGA can have profoundly adverse effects . . . excessive wheat consumption may play a significant role here . . . [and] there's evidence suggesting that gluten sensitivity may be at the root of many neurological and psychiatric conditions."

—Dr. Joseph Mercola, founder of the World's No. 1 Natural Health Website www.mercola.com

diabetes, a potentially serious condition that can lead to heart failure, kidney failure, limb amputation and blindness.

Wheat Lectins and Exorphins affect Sensitive Individuals

There are other components of wheat which can adversely affect the body in sensitive individuals; these include gliadin, gliadomorphin (exorphins, or group of opioid peptides that form during digestion of the gluten protein), and enzyme inhibitors.

Modern strains of wheat are poorer in minerals and contain more of the gluten protein than strains from 40 years ago; in fact, recent research has revealed that today's flour has nearly double the level of wheat proteins known as omega-gliadins. These gliadins can trigger inflammatory reactions in the gut of sensitive people, including a condition called wheat-dependent exercise-induced anaphylaxis, something that was unknown 20 years ago when most bread was made by a different process (symptoms may include pruritus, hives, flushing, wheezing, and GI involvement, including nausea, abdominal cramping, and diarrhea, and leading to cardiovascular collapse.)

Bread used to be made in a lengthy two-stage process, which took from 12 to 16 hours, and gave enough time for the dough to ripen, making it easier to handle and tastier to eat. Now this step has been skipped in order to increase the speed of bread-making, saving time and money. But it has been discovered that this "proving" time was important because as the dough fermented, it neutralized some parts of the wheat proteins that were most likely to trigger inflammatory reactions to gluten and cause other issues in the intestines in sensitive individuals. (You can read more about this at: www.dailymail.co.uk/femail/food/article-1298227/Tescos-misleading-claims-bread-just-tip-iceberg)

But it is wheat lectin, or "wheat germ agglutinin" (WGA), that can be the biggest trouble-maker for people who eat wheat. Many seeds of the grass family, such as wheat, rice, spelt, barley, and rye, have exceptionally high levels of defensive glycoproteins known as lectins, designed as a plant poison so that animals and insects will not eat the seeds of the plant. Lectins are carbohydrate-binding proteins which are resistant to cooking and digestion. WGA is a particularly resilient and problematic lectin that is not eliminated through sprouting. These lectins also cannot be digested by stomach acids and enzymes and so pass on through to the gut where they cause inflammation and "leaky-gut" syndrome. This creates a hyper-immune response that does not show up in allergy testing.

Wheat lectins have been shown to be pro-inflammatory, immunotoxic, neurotoxic, cardiotoxic, and cytotoxic; in fact, WGA lectin may induce programmed cell death (apoptosis). Lectins also cause leptin resistance, which means that the hunger signal is suppressed and a person will continue eating even when the body has had more than enough nutrients.

WGA lectin is highest in whole wheat, especially sprouted whole wheat, so those who are sensitive to WGA may find they can eat small amounts of highly refined white flour, but not whole-wheat flour products.

Wheat Sensitivity and Gluten Intolerance

Grains such as wheat, rye, barley and to some degree oats, cause digestive problems for a great many people. One of the biggest culprits is gluten, an elastic, rubbery protein which binds the dough in bread and other baked goods and produces a spongy consistency. But these grains also contain a number of other proteins—such as albumin, globulin, gliadin and glutenin (gluten)—that can result in adverse reactions, including allergies. These wheat proteins vary in content depending on the type of wheat.

Wheat consumption has been shown to inhibit the production of serotonin. Neurotransmitters such as serotonin can be found not just in the brain; in fact, the largest concentration of serotonin, which is involved in mood control, depression and aggression, is actually found in the intestines, showing a definitive link between wheat allergies, digestive problems and mental health issues, including "brain fog."

Dr. William Davis, a Wisconsin-based cardiologist, reports that he has helped thousands of patients by having them remove all wheat from their diets. He says the results are astounding, not only with heart and circulatory problems, but also with a variety of other ailments such as skin rashes, arthritis, insomnia, diabetes, dementia, and brain damage. "Most people are allergic, to some degree, to wheat and do not even realize it," he writes.

The difference between Wheat Sensitivity and Gluten Intolerance:

• **Wheat Sensitivity** can be caused by any of the proteins in wheat that can trigger an immune response, including albumin, globulin, gliadin, gluten, and wheat germ agglutinate. Sensitivity to these proteins can affect both the brain and the gut, causing problems with the mind, mood and behavior. It is believed to affect about 35 percent of the population and is often the cause of chronic sinus problems. The proteins present in wheat may cause different reactions in people who have a sensitivity to wheat, and often the reactions are not apparent until quite a while after the food has been eaten, even a few days, unlike a true food allergy, where the reaction is immediate. Some people have been known to get a form of asthma

(Baker's asthma) from inhaling wheat flour, and this affects up to 30 percent of individuals in the baking industry. Wheat-sensitive allergic individuals typically produce IgE antibodies to grain proteins, but some develop gluten-specific IgE antibodies. Allergy/sensitivity to wheat may occur in any individual, unlike celiac disease, which is hereditary. Some health care professionals believe that one person in 25 has a wheat sensitivity, though others put that figure closer to one person in two—or a staggering 50 percent of the population.

• **Gluten Intolerance,** though many consider it to be a wheat allergy, is actually a separate issue. Called celiac disease, it is a genetic gastrointestinal disorder characterized by intolerance to gliadin, a gluten protein found in wheat, barley and rye, and it is believed that about one out of 100 people in the US suffers from it. These people must observe a strict gluten-free diet to remain healthy, otherwise they risk triggering an immune reaction that damages the small intestine and prevents absorption of nutrients. A blood test can confirm the diagnosis. Symptoms include nausea, diarrhea, constipation and abdominal pain, as well as an array of non-gastrointestinal symptoms, such as fatigue, osteoporosis, anemia, infertility, depression, organ disorders, and more. Patients with celiac disease develop gliadin-specific IgA and IgG antibodies.

Is There a Connection Between Blood Type and Wheat Sensitivities?

Although there has been some controversy about this subject, I have learned, based on my own experience and observations over the past 20 years, that many people with type O blood do best if they stick to a wheat-free diet. This is the diet recommended by Dr. Peter D'Adamo in his book *Eat Right For Your Type,* and is also known as the Paleo or Paleolithic diet, or the Caveman diet. D'Adamo's book describes the extensive research done by himself and by his father, also a physician, when examining the medical records of thousands of their patients over many decades. And one of these recommendations is that people with type O blood should not eat wheat products.

Dr. D'Adamo says, "Type Os do not tolerate whole wheat products at all, and should eliminate them completely from their diet. Wheat products are a primary culprit in type O weight gain . . . eating gluten is like putting the wrong kind of octane in your car. Instead of fueling the engine, it clogs the works."

Wheat is in just about Everything Including Pizza and Pasta

Americans seem to have gladly adopted the cuisine of Italy, consuming pizza and pasta with greater and greater gusto. But pizza in fact originated as a snack food, and pasta evolved as a filling and cheap first course in the days when many people could afford only small amounts of animal protein for the next course. These foods are now considered appropriate for a main meal, but when they are made from highly-processed wheat, they are not nutritious foods.

When making pizza and pasta at home, it's best to use organic flour or organic wheat products, and when eating out, try asking for food made with organic wheat. If enough of us ask, one day restaurants and fast-food outlets will realize it's good business to provide it for us. After all, it could actually increase their business. So remember, when you order your pizza with all the toppings, often called "garbage pie," you might just be getting what you order—garbage.

Alternative Grains and Seed-Like Grains

Eating wheat-free means trying new grains. Fortunately, there is now a good selection of breads, pasta and baked goods made from non-wheat grains available at most health food stores and more enlightened supermarkets, such as Trader Joe's and Whole Foods Market.

Grains and grain substitutes that are safe for people with wheat allergies include amaranth, arrowroot, buckwheat, corn, millet, quinoa, rice, and tapioca. Spelt and kamut are ancient grains related to modern wheat and are not safe for people with wheat allergies, though people with a mild wheat allergy may be able to tolerate them to a degree. Researchers have found that spelt may be easier for humans to digest than regular wheat. Oats seem to have the same problems for most people as other gluten grains, but some can tolerate it on occasion.

Each person needs to find out for themselves how they tolerate wheat; if you have unexplained symptoms, one suggestion is to not eat wheat products for two weeks and then see how you feel. If troublesome symptoms, such as a stuffy nose, fatigue after eating, painful joints, or "brain fog," have lessened, maybe wheat was the culprit. But be careful, wheat is in a surprising number of packaged and processed foods, and you need to make sure you eat NONE during this test. Chronic sinus issues are most often caused by a sensitivity to wheat, and often to milk as well.

For those who are obese and have problems losing weight, the first thing to do is to cut out grains altogether and increase protein intake. Usually, there are dramatic results.

The Hall of Shame

The McDonald's Hamburger Bun

It was only when I was doing the research for the chapter on Fast Foods that I realized that the worse part about a McDonald's hamburger was the bun, and all the while the beef—"loaded with unhealthy saturated fat"—was getting the bad rap. In fact, the beef is the most nutritious item in the hamburger, along with the tomato slice. Here's what's in the bun, according to McDonald's web site:
"Enriched flour (bleached wheat flour, malted barley flour, niacin, reduced iron, thiamin mononitrate, riboflavin, folic acid, enzymes), water, high fructose corn syrup, sugar, yeast, soybean oil and/or partially hydrogenated soybean oil, contains 2% or less of the following: salt, calcium sulfate, calcium carbonate, wheat gluten, ammonium sulfate, ammonium chloride, dough conditioners (sodium stearoyl lactylate, datem, ascorbic acid, azodicarbonamide, mono- and diglycerides, ethoxylated monoglycerides, monocalcium phosphate, enzymes, guar gum, calcium peroxide, soy flour), calcium propionate and sodium propionate (preservatives), soy lecithin." It calibrates at 2,000, the level of colon cancer.

Wheat and Wheat Products

The Bottom Line

THE GOOD: Organically-grown fresh wheat berries and stone-ground whole flour (for those who do not have allergies or sensitivities to wheat and other grains)

THE BAD: Commercially-processed "whole grain" breads which almost always contain sugar and hydrogenated fats

THE DOWNRIGHT DANGEROUS: Conventionally-grown and processed wheat products and baked goods—they are poison to the body, especially when combined with sugar.

CHAPTER 9

Baked Goods

"If I'd known you were coming I'd have baked a cake . . ."
—Eileen Barton song from the 1950s

IN COUNTRIES AROUND THE WORLD, cakes have traditionally been part of celebratory events—for birthdays, weddings, baptisms, religious holidays, and other life-changing events such as retirement. Made from a combination of flour, eggs, butter, honey, spices, and a variety of nuts and dried fruit, they were a delicacy reserved for special occasions.

In the "old days," before highly-processed foods were on the market, these special treats, made from healthy ingredients and eaten in moderation, did not cause a problem in the diet. But nowadays, the vast majority of the baked goods that we can buy, including cookies, cakes, muffins, pastries and donuts, are made with bleached white flour, sugar, and refined vegetable oils—a perfect storm of unhealthy ingredients that create the most dangerous foods that we eat on a regular basis.

If a refined product like wheat flour is bad for us to eat, its negative nutritional value is magnified when it is combined with other substandard ingredients. And this can be seen on the chart opposite—baked goods made from organic and natural ingredients calibrate at the highest level of health, while those made with a combination of processed ingredients are the worst things we can feed our body, calibrating at the lowest level of any food group. And it is the consumption of foods such as these that cause serious health problems over the long term. They are cheap, they are addictive, and they are everywhere—tempting us in coffee shops, supermarkets, convenience stores, fast-food chains, vending machines, and even gas stations.

It was the invention in the late 1900s of high-speed milling machines for mass producing white flour that led to baked goods becoming so ubiquitous in the diets of industrialized nations. This refining process turned a fragile food—freshly-ground whole wheat flour—into a commodity with an almost infinite shelf life. But the processed food industry has got so used to raking in huge profits by using cheap ingredients that they are unlikely to want to use high quality raw materials as it would make their foods more expensive to produce and thus reduce their profits.

Before the days of bleached flour, battery eggs, and high fructose corn syrup, most people ate baked goods made from wholesome ingredients, and we can still make them that way—imagine the joy of eating a cheesecake made from organic ingredients—fresh eggs, rich raw cream cheese, and honey! No guilt there. But today, home-made baked goods are often made from a boxed mix or with bleached flour, so they are no healthier for us than bought products. But we can strive to use organic flour when baking at home, and the next time we go to a bakery to order a celebration cake, we can ask them to make it with organic flour. If they say they can't do that, we can bring them organic flour—we have to let businesses know that we are serious about finding safe and healthy food sources for ourselves and our families.

But even if a cake or pastry is made from organic ingredients, it's still a refined carbohydrate. Over-consumption of baked goods can cause weight-grain and lead to metabolic syndrome, a pre-diabetic disorder, and eventually to diabetes, and many people are addicted to wheat and sugar, which can cause a compulsive eating cycle.

"While we savor the tantalizing taste of a sweet roll, our bodies respond alarmingly as if a foreign invader arrived declaring war. Foods loaded with sugars and simple carbohydrates, or processed with omega-6 oils for long shelf life, have been the mainstay of the American diet for six decades. These foods have been slowly poisoning everyone."

— Dr. Dwight Lundell, heart surgeon, former Chief Resident at Yale University Hospital, author of **The Cure For Heart Disease** *and the e-book,* **The Great Cholesterol Lie**

Comparative Vibrational Levels of Health and Disease States	Bovis	Comparative Nutritional Levels of **Baked Goods: Cakes, Cookies, Muffins, & Pies**
10,000 = Level of Optimal Health e.g. a healthy newborn baby / hunter/gatherer tribes	10,000	Baked goods made from organic ingredients, sweetened with raw honey, maple syrup, or stevia
	9,500	
	9,000	
	8,500	
	8,000	
	7,500	
	7,000	
	6,500	Baked goods made from organic ingredients, sweetened with Xylitol or Maltitol
AVERAGE LEVEL OF HEALTH IN USA Inflammation	6,000	
Arthritis starts to manifest	5,500	
Heart Disease starts to manifest	5,000	
Cancer cells form: Breast, Prostate, Lung, Colon, Pancreas	4,500	
Diabetes • Osteoporosis	4,000	Walker's Shortbread • Cadbury's Chocolate Finger Biscuits
Lymphoma • Leukemia • Dementia	3,500	
Congestive heart disease Brain cancer • Multiple sclerosis	3,000	Walker's Ginger Biscuits • Average supermarket bakery muffins
Breast cancer metastasizes	2,500	Mrs. Fields Gourmet Brownies • Sara Lee Cheesecake • Cheescake Factory Cheesecake
Prostate cancer metastasizes • Common cold/ flu	2,000	Mrs. Fields Gourmet Chocolate Chip Cookies • Sara Lee Pound Cake
Melanoma	1,500	Keebler's Oatmeal Cookies • Hostess Fig Bars • Hostess Coffee Cake • Starbucks Butter Croissant
Metastatic bone and lung cancer	1,000	Dunkin' Donuts • Graham Crackers • Entermann's Crumble Cake • Hostess Mini Muffins • Drake's fruit pies Little Debbie Oatmeal Creme Pies • Keebler's & Famous Amos chocolate chip cookies
	500	Oreo Cookies • Starbucks Danish Pastry, Chocolate Donut • Hostess Donettes & Cup Cakes Little Debbie Creme Pies, Coffee Cake, Peanut Butter Bars • Teddy Grahams • Mrs. Smith's pies
	50	Pepperidge Farms cookies & cakes, e.g. Milano, Geneva, & Red Velvet Cake • Hostess HoHos, Twinkies, Ding Dongs, Suzy Q's, Zingers • Drake's Ring Dings, Devil Dogs, Funny Bones
Decay and Death	0	

BETTER HEALTH / WORSENING HEALTH

Measured in Bovis Units of Life Force Energy

Baked Goods Made from Processed Ingredients Count as Negative Nutrition

The main ingredient of baked goods, refined and bleached wheat flour, is a mass-produced food product that has been so highly processed that it is devoid of any vitality and so can be classified as "anti-nutrition." Food producers love it because it lasts indefinitely on the shelf, and products made from this flour, such as packaged cakes and cookies, can last literally for years. But baked goods made from these ingredients are seriously bad nutrition, a cheap thrill for the taste buds that gives a rush of short-lived energy, leaving a person craving more. For someone doing an active job maybe they aren't so dangerous, but are inappropriate for those in sedentary jobs.

Refined carbohydrates are energy foods, but we also need protein and quality fats to build and repair body tissue. If we eat only energy foods, our body does not get what it needs to build muscles and keep bones and teeth healthy, and the excess glucose and fructose will be stored as fat. And when we eat too many of these refined high-carbohydrate foods, we create an acidic environment in the body, forcing it to rob the bones and teeth of alkali minerals, such as calcium and potassium, to "buffer" the acidic levels in the blood. This is how an imbalanced diet causes the breakdown of the body. We simply must not eat these kinds of foods with impunity—the price we pay with our health is simply too high.

Baked Goods, Obesity and Addiction

> "When you eat sugar it triggers production of your brain's natural opioids—a key ingredient in the addiction process. Your brain essentially becomes addicted to stimulating the trelease of its own opioids as it would to morphine or heroin."
> —*Dr. Joseph Mercola, www.mercola.com*

One of the causes of obesity is thought to be an addiction to refined carbohydrates. Though the "drug of choice" may vary, the most common are wheat and sugar, and they are BOTH found in baked goods. According to the American Obesity Association, about 127 million Americans are categorized as being overweight, and of these, 60 million are estimated to be obese. It is estimated that obesity causes at least 300,000 premature deaths in the U.S. each year, with healthcare costs of approximately $100 billion.

Dr. Michael Rosenbaum, a pioneer in the field of Nutritional Medicine, believes that in some people food has a profound effect on the limbic portion of the brain, which acts as the control center of emotions and memory. And Dr. William Philpott, a clinical ecologist and founding member of the Academy of Orthomolecular Psychiatry, believes that allergens in food can trigger a rise in enkaphalin, a naturally occurring narcotic in the brain. Enkaphalin is an opiate narcotic produced by the body similar to the narcotics that can be taken into the body.

Another researcher, Dr. Marshall Mandell of Norwalk, Connecticut, found when treating hospitalized schizophrenic patients that more than 90 percent of them were addicted to one or more common substances. Using a test group of patients, he found that 88 percent of them were addicted to and/or were allergic to wheat, 60 percent to milk, and 50 percent to corn.

It has also been found that the digestion of certain food proteins can produce substances that have opiate or narcotic properties. There are a number of regulatory peptides created in the digestive tract that feed back to the brain to form the brain-gut axis. When digested, particles of milk and wheat proteins can act like endorphins, the body's own narcotics, which are known as "exorphins." It seems that exorphins are addictive in some people, and that the effects on the brain of exorphins may contribute to mental illness and appetite disorders.

Other food proteins, such as gluten, can also result in the production of substances that act like an opiate or narcotic. In one experiment, hydrolyzed wheat gluten was found to prolong intestinal transit time and this effect was reversed by the administration of naloxone, a narcotic-blocking drug. Researchers also think that deficiencies in the bowel production of natural endorphins might be associated with cravings and compulsions to eat certain foods.

Carbohydrate addiction can also be caused by excess insulin, which is released by the pancreas into the blood stream when carbohydrate foods are eaten. Too much insulin in the blood stream results in an irresistible and frequent desire to eat—the scientific term is post-prandial reactive hyper-insulinemia, which means too much insulin is released after eating. Hyper-insulinemia stems from insulin resistance, an imbalance of blood glucose and insulin levels. If left unchecked, insulin resistance can lead to obesity and metabolic syndrome, or syndrome X, which can lead to a heart attack or stroke. Other symptoms include polycystic ovarian syndrome, a leading cause of female infertility, as well skin conditions, excess body and facial hair, and male-pattern baldness in women.

Baked goods are also implicated in some neurological diseases and ADD/ADHD in children. Wheat, dairy, and soy contain high levels of glutamic and aspartic acid, which makes them all potentially excitotoxic, a pathological process where these acids cause an over-activation of nerve cell receptors. This over-activation can lead to nerve and brain injury and may contribute to neuro-degenerative conditions such as multiple sclerosis, Alzheimer's, Huntington's disease, and other nervous system disorders such as epilepsy, ADD/ADHD, and migraines.

Refined Carbohydrates and Diabetes

Diabetes is a serious disease that causes more deaths a year than breast cancer and AIDS combined. Diabetes contributes to more than 230,000 deaths in the U.S. each year, and two out of three people with diabetes will eventually die from heart disease or stroke. Being overweight is a risk factor for developing this disease, but an unbalanced diet is the biggest cause. The average American now consumes 141 pounds of sugar per year, and diabetes cases have risen to over 25 million annually, with cases of pre-diabetes now accounting for an additional 79 million people. It seems there must be a correlation in these figures, but a quote on the website of the American Diabetes Association (ADA) website reads: "Myth: Eating too much sugar causes diabetes. Fact: No, it does not. Type 1 diabetes is caused by genetics and unknown factors that trigger the onset of the disease; type 2 diabetes is caused by genetics and lifestyle factors."

They are correct about type 1 diabetes, which used to be called Juvenile Diabetes, but adults get type 2 diabetes, or Adult-Onset Diabetes. "Lifestyle factors" includes diet, because the truth is, eating too much sugar *does* cause diabetes—in fact, it used to be called "sugar diabetes." Reading a quote like that makes you wonder if the ADA is funded by the processed food industry. And in fact, Integrity in Science reports that this is the case: "The American Dietetic Association has received funding from numerous companies and receives underwriting for 'fact sheets' on topics related to the companies' products. Major ($100,000+) donors include: Kellogg, Kraft Foods, Weight Watchers International, Campbell Soup, National Dairy Council, Nestlé USA, Ross Products Division of Abbott Labs., Sandoz, Coca-Cola, Florida Department of Citrus, General Mills, Monsanto, Nabisco, Procter & Gamble, Uncle Ben's, Wyeth-Ayerst Labs. (Nov-Dec 1996, ADA Courier)."

So, since we can't trust the information on the ADA website, here are the facts: a person gets type 2 diabetes when they have so much sugar in their blood that their body can't metabolize it. Unlike in type 1 diabetes, where the body does not make insulin and it has to be injected, in type 2 diabetes, the body does make insulin, but it may not be enough or cannot be properly used by the body. Either way, too much glucose stays in the bloodstream.

And it's not just in America. The way the developing countries of the world have also embraced the consumption of processed foods and refined carbohydrates is causing far-reaching health problems; diabetes is a rising concern in China and India as they adopt Western-style eating habits. American fast-food outlets have proliferated at an astonishing rate in both countries, and the rates for diabetes are sky-rocketing. It's been reported that diabetes, stroke, and other non-communicable diseases deprive India of more than $23 billion a year in income, and the Director-General of the World Health Organization has said, "People in Asia are developing diabetes in larger numbers and at a younger age than in Europe and North America, and they are dying sooner."

The Hall of Shame

American manufacturers of baked goods, such as Pepperidge Farm, Sara Lee, and Drake's Cakes, appear to use the lowest quality ingredients and produce food that is incredibly dangerous to our health. These companies seem to have absolutely no regard for the health of the consumer, only for the health of their balance sheet.

Baked Goods

The Bottom Line

THE GOOD: Baked goods made from organic ingredients (flour, eggs, butter) and natural sweeteners such as honey and maple syrup *eaten in moderation*

THE DOWNRIGHT DANGEROUS: All baked goods made with non-organic wheat flour, sugar and/or HFCS, and refined vegetable oils

CHAPTER 10

Sugar and Sweeteners

"Of all the foods capable of inflicting damage in your body, sugar is one of the most damaging of all. Sugar is an extremely potent pro-inflammatory agent that speeds up the aging process. It also promotes the kind of dangerous growth of fat cells around vital organs which is the hallmark of diabetes and heart disease."

— *Dr. Joseph Mercola, author of* **Sweet Deception**

SUGAR IS A SWEET, SEDUCTIVE KILLER, a highly refined substance that is not a natural part of our diet. But this should come as no surprise to most people—many books and articles have been written on the subject, and recently, Dr. Robert Lustig's announcement that sugar should be classified as a slow-acting poison has attracted great media attention, with his lecture, "Sugar: The Bitter Truth," attracting more than two million viewers on YouTube. And in fact he is right—sugar calibrates at the level of 50 on the food quality scale, just a notch above weed-killer.

All the charts in this book give a clear picture of just how dangerous sugar is—when you add sugar to any food, it plummets in nutritional value. Other chapters in this book have been about the quality of food, with the idea that if you eat high quality food, you will have high quality health—but with sugar, it's not an issue of quality as there is no such thing as "good sugar." All refined sugar is bad for us, and artificial sweeteners are just as bad, maybe worse. Sugar wreaks havoc when we eat it, and the more we eat, the more havoc it causes. Ah, but it tastes so sweet! And that's the problem—sugar is highly addictive. It is not dangerous in small quantities, but we don't eat it in small quantities, we indulge in huge amounts. The average person in the U.S. now consumes between 150 and 180 pounds of sugar per year—that's almost half a pound of refined sugar EVERY DAY. That's not the result of indulging in a few squares of chocolate or a couple of cookies, that represents a serious addiction, a virtually continuous infusion of refined sugar.

And in fact, sugar cannot be considered a food, as it has no nutritive value. Yes, it has calories, which give energy, but calories don't equal nutrition. The FDA classifies sugar as a food additive, regarding it as GRAS (generally recognized as safe). Sugar is now found in just about every processed and convenience food product on sale in food markets. This wide-spread use of sugar goes hand-in-hand with the low quality of mass-produced food, which not only is lacking in nutritional content, but also lacking in taste, and for this reason, flavor enhancers, including sugar and high fructose corn syrup, are added to virtually all processed foods to make them palatable.

Science has now proven that the amount of sugar we are consuming is having a devastating effect on our health, causing serious problems such as heart disease, diabetes, cancer, arthritis, and dementia. Sugar, like alcohol, can kill in the long term. Several books have been written about the dangers of sugar in our diet, including *The Sugar Blues* by William Dufty, *Pure, White and Deadly* by John Yudkin, *The Sugar Fix* by Dr. Robert J. Johnson, and more recently, *The Real Truth about Sugar,* a summary and analysis of Dr. Robert Lustig's YouTube lecture. So people are getting the picture. But only very slowly. It's important to *really understand* how deadly sugar can be and how we can learn to avoid it in our diet. This is a long chapter, but the information is important because often a craving for sweet foods can only be resisted or conquered by a true understanding of the effects sugar has on our health. But first, let's get an idea of how and why sugar has become so ingrained in our culture and our diet.

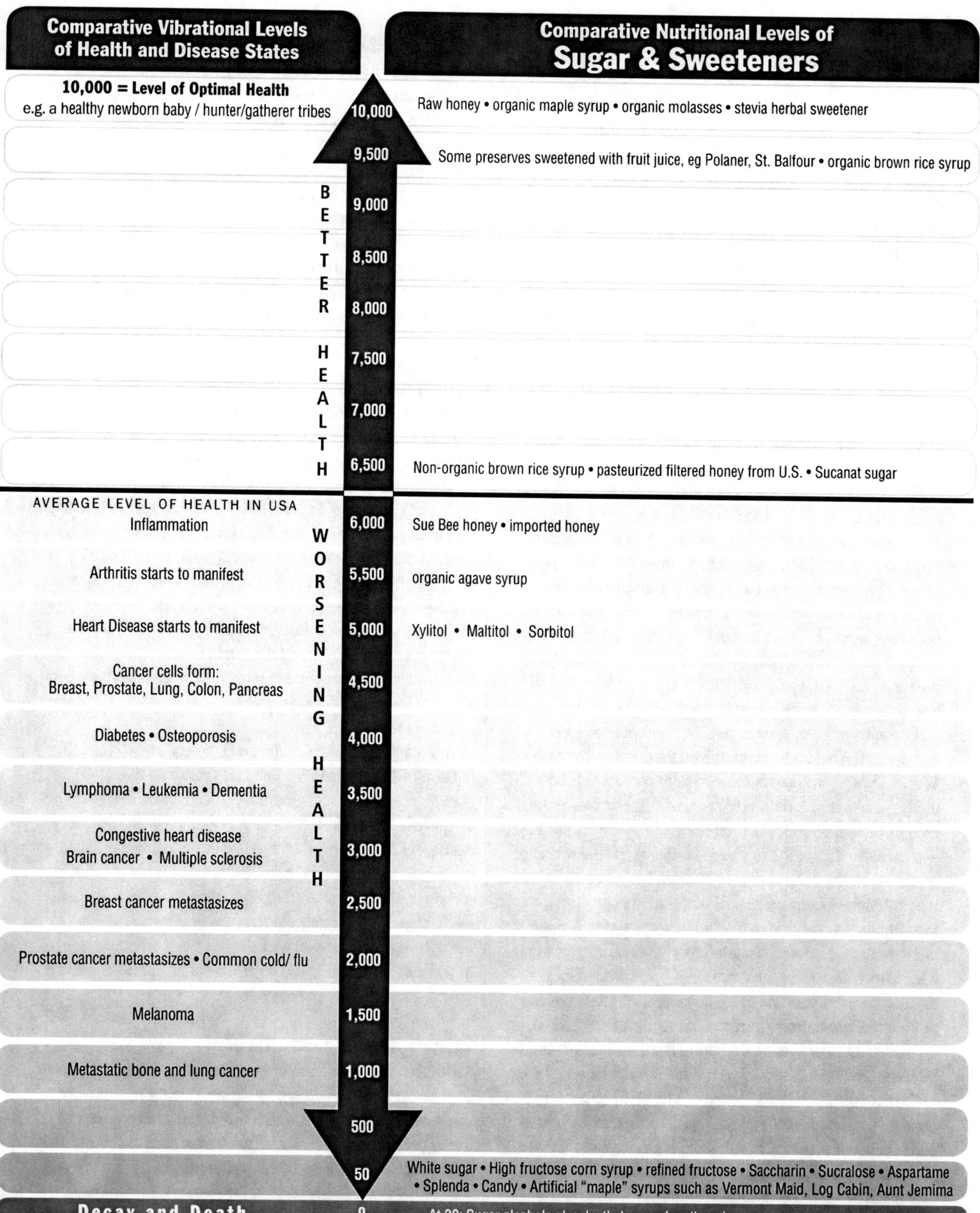
Comparative Vibrational Levels of Health and Disease States
Comparative Nutritional Levels of Sugar & Sweeteners
10,000 = Level of Optimal Health
e.g. a healthy newborn baby / hunter/gatherer tribes
10,000
Raw honey • organic maple syrup • organic molasses • stevia herbal sweetener
9,500
Some preserves sweetened with fruit juice, eg Polaner, St. Balfour • organic brown rice syrup
9,000
8,500
8,000
7,500
7,000
BETTER HEALTH
6,500
Non-organic brown rice syrup • pasteurized filtered honey from U.S. • Sucanat sugar
AVERAGE LEVEL OF HEALTH IN USA
Inflammation
6,000
Sue Bee honey • imported honey
Arthritis starts to manifest
5,500
organic agave syrup
Heart Disease starts to manifest
5,000
Xylitol • Maltitol • Sorbitol
Cancer cells form:
Breast, Prostate, Lung, Colon, Pancreas
4,500
Diabetes • Osteoporosis
4,000
Lymphoma • Leukemia • Dementia
3,500
Congestive heart disease
Brain cancer • Multiple sclerosis
3,000
WORSENING HEALTH
Breast cancer metastasizes
2,500
Prostate cancer metastasizes • Common cold/ flu
2,000
Melanoma
1,500
Metastatic bone and lung cancer
1,000
500
50
White sugar • High fructose corn syrup • refined fructose • Saccharin • Sucralose • Aspartame
• Splenda • Candy • Artificial "maple" syrups such as Vermont Maid, Log Cabin, Aunt Jemima
Decay and Death
0
At 30: Sugar alcohols glycol, ethylene and methanol
Measured in Bovis Units
of Life Force Energy

A Brief History of the Sugar Trade

"No other product has so profoundly influenced the political history of the Western world as has sugar."
—*William Dufty, from his book* **Sugar Blues**

White sugar as we know it comes from sugar cane and sugar beets. Sugar cane grows in tropical countries and is thought to have originated in India, where it was chewed for its sweet juice. I remember being taken to a traditional opera in Hong Kong by my Chinese nanny in the 1950s and being given a stick of sugar cane to chew on during the performance. But you'd have to chew a heck of a lot of sugar cane to get anywhere near the amount of sugar that you'd get in a can of Coke!

For thousands of years of human evolution, refined sugar was not part of the human diet. People ate fresh and dried fruits and used honey and natural syrups as sweeteners, and stayed healthy as these foods were not addictive. But about 2,000 years ago, people discovered that this cane could be crushed to yield a sweet juice, in the same way that American Indians learned to utilize the syrup of the maple tree. In 325 BCE, Alexander the Great's admiral Nearchus related that "the reed in India yields honey without bees," and the ancient Greek writer Herodotus wrote about "honey made by the hands of men." But fresh sugar cane juice would not keep without fermenting, and around 600 CE, in Persia, a method was developed of heating and refining the cane juice so it would crystallize into a solid form. This allowed cane sugar to be stored indefinitely and easily transported and traded, and so rock sugar became a valuable commodity. Europeans started trading with the Persians and by the early 14th century, Cyprus had become a major producer of sugar using the labour of Syrian and Arab slaves. This inflamed the envy of Europeans and they soon realized that it would be easier and cheaper to grow the sugar cane rather than import the end product from the pagan lands of the East. Early records show that in 1306, a diplomatic appeal was sent to Pope Clement V that argued: "In the land of the Sultan, sugar grows in great quantities and from it the Sultans draw large incomes and taxes. If the Christians could seize these lands, great injury would be inflicted on the Sultan and at the same time Christendom would be wholly supplied from Cyprus . . . As regards Christendom, no harm would follow." As an assurance, these may have been the most mistaken words of all time, as this signalled the beginning of the European slave trade, a horror which was to last for six hundred years and encouraged political corruption, organized crime, and immense human suffering.

The first European sugar cane plantations were set up in Spain, and in 1420, the Portuguese introduced the sugar cane to Madeira and the Canary Islands. In 1444, Henry the Navigator of Portugal is recorded as having captured 235 slaves in Lagos, West Africa, and took them to the sugar plantations in Seville. Ten years later, the Pope personally gave his blessing, giving authority to "attack, subject, and reduce to slavery the Saracens, Pagans, and other enemies of Christ."

By 1456, Portugal had control of the European sugar trade and most of the countries of Western Europe were profiting from sugar. After the discovery of the New World, the Spaniards established sugar-works in Hispaniola, and in 1641 sugar cane was transplanted to Barbados, and from there to the other islands of the West Indies. The slave trade triangle was now in full operation, with ships transporting slaves from Africa to the West Indies, delivering sugar, rum and molasses to North America and Europe, and returning to Africa to pick up more slaves.

British historian Noel Deerr has written, "It will be no exaggeration to put the toll of the Slave Trade at 20 million Africans, of which two-thirds are to be charged against sugar." In the early 1800s, when Britain had become the center of the sugar industry, the British government issued a statement saying, "The pleasure, glory, and grandeur of England has been advanced more by sugar than by any other commodity. The impossibility of doing without slaves in the West Indies will always prevent the traffic being dropped." However, the tide was beginning to turn—France outlawed slavery in 1807, the British in 1833, and other European countries soon followed. But America stepped into the breach, cultivating sugar in Cuba and the Southern states, and developing a taste for the substance that overtook even the British. Soon Americans were consuming more sugar per capita than any other nation in the world.

This is a horrific tale of profiteering, misery, and corruption, but also of addiction, as this trade was obviously the result of strong demand. As time went by, this addiction did not go un-noted—Dr. Robert Boesler, a New Jersey dentist, wrote one hundred years ago, in 1912: "Modern manufacturing of sugar has brought about entirely new diseases. The sugar of commerce is nothing else but concentrated crystallized acid. If, in former times, sugar was so costly that only the wealthy could afford to use it, it was of no consequence . . . but today, when, because of its low cost, sugar has caused a degeneration of the people, it is time to insist on a general enlightenment."

Why is Sugar Addictive?

Sugar acts on the brain much like addictive narcotics which affect our brain's natural opiate system. Opiates are the pleasure chemicals released in our brains, which the human body produces to use as neurotransmitters. The drugs derived from the poppy plant, such as opium, morphine, heroin, and oxycodone, act in the same way. All these substances bind to the same receptors as naturally-occurring opioids to produce the neurotransmitter dopamine, the body's own feel-good chemical that is responsible for our motivation and reward systems. After eating sugar, glucose levels rise and the brain produces more dopamine, which drenches the brain in "happy hormones."

Many people can't stop eating sugar once they start: they crave sugary foods, they need more and more to feel satisfied, and they experience withdrawal if they stop eating them—the definition of an addictive drug.

Scientific studies have proven the addictive nature of refined sugar. Dr. Serge Ahmed, a researcher in Bordeaux, France, has been working on experiments with rats, giving them the choice between cocaine and sugar. The rats ended up choosing the sweet taste of sugar over cocaine. And in their paper on "Evidence for Sugar Addiction" in *Neuroscience and Behavioral Reviews*, researchers N.M Avena, P. Rada, and B.G. Hoebel wrote: "Sugar is noteworthy as a substance that releases opioids and dopamine and thus might be expected to have addictive potential." Their study showed evidence to support the hypothesis that rats can become sugar dependent—when laboratory rats were given intermittent access to a sugary drink, they exhibited typical addictive behaviors almost immediately: bingeing when sugar was available, and showing symptoms such as withdrawal, anxiety, and depression when it was not.

Most people living in modern societies are addicted to sugar whether they are aware of it or not, often using it as a form of self-medication to temporarily boost their mood and energy. Withdrawal symptoms can include moodiness, irritability, breaking into a sweat, and becoming light-headed. You are most probably addicted to sugar if you can't go for one day without it—that is, without ANY sugar, and with no foods containing sugar. It's a hard thing to do. Many people say to me, Oh, I don't eat sugar, meaning, *I don't load it into my tea or coffee by the spoonful.* But they do eat baked goods, bread, crackers, ice cream, muffins, peanut butter, jam, soft drinks, canned soups, tomato ketchup, and many other processed foods containing sugar, but they don't count it because they don't see it. Like the 10 spoonfuls of sugar in a can of Coke—just because you can't see it, doesn't mean it isn't there. I was making sugar syrup the other day for my hummingbird feeder and measured out four spoons of sugar into a jug. As I poured in boiling water to dissolve it and watched the pile of sugar disappear into the clear liquid, I was suddenly struck by what a dangerous substance it really is—because it's invisible.

But we all need to be aware that damage is being done and sugar consumption can lead to serious consequences such as diabetes, heart disease, cancer, arthritis, osteoporosis, gout, and other degenerative diseases. The simple answer is to cut out sugar from our diets, but sugar is so addictive that people don't want to hear that. I've had people tell me that they would rather die than give up their morning muffin or afternoon cookies.

Glucose and the Glycemic Index

Table sugar, or sucrose, is made up of more-or-less equal parts of glucose and fructose. Glucose is the most simple of sugars and is an essential energy source for the cells in the body. The body needs glucose, but it doesn't need refined sugar—it can get its glucose from much more nutritious sources.

Glucose is classified as a simple carbohydrate and is absorbed very quickly by the body, while complex carbohydrates, such as those in whole grains and beans, take longer to be absorbed.

All the sweeteners we eat are made up of combinations of simple carbohydrates, which include glucose; fructose, or fruit sugar; lactose, or dairy sugar; sucrose, which comes from plants such as sugar cane and sugar beets; and maltose, which is produced by germinating seeds such as barley, and from caramelized glucose. Galactose is another simple sugar that is found in dairy products and sugar beets. All of these are absorbed directly into the bloodstream through the intestinal lining.

The Glycemic Index is a way of measuring how fast a food is absorbed by the body. Glucose has a glycemic index of 100, meaning that it is absorbed very quickly. The Glycemic Index is useful for those with blood sugar problems and diabetes, but it does give the false impression that sugars that rate low on the index are healthier, such as fructose. Because fructose ranks low on the index, it was thought that it was less damaging than sucrose but that has been found to not be the case. Another example is agave nectar, which consists primarily of fructose with a lesser amount of glucose, so it's actually less healthy than pure sugar because of its high fructose content.

How Eating Simple Sugars Can Cause Diabetes

So if simple sugars feed the body's cells, why is eating refined sugars such a problem? It is because the body is constantly working to balance the level of sugar in the blood, and also its pH, or acid/alkali balance. If our blood contains too much sugar, or is too acid or too alkaline, we will die. It's literally a life-and-death balancing act that the body is constantly engaged in. When we eat simple carbohydrates, i.e. sugar, the body uses insulin to deal with it, getting it out of the blood stream as quickly as possible and shunting it into various organs and cells. This system works pretty well unless we regularly eat large amounts of sugar—then we can overwhelm the system and become "insulin resistant," meaning we keep pumping more and more insulin into our blood stream to deal with the sugar. This puts a bigger strain on the body and leads to type 2 diabetes. All sugars, including honey, maple syrup, table sugar and fruit sugar, have this effect on the body. The only sweeteners that don't have this effect are the herb stevia, and the sugar alcohols xylitol, maltitol, and sorbitol, which is why they are safe for diabetics. However, of all the sugars, it is sucrose and high fructose corn syrup that have the most devastating effect on the body, and the reason is: fructose.

The Dangers of Fructose

Fructose is now the number one source of calories in the U.S. Most of this comes from high fructose corn syrup (HFCS), which is cheap and plentiful and is used to sweeten a vast array of foods, from canned soups, ketchup, and baked goods to processed and packaged foods. Most infant formulas contain sugar or HFCS, which explains how six-month-old babies can be obese, and even some foods labelled "natural" often contain fructose as a sweetener. There is now a new disease called non-alcoholic fatty liver disease caused by the overconsumption of fructose. It now affects one third of all Americans, with even young children beginning to show symptoms.

Table sugar contains fructose—it is about 50 percent glucose and 50 percent fructose (or to be really specific, 48 percent fructose, 47 percent glucose, and 5 percent sucrose.) The reason this is a problem is that glucose and fructose are metabolized differently in the body—glucose is absorbed in the intestines and then into the blood stream where it is used for energy by the cells, while fructose is metabolized in the liver and the excess is stored as triglycerides, or fat globules in the blood, which mostly ends up as fat. But when too much fructose arrives at the liver, the liver can become overwhelmed, and so it shunts even more triglycerides around the body. When the blood is saturated with these fat globules, they are deposited in abdominal tissues, forming unsightly lumps of fat which include beer bellies, protruding behinds, and man-breasts.

Scientific studies have shown that fructose is metabolized in the body just like alcohol and affects the liver just like alcohol—but as it does not affect the brain, the effects are not immediately apparent. There's no missing the effects of drinking a six-pack of beer, but you could drink a six-pack of Coca Cola and not show any immediate ill effects. The damage caused by fructose is insidious, it happens over time. But we all need to be aware that damage is being done and can lead to serious consequences.

High fructose consumption is also the cause of metabolic dysfunction, which is one of the causes of obesity. According to Dr. Robert Lustig, the diseases related to metabolic dysfunction account for 75 percent of the healthcare costs in the U.S. The classic signs of metabolic syndrome include abdominal obesity ("beer belly"), elevated triglycerides, elevated blood sugar, and high blood pressure. This leads to type 2 diabetes, non-alcoholic fatty liver disease, hypertension, polysystic ovarian syndrome, which affects 10 percent of American women, cancer, heart disease, and dementia.

Fructose is also dangerous because it tricks the body into gaining weight by turning off the body's appetite-control system. Fructose does not stimulate insulin in the way that glucose does, which in turn does not suppress ghrelin (the "hunger hormone,") and therefore does not stimulate leptin (the "satiety hormone,") with the result that people don't know when to stop eating.

Scientists from the University of California Davis did a controlled study showing the effects of fructose. They reported: "Over 10 weeks, 16 volunteers on a strictly controlled diet, including high levels of fructose, produced new fat cells around their heart, liver and other digestive organs. They also showed signs of food-processing abnormalities linked to diabetes and heart disease. Another group of volunteers on the same diet, but with glucose sugar replacing fructose, did not have these problems."

Fructose can also fuel cancer cells. A study performed by UCLA's Jonsson Comprehensive Cancer Center showed that pancreatic cancer cells used fructose and glucose in different ways, concluding that the cancer cells utilized fructose to multiply more readily than glucose. "These findings show that cancer cells can readily metabolize fructose to increase proliferation," said Anthony Heaney of the study's team.

Fructose is found in fresh fruit, and some nutritional experts caution against eating more than three pieces of fruit a day, due to the high general intake of fructose in the American diet. They also advise severely limiting fruit juice, which is often just a source of empty calories.

The Truth About High Fructose Corn Syrup

There's been a lot in the news lately about how HFCS is more damaging than sugar. In fact it is—and it's because HFCS has a higher percentage of fructose than sugar, being 55 percent fructose and 45 percent glucose. That extra 10 percent of fructose puts an even greater strain on the liver.

HFCS is used in so many foods because it is a cheap product as a result of farming subsidies. Since the mid 1990s, the U. S. federal government has subsidized corn growers by $40 billion.

Scientists have repeatedly proven that all forms of fructose found in thousands of food products and soft drinks can negatively impact human metabolism and are contributing to the growing obesity epidemic, but the Corn Refiners Association, a large organization that represents the corn refining industry, continues to assert that HFCS is completely safe and perfectly "natural."

But HFCS is anything but "natural." HFCS does not exist in nature—it is a chemically-converted, unnatural corn-based sweetener. Another thing to know about HFCS is that about 86

Ten Reasons to Avoid Refined Sugar

1. Cancer: Sugar is the main food of cancer cells. Every form of cancer cell requires 10 to 50 times more glucose than normal healthy cells (the Warburg effect.) Eating sugar is like giving fertilizer to cancer cells—it makes them grow and proliferate.

2. Heart Disease: Sugar-containing foods cause hardening of the arteries and heart disease. Eating refined carbohydrates causes the pancreas to secrete higher than normal amounts of insulin, which is irritating to blood vessel linings and can lead to coronary artery disease.

3. Endocrine Fatigue: Sugar depletes the adrenal glands, causing adrenal exhaustion, chronic fatigue, and memory loss. A combination of sugar and caffeine are a double-whammy to the adrenal glands. Add stress to the mix, and you are heading for trouble.

4. Diabetes: Excess sugar in the diet creates fluctuating sugar levels in the blood, causing insulin problems and eventually diabetes. Diabetes can lead to renal failure, blindness, circulation problems and heart disease. People with diabetes age one-third faster than non-diabetic people because of the toxic effects of sugar.

5. Loss of immunity: Sugar depresses the immune system by reducing the effectiveness of white blood cells and killer cells in the blood. If you feel you are coming down with a cold or the flu, DON'T consume sweet foods.

6. Acidosis: Sugar is highly acidic. Excess sugar intake increases the likelihood of acidosis, an acid condition in the body which creates prime circumstances for the growth of disease organisms and degeneration. Blood is constantly seeking a balanced pH, so when it is too acidic, it seeks alkaline substances to balance it. To do this, it leaches minerals and vitamins from the bones, teeth and other organs, leading to vitamin deficiencies, arthritis, and tooth decay.

7. Candidiasis: Sugar feeds the "bad" bacteria in the gut, causing a build-up of the yeast *Candida albicans*, resulting in candidiasis, a systemic fungal infestation. Some of the symptoms are "brain fog," sinus problems, food allergies, and chronic constipation and bloating. Candidiasis is prevalent in people who are addicted to sugar and who have taken more than a few courses of antibiotics. Antibiotics kill off the "good" bacteria in the gut as well as the "bad" bacteria in the body.

8. Tooth Decay: We all know this one, and it may not seem such a big deal—until you get a bill from the dentist. Xylitol is an excellent sugar-substitute which looks and tastes like sugar, but has a third less calories, and it does not cause tooth decay; in fact, it is actually good for the mouth/nasal area and is used in chewing gum. As an ironic note, tooth decay is the only detrimental effect of sugar accepted by the American Medical Association.

9. Obesity: Refined sugar supplies empty calories as well as an unhealthy dose of fructose, which is a major cause of obesity. Being overweight is a symptom of metabolic syndrome, which means you are at a high risk for diabetes, heart disease and cancer, and also makes you less likely to want to exercise. The idea that a calorie is a calorie has become common wisdom—calories in minus calories out equals weight gain or loss. But in fact that is not true. A calorie from fat is not metabolized and stored in the body in the same way that a calorie from fructose is. So, when it comes to obesity, it's WHAT we eat that is important, not how many calories we consume.

10. Wrinkles and Aging Skin: If all these reasons for avoiding sugar fail to deter you, this one will do it for sure! Sugar causes the skin to age by a process called glycation, a condition where glucose attaches to the proteins of collagen, making skin stiff and inflexible, leading to wrinkling and aging. Glycation also adversely affects the tiniest capillaries in the body, especially the eyes and the brain; in fact, Alzheimer's has been called "diabetes of the brain." And beware that fructose has 10 times the glycation activity of glucose.

percent of the corn grown in the U.S. is genetically modified, and a large proportion of that goes into making HFCS. So there's no question that most HFCS on the market contains GM ingredients, and should be avoided for that reason alone. There are no warning labels on the products that contain it, so we should assume that ALL high fructose corn syrup is genetically modified.

Sugar Causes Glycation, Which Causes Wrinkles in the Skin

> "One of the biggest hidden threats to our health is the consumption of all forms of sugar. In addition to its detrimental effects on the body's proper pH balance, a major problem stemming from sugar consumption has to do with a chemical process called glycation."
> — *Dr. David Williams, editor of Alternatives newsletter*

Glycation is a chemical reaction that occurs in the body when the sugar in the blood (glucose) combines with certain amino acids found in proteins. This reactive process creates by-products known scientifically as "advanced glycation end-products," or AGEs. When proteins in blood vessels undergo glycation, they become stiffer and less flexible, leading to higher blood pressure, plaque formation, blood flow blockages, heart and artery disease, and eventually, stroke or heart attack. The smallest blood vessels, such as those in the back of the eye, the kidney, and the brain, are the most easily affected as they need a constant supply of glucose. Glycation can also lead to diabetes, cancer, and deafness, and is a significant contributor to Alzheimer's disease. AGEs also causes high levels of inflammation, which greatly contributes to aging.

Glycation also causes permanent wrinkles in the skin by affecting collagen—this can be seen in certain people who have "corrugated" skin on their faces; you can be sure they have a sugar addiction. Dr. Nicholas Perricone has written about this in his book *The Wrinkle Cure:* "If you have ever wondered why fast food is constantly cited as a cause of skin problems, the answer lies in a biological process called glycation. Glycation . . . is a major cause of the visible signs of aging." He goes on to say that fructose has 10 times the glycation activity of glucose.

You can observe a form of glycation in the kitchen during baking when sugar combines with certain amino acids in grain proteins and causes bread and pastries to turn brown, and also when meat is grilled, coffee is roasted, and sugar is caramelized. This is why many nutritional experts warn against eating barbecued, grilled, and fried foods. You can also picture glycation occurring when the clear, runny portion of a raw egg, which is mostly protein, is heated—it quickly and permanently transforms from a runny, clear liquid to a solid white mass. This is similar to the effects of glycation in the body—it can affect proteins in tissues *forever,* and unfortunately, the long-term health consequences can be disastrous.

How to Kick the Sugar Habit in Seven Days

This might seem impossible while you are in the throes of sugar addiction, but rest assured that once sugar is out of your system, you won't crave it any more.

Be aware that if you have a serious sugar addiction you will also have to stop eating honey and maple syrup and other natural sweeteners until you get rid of your cravings. This is where stevia and xylitol are really useful. Also cut down on fruit—those with a severe sugar craving often substitute fruit instead, and the same goes for fruit juice, it's just pure sugar. Alcohol too—an occasional glass of white wine is the best choice if you are trying to kick the sugar habit. It's also best to avoid refined wheat products, such as bread and pasta, during this time, as wheat and sugar addictions generally go hand-in-hand and refined wheat is absorbed as fast as sugar into the blood stream.

First, cut down on sugar gradually, and don't eat any processed foods that contain it, such as tomato ketchup, cocktail sauce, canned soups, peanut butter, packaged bread—well, just about all processed foods. Then banish sugar and all the foods that contain it from your house. Stock your pantry and refrigerator with healthy foods, especially foods that satisfy you. Fatty foods are the most satisfying, which is why it's impossible to kick a sugar addiction when you are on a low-fat diet. We actually need far more fat (healthy fat, that is) in our diets than the medical profession has been telling us, up to 50 percent in fact. Animal products, avocado, raw nuts, and foods cooked in butter and olive oil are all satisfying and healthy. I remember that when I was kicking the sugar habit, I would roast an organic chicken and eat the entire thing, scraping the bottom of the pan for all those delicious caramelized juices so I would feel full.

Do whatever it takes, eat whatever, whenever and however much you need for you to feel full, just so long as it doesn't contain sugar or wheat. Take it one day at a time. When you have got through a day without eating sugar, congratulate yourself, and know that you can do it for another day, and then another—and then, after seven days, sugar will be out of your system and your craving will be just about gone.

It's best to start the day with protein, such as scrambled eggs, and eat enough so you feel full and won't be tempted to eat a mid-morning snack. For lunch, have a hearty meal of protein and vegetables (root vegetables are very filling,) and eat enough to get you through to 4 p.m. Now we have reached the dangerous time! Don't give in and eat cookies, a pastry, or candy bar—make sure you have a healthy snack on hand, such as nuts, corn chips and guacamole or salsa, carrot sticks and hummus, celery sticks or apple slices with cheese or peanut butter (not the sweetened kind), or chicken-liver or fish pate with rice crackers. And for dinner eat more protein and vegetables until you are full.

You can't fight a food addiction if you are hungry, so fill yourself up with healthy food. You won't gain weight—obesity is mainly caused by refined carbohydrates and fructose, not protein and vegetables. But beware that just a taste of sugar can bring the craving right back, so be vigilant. Once you have got rid of your craving for sugar, you may eat honey and maple syrup in moderation.

Kicking the sugar habit is such a worthwhile thing to do because, finally, you will be in control of your food, your food won't be in control of you. "Just say no" is the best thing to say to sugar.

Natural Sweeteners

We tend to associate sugar with sugar cane and sugar beets, but different forms of sugar are found abundantly in the vegetable world, including nectar from flowers, which bees make into honey, and sap, from which we get maple syrup. These sweeteners are healthier than refined sugar, as they contain enzymes and trace amounts of vitamins, minerals, amino acids and other beneficial elements, but they still affect blood sugar levels and so should be eaten in moderation. For someone who has blood sugar issues, such as diabetes and metabolic syndrome, or Candidiasis, it's best if they avoid honey and maple syrup and instead substitute the herb stevia or the sugar alcohol xylitol.

Honey

The U.S. consumes about 400 million pounds of honey a year, which is around 1.3 pounds a person. About 35 percent of this is consumed in homes, restaurants and institutions, while the remaining 65 percent is used by the food industry for baked goods, sauces, beverages, and hundreds of different processed foods—think of Honey-Nut Cheerios, for instance.

As with all nutritive sweeteners, honey consists mostly of sugars with trace amounts of vitamins and minerals. Bees convert nectar, a sugar-rich liquid produced by plants, into honey by adding an enzyme which breaks down the complex sugars into simple sugars. Nectar is produced in glands of flowers called nectaries which attracts pollinating animals. Common nectar-consuming pollinators include bees, butterflies, moths, hummingbirds, and bats. Nectar is a combination of sucrose, glucose, and fructose; honey bees transform these sugars into honey by a process of regurgitation until they are partially digested. The sugar content of honey is mainly fructose (about 38.5 percent) and glucose (about 31 percent), with the remaining sugars consisting of maltose, sucrose, and other complex carbohydrates.

Fresh honey is a supersaturated liquid, containing more sugar than the water can typically dissolve at ambient temperatures. An excellent preservative, honey, and objects immersed in honey, have been preserved for decades and even centuries. Most microorganisms do not grow in honey because of its low water content, but honey sometimes contains dormant endospores of the bacterium *Clostridium botulinum*, which can be dangerous to infants. The AAP Pediatric Nutrition Handbook advises, "Infants younger than 12 months should avoid all sources of honey."

Raw honey is honey taken directly from the beehive, extracted from the honeycomb, strained and bottled, without being heated. This raw product contains some pollen and may contain small particles of wax. Local raw honey is sought after by allergy sufferers as the local pollen contained in the honey is thought to lessen a sensitivity to hay fever. Excessive heating can reduce the nutritional value of honey—heating up to 98.6 °F causes loss of nearly 200 components, some of which are antibacterial, and heating up to 104 °F destroys invertase, an important enzyme.

Raw honey has anti-bacterial properties and has been a traditional topical treatment for infected wounds for over 2,000 years. Around 50 AD, the ancient Greek physician Dioscorides described honey as being "good for all rotten and hollow ulcers." Today, laboratory studies have shown that honey has an antimicrobial action against a broad spectrum of bacteria and fungi, and it has been "rediscovered" by the medical profession, particularly in cases where conventional methods are failing, such as bed sores and open wounds. Most importantly, it can be effective on antibiotic-resistant strains of bacteria, including MRSA (Methicillin-resistant *Staphylococcus aureus*, a bacterium responsible for several difficult-to-treat infections in humans.) Manuka honey has a long-standing reputation in New Zealand folk-lore for its antiseptic properties and is available at health food stores and by mail order.

But make sure when you buy honey that you are buying a quality product, preferably locally produced. That may be easier said than done, however—the USDA reports that U.S. beekeepers can only supply about a 48 percent of this country's demand, and the remaining 52 percent is imported from 41 other countries. Andrew Schneider, a Pulitzer Prize-winning investigative reporter, wrote a revealing article for *Food Safety News* and The Food Watchdog.com entitled, "Asian Honey, Banned in Europe, Is Flooding U.S. Grocery Shelves," in which he reports that a third or more of all the honey consumed in the U.S. is likely to have been smuggled in from China and may be tainted with illegal antibiotics and heavy metals—and much of it may not even be honey at all, but flavored sugar syrup masquerading as honey.

Maple Syrup

Maple syrup has a unique flavor, and is only produced in North America. It is made from the sap of the sugar maple, red maple, or black maple, though other species of maple can also produce syrup. In cold climates, these trees store starch in their trunks and roots before the winter, and this starch is then converted to sugar that rises in the sap in the spring. Maple syrup is collected by boring holes into the tree trunks and collecting the exuded sap. The sap is processed by heating to evaporate much of the water, leaving a concentrated syrup.

Maple syrup consists primarily of sucrose and water with small amounts of other sugars such as fructose and glucose. It also contains small amounts of minerals, amino acids, and a variety of volatile organic compounds, all of which contribute to its flavor. Organic acids, most notably malic acid, makes the syrup slightly acidic. Scientists have discovered 34 new compounds in pure maple syrup, five of which have never before been seen in nature. Among these is quebecol, a phenolic compound created when the maple sap is boiled to create syrup.

Maple syrup is a delicious and nutritious natural sweetener, but make sure you only buy genuine maple syrup—the artificial varieties are merely flavored corn syrup and calibrate at the same level as sugar. Maple syrup is expensive, but it's worth it, and because it's expensive, we are encouraged to use it in moderation. Just a drizzle will do!

Brown Rice Syrup

Brown rice syrup is derived by culturing cooked rice with enzymes (usually from dried barley sprouts) to break down the starches, then straining off the liquid and reducing it by cooking until it thickens. Brown rice syrup is used to sweeten some drinks, such as rice milk, and can be bought in bulk at health food stores. The breakdown of brown rice syrup is 45 percent maltose, 3 percent glucose, and 52 percent maltotriose, a complex trisaccharide. While glucose has a glycemic index of 100, maltose actually has a glycemic index of 105, so it is sweeter than glucose and is absorbed into the blood stream even faster. Maltotriose has a glycemic index somewhere in the 60s, about the same as whole, cooked brown rice. The result is that, combined, these sugars have a GI index higher than table sugar, so people with blood sugar concerns and Candidiasis should avoid brown rice syrup. It is a healthier choice than table sugar, but, as with all sweeteners, it should be eaten sparingly.

Sucanat

Sucanat, a brand-named product, is a whole cane sugar that is made by crushing freshly-cut sugar cane, extracting the juice, and heating it in a large vat to form small brown grainy crystals. It is essentially pure dried sugar cane juice, so it does retain certain nutrients. Unlike refined and processed cane sugar, Sucanat contains much of the molasses that would otherwise be removed in the refining process, similar to panela and muscovado, which gives it a strong flavor. It was first introduced in 1978 and is a registered trademark of Ragus Holdings, Inc. The name is a contraction of "sucre de canne naturel," or natural cane sugar, and it is produced in Costa Rica. It registers high on the glycemic index as it is a cane sugar.

Agave Syrup

Nutritional experts are now warning against regarding agave syrup as a healthy sweetener since it is a highly processed substance. Agave nectar is commercially produced in South Africa and Mexico from several species of the agave plant. Agave nectar is 1.4 to 1.6 times sweeter than sugar, and is also sweeter than honey, though less viscous. Because it dissolves quickly, it can be used as a sweetener for cold beverages such as cocktails, smoothies and iced tea. It is also commonly used as an alternative to honey by vegans. Agave consists primarily of fructose and glucose, ranging from 90 percent fructose and 10 percent glucose to around 50 percent of each, depending on the raw product and the processing. But either way, its high fructose content makes it an undesirable sweetener.

Coconut Nectar

Coconut nectar is a highly nutrient-rich "sap" produced when the coconut tree is tapped. Nectar made from this natural sap is a raw, enzymatically alive product, minimally evaporated at low temperatures. It is low on the glycemic index and is a source of amino acids and minerals. It has a naturally sweet, mild flavor and can be used as a sweetener on pancakes, over cereal, in tea and smoothies, and in dessert recipes. It is nutritionally superior to Agave syrup.

Artificial Sweeteners

> "Today, you find artificial sweeteners in everything from yogurt to baked goods. Big business continues to tell you that they're 'sugar-free,' they're 'a healthy alternative to sugar.' Tragically, the truth is this: artificial sweeteners such as Splenda and Nutrasweet are NOT healthy—or safe."
>
> —*Dr. Joseph Mercola, from his book* **Sweet Deception**

Although the food industry insists that artificial sweeteners are safe, there is much evidence to the contrary, and virtually all nutritional experts consider them to be dangerous. But these sweeteners are attractive to food manufacturers as they are cheaper to use than sugar or HFCS due to the smaller quantities required, but they do have a characteristic aftertaste that some people find unpleasant.

The FDA-approved non-nutritive sweeteners are sucralose, aspartame, saccharin, acesulfame potassium, and neotame. The herb Stevia has recently been added to this list. Cyclamate is approved as a sweetener in over 55 countries, though it is banned in the U.S.

Sucralose, sold under the brand name Splenda, owned by the British company Tate & Lyle, is simply chlorinated sugar; in chemical terms, it is a chlorocarbon. Few scientific studies have been performed on the effects of sucralose in humans, and the majority of the studies were on animals. Many problems were found, even though they were ultimately dismissed, including brain lesions, decreased red blood cell count and anemia, enlarged and calcified kidneys, increased mortality, male infertility, and spontaneous abortions in rabbits. Because sucralose, unlike aspartame, retains its sweetness after being heated and has at least twice the shelf life of aspartame, it has become more popular as an ingredient.

The latest research is showing that artificial sweeteners such as Splenda and Nutrasweet can cause inflammatory bowel disease (IBD), a serious autoimmune disease, by inactivating digestive enzymes and altering gut barrier function. In 1991, Canada was the first country to approve the use of sucralose as a sweetener in such products as breakfast cereals, beverages, desserts and bakery products, and it is now suspected to be the cause of a dramatic increase in cases of IBD. A study published in 2008 in the *Journal of Toxicology and Environmental Health* showed that Splenda reduced the amount of good bacteria (probiotics) in the intestines by 50 percent, and also increased the pH level. It is thought that many consumers may suffer ill effects from artificial sweeteners such as Splenda without realizing that their problems are related to their consumption of artificially sweetened foods and beverages. And the truth is, the long-term damage of sucralose consumption is largely unknown.

Nutrasweet contains aspartame, which is derived from aspartic acid and is approximately 200 times sweeter than sugar. Though FDA officials describe aspartame as being "one of the most thoroughly tested and studied food additives the agency has ever approved," research has shown that the amino acids in aspartame can attack cells, even crossing the blood-brain barrier to attack brain cells, creating a toxic cellular over-stimulation called excitotoxicity, and that long-term consumption of aspartame leads to oxidative stress and vascular congestion. In 2012, a study out of Harvard, the longest ever human aspartame study, spanning 22 years, found a clear association between aspartame consumption and non-Hodgkin's Lymphoma and leukemia in men. The study also found that leukemia was associated with diet soda intake in both men and women. Most people don't make the connection between their headaches, fatigue, anxiety attacks and other symptoms as being caused by artificial sweeteners.

Saccharin is the most popular artificial sweetener after sucralose and aspartame. The use of saccharin, first discovered in 1878 by a chemist working on coal tar derivatives, has always been controversial, but the EPA has officially removed saccharin from their list of hazardous commercial chemical products, and in 2010, stated that saccharin is no longer considered a potential hazard to human health. Saccharin is often used together with aspartame in diet carbonated soft drinks as aspartame's sweetness has a relatively short shelf life. In the United States, the most popular brand of saccharin comes in the pink packets of "Sweet 'N Low."

Neotame is an artificial sweetener made by NutraSweet that is between 7,000 and 13,000 times as sweet as table sugar. It was approved by the FDA for general use in 2002.

Although these artificial sweeteners contribute no calories, or food energy, to the diet, they can still trigger the release of insulin, which does not make them a good choice for diabetics and other people concerned about blood sugar levels.

The Sweet Herb Stevia

The herb Stevia comes from a species of plants native to South America, Central America, and Mexico. These plants were first investigated by Spanish botanist and physician Petrus Jacobus Stevus (Pedro Jaime Esteve). The leaves of the stevia plant have 30 to 45 times the sweetness of table sugar. Human use of the sweet species *S. rebaudiana* originated in South America and the leaves have been traditionally used for hundreds of years in Paraguay and Brazil to sweeten local teas, medicines, and as a "sweet treat." Stevia has a negligible effect on blood glucose, and it is thought it may even enhance glucose tolerance, therefore it is an excellent natural sweetener for diabetics and others on carbohydrate-controlled diets.

In 1991, after allegedly receiving an anonymous industry complaint, the FDA labeled stevia as an "unsafe food additive" and restricted its import. Stevia remained banned until after the 1994 Dietary Supplement Health and Education Act forced the FDA to revise its stance to permit stevia to be used as a dietary supplement, although not as a food additive. In 2008, the FDA gave a "no objection" approval for GRAS (generally recognized as safe) status to Truvia (developed by Cargill and The Coca-Cola Company) and PureVia (developed by PepsiCo and the Whole Earth Sweetener Company, a subsidiary of Merisant), both of which use a substance derived from the Stevia plant, and Coca Cola and PepsiCo have now introduced products that contain this herb.

Sugar Alcohols Are a Safe Alternative

Sugar alcohols are useful sugar substitutes which taste like sugar but provide fewer calories than sugar because they are not completely absorbed in the body. Those now on the market include maltitol, xylitol, mannitol, and sorbitol.

Maltitol has 0 grams of carbohydrates per serving and is endorsed and recommended by National Diabetes Outreach. Maltitol and sorbitol are used to sweeten diabetic chocolate, as sugar alcohols do not affect blood sugar. Xylitol seems to be the best tolerated of the sugar alcohols—it is as sweet as sucrose but has only two-thirds the calories. Xylitol is found in the fibers of many fruits and vegetables, including berries, oats, and mushrooms, as well as fibrous material such as corn husks, sugar cane bagasse, and birch bark.

These sugar alcohols do not contribute to tooth decay, do not brown or caramelize when heated, and they do not feed yeast, so cannot be used in baking where yeast needs to rise. It is for this reason that sugar alcohols can be eaten in place of sugar by people suffering from candidiasis, a systemic yeast infection caused by an overgrowth of *Candida albicans. Candida albicans* is a naturally-occurring organism that lives in the mucus membranes of the body and is normally kept in balance by beneficial bacteria called probiotics. But a dose of antibiotics can kill the beneficial bacteria, allowing for *Candida albicans* to grow uncontrollably. This is then exacerbated by eating refined sugar, yeast's favorite food, and the infection continues to grow.

High intakes of some sugar alcohols can lead to abdominal gas and diarrhea, and any foods that contain sorbitol or mannitol must include a warning on their label that "excess consumption may have a laxative effect." The American Dietetic Association advises that intakes of more than 50 grams per day of sorbitol or more than 20 grams per day of mannitol may cause diarrhea. Some individuals experience symptoms even after a single-serving quantity, but with continued use, most people develop a degree of tolerance to sugar alcohols and no longer experience these symptoms.

The simplest sugar alcohols are ethylene glycol and methanol—sweet, toxic chemicals used in antifreeze.

Sugar and Sweeteners

The Bottom Line

THE GOOD: Used in moderation: raw honey, organic maple syrup, organic brown rice syrup, and organic molasses • the herb stevia

THE NOT-SO-BAD: Agave syrup • Sucanat • Xylitol, maltitol and sorbitol

THE DOWNRIGHT DANGEROUS: Refined white sugar, refined fructose, and high fructose corn syrup, and products that contain them • artificial sweeteners such as Splenda and Nutrasweet, and products that contain them • candy

CHAPTER 11

Meat and Poultry

"You eliminate saturated fats from your diet at your own peril, as doing so will actually increase, not decrease, your risk of heart disease, particularly if you replace them with carbohydrates, which are the true dietary villain you need to be avoiding."

— *Dr. Joseph M. Mercola, founder of www.mercola.com one of the Internet's most visited health information sites*

HISTORICALLY, AMERICANS HAVE ALWAYS BEEN a nation of meat-eaters. In the 19th century, records show that meat, often beef, was eaten three times a day, for breakfast, lunch and dinner. But now it has become the fashion in the U.S. and much of the Western world to view fat, and especially saturated fat, as a problematic part of our diet, blaming it for an epidemic of heart disease supposedly caused by high blood cholesterol levels.

The irony of this supposed link between heart disease and a high fat diet is that since the 1960s, the American public ate about half as much lard, less butter, and less animal fat than before, but ate more margarine, vegetable shortening and salad oils. The result is that cases of heart disease increased even though vegetable-fat consumption per capita in America doubled and the average consumption of all animal fat dropped. This leads us to the conclusion that the epidemic of heart disease may in fact have been *caused* by the increase in vegetable fat consumption and decrease in the consumption of animal fats, and not the other way around. And in fact, many medical experts believe that the dramatic rise in degenerative diseases in Western society can be correlated with an increased consumption of refined vegetable oils and a corresponding reduction in saturated fats. This has been confirmed by the latest research from the Netherlands and Denmark showing that replacing saturated fats in the diet with carbohydrates such as bread, pasta and rice will actually *increase* the risk of heart disease, not reduce it.

And in fact, a close examination of the scientific research over the past 50 years that claims to prove a link between dietary fat and disease shows a lack of scientific oversight and a casual acceptance of wishful thinking and erroneous assumptions. Despite evidence to the contrary, the American Medical Association started a campaign in the 1970s arguing that a low-fat diet was a healthy diet. Unfortunately, they are still maintaining that theory today, although more than 900 scientific studies have proven otherwise. In fact, cardiologist Dr. Ernest N. Curtis, author of *The Cholesterol Delusion*, has called the belief a "delusion," meaning that it is a false belief held with conviction *despite* solid evidence to the contrary. The idea behind this "delusion" seems to have been to create a mythology that saturated fat, especially from animal sources, is bad for us, but this myth and the resulting advice that we should consume low-fat foods, less animal fats, and more carbohydrates and vegetable oils has caused immense harm and suffering, indeed, disease and death, in millions of people instead of saving lives.

We are still being bombarded with advertisements and articles in the media that lead us to believe that fats in our diet are bad for us and will make us "fat." But after 40 years of having cut down drastically on fat in our diets, Americans are no healthier and the country is now facing an epidemic of obesity and degenerative diseases that is creating a crisis for the U.S. health care system. A by-product of this erroneous belief that saturated fat is unhealthy has led to a proliferation of alternative diets such as vegan and raw food diets, which can be dangerous, especially for those people whose physical makeup needs a high animal protein intake. No one could fault a person for choosing not to eat animals for ethical reasons, but avoiding meat for health reasons is not a wise choice since animal protein is an essential part of our diets. But that is true only for free-range, organically-fed and wild animals, not factory-farmed meat and poultry, which is best avoided both for nutritional and ethical reasons, especially since factory-farmed animals are fed corn, virtually 100 percent of which is genetically modified, so when we eat these animals, we are also eating dangerous GM substances.

Why Eating Meat is Good For Us and Why We Were Told it Was Bad

> "From the inception of the diet-heart hypothesis in the early 1950s, those who argued that dietary fat caused heart disease accumulated the evidential equivalent of a mythology to support their belief. These myths are still passed on faithfully to the present day."
> — *Gary Taubes, author of* **Good Calories, Bad Calories**

The idea that cholesterol causes disease comes from a set of closely related theories known as the Lipid Hypothesis, the Cholesterol Theory, and the Diet-Heart Theory. These theories claim that too much cholesterol in the blood is the major cause of hardening of the arteries, and that too much saturated fat and cholesterol in the diet raises the cholesterol level, leading to heart attack and stroke.

The medical literature concerning saturated fats and cholesterol levels in the blood has been minutely examined and documented by Gary Taubes in his book, *Good Calories, Bad Calories*, in which he exposes the medical, food processing and pharmaceutical industries for perpetuating convenient myths designed to make people sick and profit from them. As he relates in his book, one of these myths was that a pandemic of heart disease had ravaged the country since World War II, and another "told of how a nation turned away from cereals and grains to fat and red meat and paid the price in heart disease. The facts did not support these claims, but the myths served a purpose, and so they remained unquestioned."

Dr. Ernest N. Curtis, a California cardiologist, studied the research done on these theories and noticed a pattern of deceit and manipulation that included using dubious data and statistics, unscientific reasoning, and "statistical massaging" designed to make trivial differences seem significant, with a number of these studies bordering on outright scientific fraud. "If you examine the statistics closely," he explains, "You will see that the incidence of heart attacks is spread pretty evenly throughout the entire range of cholesterol levels." One researcher, George V. Mann, ScD, M.D., professor of Biochemistry at Vanderbilt School of Medicine, went so far as to call the Diet-Heart Theory "the greatest scientific fraud of the 20th century—perhaps any century."

This theory can be traced back to the late 1940s when a physiologist named Ancel Keys, who developed the K-rations during WW II, decided that heart disease was caused by dietary cholesterol—even though autopsy examinations failed to demonstrate that people with high cholesterol levels had arteries that were any more clogged than those with low levels, and that researchers in 1937 had shown that dietary cholesterol has very little effect on the amount of cholesterol in the blood. But Keys was convinced that eating too much cholesterol-containing food would elevate blood cholesterol levels, causing heart disease. He insisted that ALL fats raised cholesterol levels, and if it did that, the way to reduce cholesterol levels was to eat less fat. Thus began the crusade against dietary fat, and especially animal (saturated) fats.

In his book, Taubes explains how researchers whose scientific work showed that there was no relationship between high cholesterol levels and heart disease were ridiculed, and so Keys' theory prevailed, even though *Time* magazine in 1961 featured Keys on its cover with a four-page story noting that his theory was "still questioned by some researchers with conflicting ideas of what causes coronary disease."

Despite 50 years of studies and more than $900 million spent on research, there has been no conclusive evidence that a diet high in animal fats has a significant effect on cholesterol levels in the blood. But the truth is gradually being accepted by mainstream America: in 2011, nutrition experts from the Harvard School of Public Health (HSPH) told food industry leaders at the seventh annual World of Healthy Flavors Conference that "it is time to end the low-fat myth." The conference, co-hosted by the Culinary Institute of America and HSPH, each year brings together nutrition researchers with representatives from schools, supermarkets, and food industry giants to share strategies for offering Americans healthier menu options. The nutrition experts encouraged audience members to avoid "low-fat" terminology and thinking, "since diets low in fat are often high in sodium and carbohydrates from sources such as white flour and rice, refined snacks, and sugary drinks." Instead, the panelists said, chefs should focus on cutting trans fats from their menus and educating consumers about seeking out healthy fats.

The Big Pharma Connection

Trying to find evidence of the supposed dangers of cholesterol in our diet and the benefits of low-fat diets has long been a goal of the scientific community and the corporate interests that finance them—the reason being that statins, drugs that lower cholesterol levels, are one of the most widely prescribed drugs in the world. In the U.S., a staggering one in four people over the age of 45 is now taking this drug. But they are not safe: to date, there have been hundreds of studies performed showing the adverse effects of statins, which include muscle problems, heart failure, diabetes, birth defects, and increased cancer risk.

Statins act by blocking a crucial enzyme in the liver responsible for making cholesterol. But this enzyme also makes Coenzyme Q10 (CoQ10,) which is essential for cell health, so it's no surprise that many potentially dangerous side effects go hand-in-hand

Comparative Vibrational Levels of Health and Disease States	Bovis Units	Comparative Nutritional Levels of **Meat & Poultry**
10,000 = Level of Optimal Health e.g. a healthy newborn baby / hunter/gatherer tribes	10,000	Meat, organs and fat of wild animals and naturally-raised farm animals, including bacon & ham
	9,500	Coleman beef • Bell & Evans chicken • Tour Eiffel pork pate • Pacific organic chicken stock
	9,000	Shady Brook Farms turkey • Supermarket lamb • Boar's Head head cheese • Tour Eiffel & 3 Little Pigs duck/chicken pate
	8,500	Conventionally-raised duck
	8,000	Lard (from corn-fed cattle)
	7,500	
	7,000	Smithfield Smoked Pork Picnic • Hatfield ham steak • Boar's Head ham steak
	6,500	Supermarket steak (feed-lot/corn fed) • Pacific free-range chicken broth
AVERAGE LEVEL OF HEALTH IN USA Inflammation	6,000	Purdue chicken and turkey • Butterball turkey • Shady Brook Farms turkey sausage
Arthritis starts to manifest	5,500	Oscar Mayer bacon • Plumrose bacon
Heart Disease starts to manifest	5,000	Oscar Mayer Breakfast Sausages • Average supermarket ground beef and sausages
Cancer cells form: Breast, Prostate, Lung, Colon, Pancreas	4,500	Average supermarket chicken, eg. White Gem (Stop & Shop) • average pork chops
Diabetes • Osteoporosis	4,000	Hebrew National Beef Franks • Deutschmacher Frankfurters • Tony Roma's Baby Back Ribs (pork) • Oscar Meyer hot dogs
Lymphoma • Leukemia • Dementia	3,500	Johnsonville Italian Sausage • Valley Fresh chicken breast (canned) • Armour Potted Meat
Congestive heart disease Brain cancer • Multiple sclerosis	3,000	Jimmy Dean pork sausage patties • Johnsonville brats, breakfast sausage • Libby's Vienna sausage (canned) • Boar's Head roast beef, prosciutto, pancetta
Breast cancer metastasizes	2,500	Hormel Spam • Lloyd's Barbecue Pork Spareribs • Swanson chicken (canned) • Jimmy Dean Maple Sausages
Prostate cancer metastasizes • Common cold/ flu	2,000	Canned meat: Swanson Chicken a la King, Hormal White & Dark Turkey, Snow's White Chicken • Boar's Head Bologna • Underwood Deviled Ham • Hormal canned beef patties • Bubba Burgers
Melanoma	1,500	Libby's Corned Beef Hash • Boar's Head deli meats: Ham, pastrami, turkey, roast beef, olive loaf, chicken breast • Russer smoked ham, pastrami, Bologna, Genoa Salami • Wunderbar Bologna
Metastatic bone and lung cancer	1,000	Campbell's Cream of Chicken Soup and Chicken Noodle Soup
	500	Campbell's 98% Fat Free Cream of Chicken Soup
	50	
Decay and Death	0	

BETTER HEALTH ↑ / WORSENING HEALTH ↓

Measured in Bovis Units of Life Force Energy

> "We already know that statins cause muscle weakness and chronic heart failure. But I've repeatedly mentioned that your brain could be a much bigger victim to statins. That's because the brain needs cholesterol for good health. It needs so much, in fact, that it makes its own. Statins don't just inhibit cholesterol production in your liver. They also inhibit cholesterol production in your brain."
>
> — *Dr. Robert J. Rowan,* **Second Opinion** *newsletter*

with statin drug use. This is a great irony since, while supposedly reducing the risk of cardiovascular events and heart disease, these statin drugs can actually *increase* the risk of heart disease because they deplete the body of CoQ10, which can lead to heart failure.

Dr. Stephanie Seneff, a senior scientist at MIT, reports: "Statin drugs interfere with cholesterol synthesis in the liver, but [they] also interfere with the synthesis of cholesterol in the brain . . . Indeed, a population-based study showed that people who had ever taken statins had an increased risk of Alzheimer's disease."

She predicts that the statin drug run is about to end. "The thalidomide disaster of the 1950s . . . will pale by comparison to the dramatic rise and fall of the statin industry. I can see the tide slowly turning, and I believe it will eventually crescendo into a tidal wave, but misinformation is remarkably persistent, so it may take years."

Over the past decade, cholesterol level guidelines have been changed by the medical profession at the urging of drug companies, in effect creating more "patients" who can now be treated with cholesterol-lowering drugs. It has even been suggested screening children prior to puberty and prescribing statins to kids as young as eight. Significantly, it was discovered in an investigation that eight of the nine doctors on the approval panel for these updated guidelines had financial ties to the companies making the cholesterol-lowering drugs.

We are not likely to read the truth in the popular press. Recently, a short article appeared in *Time* magazine entitled, "The Anti-Cholesterol Diet. How the right foods can lower your lipids." The opening sentence read, "Can you eat your way to lower cholesterol levels? Apparently, yes. While drugs called statins do a good job of reducing the amount of artery-clogging fats in the blood, a new study finds that it's also possible to get some of the same heart-healthy benefits just by eating foods that can mimic some of the drugs' effects." With 13 full pages of ads from drug companies in that issue of the magazine, could they report anything but? It's a salutary lesson in remembering not to take dietary or medical advice from a news magazine that is funded largely by the pharmaceutical industry.

Cholesterol is Essential for Good Health

Cholesterol is not the dietary villain it's made out to be—it is a naturally-occurring fat which is fundamentally required for good health. It is the raw material for our steroid hormones, including sex hormones, being the precursor to both the male hormone testosterone and the female hormone estrogen, which cannot be made without it.

A pearly-white fatty substance, cholesterol is manufactured in the liver and can be found in all the tissues of the body, especially the brain. In fact, 25 percent of the body's cholesterol is found in the brain. Cholesterol performs several important functions in the body, including forming and maintaining cell walls and structures and insulation for nerve cells. Bile, a fluid produced by the liver, plays a vital role in the processing and digestion of fats; to make bile, the liver uses cholesterol. Cholesterol is also important in the development of memory, and is necessary for the uptake of hormones in the brain. Myelin, the protective sheath that covers communicating neurons in the brain, is composed of 30 percent protein and 70 percent fat. Serotonin, the body's "feel-good" chemical, does not work properly when cholesterol levels drop too low.

Most importantly, our bodies need cholesterol to make vitamin D. In the presence of sunlight, cholesterol is converted into vitamin D in our skin. Exposing the skin to sunlight also allows the skin to synthesize cholesterol sulfate, and lack of this important substance has been shown to negatively affect brain function. Low levels of vitamin D can also cause impaired memory and dementia, increased risk of depression and suicidal behavior, and increased risk of cancer, Alzheimer's, and Parkinson's disease. The consequences of low cholesterol levels include disruption of the production of adrenal hormones, allergies, asthma, blood sugar problems, edema, mineral deficiencies, chronic inflammation, difficulty in healing, reduced libido, infertility and various reproductive problems. Dietary cholesterol comes from eating animal products such as beef, eggs, chicken, and dairy products.

Who are the Meat Eaters?

Largely due to the research carried out by James D'Adamo and his son, Peter D'Adamo, and the success of his book *Eat Right For Your Type,* we now know that some people are by nature meat eaters while others do better on a mixed diet. The extensive research behind these findings show that people with type O blood are typically healthier and have more energy when they eat a diet high in animal protein. They are biologically able to digest and assimilate a diet that has a much higher proportion of animal products than a person with type A blood, while those with type A blood tend to do better when they stick to a diet of poultry and fish and lots of vegetables, and with less red meat. Dr. D'Adamo believes that those with type B or AB blood can digest just about all foods, including dairy products, which are problematic for type O's and A's to digest.

People with type A blood seem to be able to survive on vegetarian diets but it's hard for a human being to *thrive* on these diets, and especially someone with type O blood. But we need to remember that we are all different, we all have different dietary needs, and meat-eaters do not need to be made to feel guilty for eating meat, and meat-eaters need to have empathy for vegetarians who choose not to eat animal products. The crime is in how we treat our domesticated animals, not whether or not we eat them.

Dr. Weston Price's Dietary Research

In his book, *Nutrition and Physical Degeneration*, Dr. Weston Price documents how he traveled the world in the 1930s examining the diets of primitive tribes in an attempt to find the source of physical degeneration in modern Western societies. His findings showed that many primitive cultures lived primarily on animal products with very little to almost no vegetable matter or fruit. He found that the tribes living in the harshest climates with the most restricted diets were actually the most robust physical specimens. The tribes he visited included the Masai in East Africa, who lived mainly on milk, meat and blood from their cows and goats; the Eskimos who lived on marine mammal flesh, organs and blubber; North American Indians who lived on elk and moose and other wild animals; and Australian Aborigines and New Zealand Maori, who lived in virtually a desert, yet thrived for millennia on a diet of small wild animals, birds, insects, grubs and rodents. In examining these peoples, he noticed that those who had adopted a Western diet, consisting mainly of imported foods such as white bread, sugar, jams, and canned foods, had a markedly lower standard of health, with tuberculosis and rampant dental decay due to malnutrition.

The Dismal Truth about Factory Farming

Now that Agribusiness and multi-national food corporations have taken over many smaller, family-run operations in the drive to maximize profits at the expense of food quality, ethics and safety, one of the consequences is that we have lost our direct connection to small businesses and family farms. Many people have never fed chickens, collected eggs, or seen a cow being milked. To them, chicken comes in a plastic-wrapped packet at the supermarket, and milk comes from a carton.

Factory farming is far removed from the way nature intended us to interact with domestic animals. On a spiritual level, we will never be forgiven if we mistreat animals. Eating factory-farmed meat is bad for our body and bad for our soul. In his movie "Food Inc.," film-maker Robert Kenner dramatically documents the horrors of factory farming and the lack of respect shown to these animals who give their lives to feed us. We must provide animals with decent living conditions, treat them with respect, and feed them healthy diets. If we don't, we are the losers. And if this means our food costs more, then so be it—it's still cheaper than the cost of getting sick. And as more of us adopt a diet of healthier food, the more prices will go down.

Two percent of U.S. livestock facilities now produce 40 percent of farm animals, and these large, corporate-owned concentrated animal feeding operations (CAFOs) have been highly promoted as the best way to produce food for the masses. But the only reason these CAFOs are able to remain profitable is because they use subsidized crops to feed the animals rather than their natural food, which is grass. Factory farms use huge amounts of soy, corn, and other grains to feed their animals, crops that are cheap to buy because of government subsidies. And because these crops are so cheap and so in demand, they have led to a monoculture in the U.S. of foods that not only end up in animal feed but also fuel the processed food industry and a fast food diet.

The book *CAFO: The Tragedy of Industrial Animal Factories* states: "Thanks to U.S. government subsidies, between 1997 and 2005, factory farms saved an estimated $3.9 billion per year because they were able to purchase corn and soybeans at prices below what it cost to grow the crops. Without these feed discounts, amounting to a 5 to 15 percent reduction in operating costs, it is unlikely that many of these industrial factory farms could remain profitable."

By contrast, many small farms that produce much of their own forage receive no government money, which on the surface makes them seem to be inefficient and uncompetitive. Government subsidies create an uneven playing field, and traditional and organic farms face an uphill battle to be competitive with the mega-farms and CAFOs which receive subsidies.

Currently, the production and sale of organic food represents about four percent of the food economy in the U.S, and local food makes up about two percent. These are tiny numbers, but they are steadily growing with the increase in organic departments in food stores, and the proliferation of small local farms and farmers' markets that are appearing in every corner of the U.S. Organic produce and animal products can fetch a premium price, and, with the option of selling direct to the consumer, it makes owning a small farm a more viable proposition these days. For the sake of our health and the environment, it's important that we patronize these farms and farm stands and do our best to eat organic and eat local. But beware—just because meat is labeled "organic" it doesn't mean it is grass-fed, as animals can be fed organic corn and it can still be legally labelled "organic."

Antibiotics in Animal Feed

Farm animals are healthiest when they eat the foods they are designed to eat. Cows have stomachs that can digest grass, pigs can digest acorns, grains, grass and other plants, and chickens and turkeys can eat grains and plants as well as bugs and worms. Problems arise when animals are fed conventional or industrial feed that is not part of their native diet. For instance, grain is not a natural food for grazing animals, which are basically grass-eating machines, and this practice can cause digestive distress and the growth of dangerous E. coli bacteria. The agricultural industry has found that treating these animals with antibiotics helps control the problem, but with industrial farms using 29 million pounds of antibiotics in 2009 alone, it could be said that agricultural antibiotic use is out of control in the U.S.

About 80 percent of all the antibiotics produced in the US are used in agriculture, not only to fight infection in farm animals, but also to promote weight gain. Unfortunately, this practice is contributing to the alarming spread of antibiotic-resistant disease. The link is so clear between continuous, low-dose antibiotics and antibiotic-resistant disease that the use of antibiotics as growth promoters in animal feed has been banned in Europe since 2006.

In 2010, in a "draft guidance" to the industry, the FDA acknowledged that overuse of antibiotics is a problem and proposed that livestock producers stop using "sub-therapeutic," or small, regular doses of antibiotics in animal feed. They wrote: "Antimicrobial drugs have been widely used in human and veterinary medicine for more than 50 years ... The development of resistance to this important class of drugs, and the resulting loss of their effectiveness as antimicrobial therapies, poses a serious public health threat."

Resistant bacteria are becoming increasingly common on farms, and, according to a 2009 University of Iowa study, 70 percent of hogs and 64 percent of workers in industrial animal facilities tested positive for methicillin-resistant S*taphylococcus aureus* (MRSA). The study pointed out that once MRSA is introduced, it could spread to other swine, as well as to their caretakers and in turn, their caretakers' families and friends.

There is also mounting evidence that the poultry industry's indiscriminate use of antibiotics induces antibiotic resistance among food-borne bacteria that commonly infect humans. One such antibiotic-resistant strain is Campylobacter, a pathogen common to chicken products. Chickens raised in confined feedlot operations are up to 460 times more likely to carry antibiotic-resistant strains of Campylobacter than organic chicken products, which are antibiotic-free. Campylobacter produces an inflammatory, sometimes bloody, diarrhea, including cramps, fever and pain. Symptoms typically last for five to seven days.

Antibiotics are found not only in conventionally-raised meat and poultry on the market, but have made their way into produce such as corn, lettuce, and potatoes via animal manure used as fertilizer. Not only are antibiotics passed on to us in meat and milk, but the run-off from factory farms puts antibiotics into the water table.

Opinion columnist Mark Bittman wrote in the *New York Times* that we need to take responsibility for finding high-quality, non-tainted and antibiotic-free food. The FDA, he wrote, is "consistently under-financed and increasingly unable to do its job, which is largely to protect the public health" and "has no money to spare, but the corporations that control the food industry have all they need, along with the political power it buys. That's why we can say this without equivocation: public health, the quality of our food, and animal welfare are all sacrificed to the profits that can be made by raising animals in factories."

Omega-3 EFAs in Pasture-Fed Meat

Omega-3 and omega-6 are types of essential fatty acids, meaning that we cannot make them on our own and have to obtain them from our diet. Omega-6 fatty acids are essential for health, but an over-abundance of omega-6 polyunsaturated fats in the diet leads to chronic inflammation, which is believed to be at the source of just about every disease we see today. Omega-6s are most abundant in vegetable seed oils such as corn, canola, and cottonseed oils, while omega-3s come from green leaves, such as the grass that cows and sheep graze on.

However, few people realize that grain-fed animals are also a major source of omega-6s. Cattle were not designed to eat grains, and one of the problems with factory-raised meat, especially beef, is that animals fed corn instead of their natural diet, grass, are high in omega-6 fatty acids, rather than the more healthy omega-3 fatty acids. And with today's diets containing more vegetable oils—because we've been told that saturated fats are bad for us—our omega fatty acid balance is way off, with a ratio more like 1:20 rather than a beneficial 1:2 or even 1:1. Health problems begin to show up when the essential fatty acid imbalance exceeds the ratio of 1:4. This means that we can safely eat twice as many omega-6 oils, such as those found in corn and canola oil, as omega-3s, like those contained in butter, eggs, and grass-fed meat, but we shouldn't go over that limit.

Meat and dairy products from animals fed a high-grain diet have up to ten times more omega-6s than products from pasture-raised animals. An article in the *Journal of Animal Science* found that ratio may be even higher, noting, "Grain-fed beef can have an omega 3:6 ratio higher than 1:20," while grass-fed beef has an omega 3:6 ratio of 1:0.16.

About two-thirds of the human brain is composed of essential fatty acids. The membranes of neurons—the brain cells that communicate with each other—are composed of a thin double-layer of fatty acid molecules. When we digest the fat in our food, it is broken down into fatty acid molecules of various lengths. Our brain then uses these fatty acid molecules as raw materials to build healthy cell membranes. These cell membranes need to be permeable so micro-nutrients can enter the cells to give the body energy, and metabolic waste products can exit. If cell membranes are built of substandard fats, such as trans-fats, they become impermeable, and then the body's health becomes compromised at the cellular level. This is why it's so important to include healthy fats in our diet.

Animal Products Are Our Only Source of Vitamin B12

Animal products contain a plentiful supply of B vitamins, water soluble vitamins that are essential for good health. Vitamin B used to be referred to as one vitamin, but now vitamin B is known to be made up of eight important vitamins usually referred to as the vitamin B complex. B vitamins are available from a variety of foods, including all kinds of meat, tuna, whole grains, potatoes, bananas, lentils, chili peppers, beans, nutritional yeast, brewer's yeast, and molasses. But it is vitamin B12 that is vitally important in the diet because it is not available from any source other than animal products. This is of particular importance to vegetarians, in whom vitamin B12 deficiency is extremely common. But since a deficiency may not show itself for a number of years, many vegetarians are unaware there's a problem until it's too late.

There are a variety of symptoms of B12 deficiency, ranging from changes in mood, such as lack of motivation or feelings of apathy, to birth defects in children. First signs can include mental fogginess, memory troubles, muscle weakness and fatigue, and can eventually lead to permanent nerve damage, depression, numbness and tingling in the hands and feet, nervousness, paranoia, hyperactive reflexes, impaired memory and behavioral changes. It is believed that after about seven years of B12 deficiency, irreversible brain damage and other problems can result. Conversely, research has shown that a high vitamin B12 level in elderly individuals may protect against brain atrophy or shrinkage, associated with Alzheimer's disease and impaired cognitive function.

Among pregnant women, nursing women and infants, the effects of vitamin B12 deficiency can be particularly devastating, causing infertility and repeated miscarriages. The National Institutes of Health state that children born to women who have low blood levels of vitamin B12 shortly before and after conception may have an increased risk of a neural tube defect, and that women with the lowest levels of B12 had five times the risk of having a child with a neural tube defect compared to women with the highest B12 levels. Women who consume little or no meat or animal-based foods are the most likely group of women to have low B12 levels, along with women who have intestinal disorders that prevent them from absorbing sufficient amounts. Recently, the news carried stories of the tragedy of an eleven month-old baby who died from complications associated with vitamin deficiencies, including B12, allegedly caused by her mother's vegan diet.

B vitamins are particularly concentrated in liver, sardines, salmon, venison, beef, lamb, shrimp, halibut, scallops, and yogurt, in order of highest to lowest amount. The Vegan Society, the Vegetarian Resource Group, and the Physicians Committee for Responsible Medicine, among others, recommend that vegetarians and vegans either consistently eat foods fortified with B12 or take a daily or weekly B12 supplement. Dr. Gabriel Cousens, a proponent of a vegan diet, has written: "Up until this time, many of us have felt that additional supplementation for live-fooders with sea vegetables or probiotic formulas was sufficient for protection against B12 deficiency. This does not seem to be the case. In macrobiotics, who primarily cook their food, we see a very high percentage of children actually having growth retardation due to low B12 intake." Cousens now recommends vitamin B12 supplementation.

Vitamin C in Animal Protein

From reading the literature, it's evident that scurvy, a vitamin C deficiency that can be fatal, was rare before the proliferation of refined sugar and flour products. Historical reports from early sailing voyages show that sailors fed a ration largely made up of refined carbohydrates with a long shelf life (e.g. rum, white flour products, jam, and sweets) suffered greatly from scurvy while at sea. On the other hand, it was noted that indigenous groups whose diets were almost entirely meat-based (Aborigines, Eskimo, Masai) never suffered from this disease. It seems that refined carbohydrates, separated by processing from their own source of vitamins and minerals which are needed for digestion, rob the body of these vitamins and minerals in order to digest the degraded food. It is this that causes the scurvy, not simply a deficiency of vitamin C-containing fruits and vegetables. William Dufty describes many historical events such as these in his informative and entertaining book, *Sugar Blues,* as does Weston A. Price, DDS, in his book *Nutrition and Physical Degeneration*, including this nugget of information:

"I should like to quote [Admiral] Donald B. MacMillan writing in 1920, recalling his time with Peary on their 1908/09 attempt on the North Pole: The men . . . 'in quest of musk-oxen, caribou, and Arctic hare: for Peary, who never had a single case of scurvy on any of his expeditions, fully appreciated the value of fresh meat as an antiscorbutic. Fresh vegetables, acids, and fruits are not necessary. This fact we have known for at least a half century, having acquired it from the experience of the American whaling captains. Scurvy stricken patients were always dispatched by them immediately to the igloos of the Eskimos, there to be restored to health by consuming raw frozen meat.' "

The evidence shows that a diet that includes quality animal protein, vegetables, fruits, and nuts is a healthy diet and does not need to be supplemented by artificial vitamins. It is the introduction of grains and sugars into this whole foods diet that causes vitamin deficiency and ill health.

Conventional vs. Sustainable Meat Production

There has been much investigation recently into the comparison between conventional and sustainable meat production, and it has been found that conventional meat production contributes to climate change in ways that sustainable livestock farming doesn't. One of the biggest issues is the land clearing necessary to grow crops to feed livestock. Other issues are the fertilizers, pesticides, and heavy machinery that burns fossil fuels used to grow and harvest these crops, and the resulting large manure piles or lagoons that emit greenhouse gases. Sustainably raised animals, on the other hand, feed on natural pasture and nourish the land with their manure. Another issue in the raging debate about whether or not we should include meat in our diet is the fact that, as shown in the Nutritional Equivalents chart on page 33, our daily animal protein consumption can be a lot less if it's of high quality—for instance, four ounces of grass-raised beef equals one pound of corn-fed beef. That's one quarter less, which is a significant amount.

Local Harvest lists farmers' markets, family farms, and other sources of sustainably grown food in your area. Some websites where you can order pasture-raised meat and poultry are: Black Wing (blackwing.com); La Cense Beef (lacensebeef.com); and Dr. Joseph Mercola (mercola.com). EatWild is a comprehensive source for grass-fed meat and dairy products in the U.S. and Canada (eatwild.com). The Weston Price Foundation has chapters all over the world and many of them are connected with buying clubs in which healthy meat products can be purchased locally.

> "It is doubtful that you can build a more sustainable agriculture without animals to cycle nutrients and support local food production. If our concern is for the health of nature . . . then eating animals may sometimes be the most ethical thing to do."
>
> —*Michael Pollan, author of* **The Omnivore's Dilemma**

Meat and Poultry

The Bottom Line

THE GOOD:
Wild and humanely-raised animals and poultry fed an appropriate, chemical-free diet, and their products (eggs, pate etc.)

THE BAD:
Grain-fed meat, even if fed organic feed • poultry fed GM grains

THE DOWNRIGHT DANGEROUS:
Products of concentrated animal feeding operations • animals fed inappropriate food, antibiotics, and chemical growth-hormones

CHAPTER 12

Fish and Seafood

CURRENT ADVICE FROM NUTRITIONISTS ABOUT EATING FISH is conflicting—eat fish because it's high in healthy fish oils, they tell us, but don't eat fish because it's high in mercury and PCBs. Then there are the concerns about over-fishing the oceans, while farmed fish has a dubious reputation—after all, it's only as nutritious as the food it's been fed. So what's a person to do? It's hard to know. But let's look at some of the issues.

There is no doubt that wild fish is the healthiest fish to eat, whether fresh or frozen, and cold-water oily fish, such as mackerel and herring, has the highest nutritional value. Many types of wild fish when canned are also high in nutritional quality, such as salmon, tuna, herring, sardines, and clams. But in recent years there has been an enormous decline in the quantity of wild fish brought into ports all around the world, bringing an end to a way of life that has sustained coastal communities for over one thousand years. With this change has come the rise of industrial-scale production of fish farming, and fish farms now provide more than 50 percent of the world's supply of seafood.

Awareness of depleted wild fish stock has grown among consumers and now some people are choosing to purchase farmed fish in an attempt to protect wild fish. But the difference in quality of various types of farmed fish can be significant, depending upon where and under what conditions it has been raised. Farmed fish from a responsible and regulated source, such as Scotland or the U.S., is a good choice, but beware of any fish or seafood farmed in Southeast Asia—all of the less healthy varieties of fish and seafood come from China, Vietnam, Taiwan, and Indonesia. Canned seafood has the country of origin on the label, so it's easy to avoid, but when buying certain seafood, such as frozen shrimp, it's a good idea to ask your fishmonger where it comes from. As for wild fish, stay away from larger predatory fin fish species, such as tuna and swordfish, in favor of smaller fish such as sardines and mackerel which have had less time to build up a high level of toxins.

Seven percent of the world's oceans are now considered to be depleted, while 52 percent are fully exploited, and one percent is considered to be recovering. One example of a recovering wild species is the Atlantic swordfish, which has been protected from extinction by regulations limiting its catch. And the 200-mile limit, a law enacted by the Third United Nations Convention on the Law of the Sea in 1982, certainly helped by giving all countries exclusive rights to fishing within 200 nautical miles of their own coastlines. But despite these efforts, many experts are concerned that a larger proportion of the world's oceans could become depleted if more isn't done. Over-fishing, discarding by-catch, and sea-floor dredging are still concerns in more than 70 percent of the world's fisheries, and acidification of the oceans is taking its toll on tropical reefs and shellfish habitat. With such dire predictions, it seems that responsible aquaculture is not just advisable but essential.

Aquaculture is the farming of aquatic organisms such as fish, crustaceans, molluscs, and aquatic plants. Different kinds of aquaculture include fish farming, shrimp farming, oyster farming, algaculture (such as seaweed farming), and the cultivation of ornamental fish. Fish farming involves raising fish commercially in tanks or enclosures, usually for food, while a fish hatchery is a facility that releases young fish into the wild for recreational fishing or to supplement a species' natural numbers. The most common fish species raised by fish farms are salmon, carp, tilapia, European sea bass, catfish and cod. Oysters and mussels are some of the more successful species grown by this method—they taste excellent and make a positive environmental contribution to the waters in which they are raised.

Developing aquaculture practices that provide a high quality product with little negative impact on the environment is imperative, otherwise we may soon see the extinction of the last wild things in our diet—and then we'll have to ask ourselves, will we be far behind?

The Truth about Farmed Fish

With fish stocks in the oceans steadily declining and global demand for seafood increasing dramatically, farmed seafood has rapidly become a huge industry worldwide.

China is now the biggest producer and exporter of seafood in the world, and the fastest-growing supplier to the U.S. China produced about 115 billion pounds of seafood last year, about 70 percent of the farmed fish produced in the world. The entire eastern seaboard of the country is lined with thousands of giant factory-style farms, but an acute water shortage and water supplies contaminated by sewage, industrial waste and agricultural runoff results in a product of questionable nutritional value. The fish farms in turn are discharging wastewater that further pollutes the water supply and more than half of the rivers in China are too polluted to serve as a source of drinking water. Farmers have learned to add illegal veterinary drugs and pesticides to the feed which helps keep their stocks alive but it leaves poisonous and carcinogenic residues in seafood, posing health threats to consumers.

In recent years, the European Union and Japan have imposed temporary bans on Chinese seafood because of illegal drug residues, and inspectors in the US recently blocked imports of several types of fish after traces of illegal drugs linked to cancer were detected in the fish.

If you choose to eat farmed fish, try to track down fish farmed with sustainable practices. Clean Fish (www.cleanfish.com) is committed to finding, sourcing and distributing the world's best wild seasonal and farmed fish, including Loch Duart Scottish Salmon, Laughing Bird Caribbean White Shrimp, and Peruvian Blue Tilapia. The founders are also committed to funding and creating new methods of feeding farmed fish, creating the equivalent of "grass farms" in the ocean, and transforming fishing practices by innovative changes in equipment and fish feed.

• Farmed Shrimp

Approximately 90 percent of all the shrimp consumed in the U.S. is farmed and imported. Shrimp farming is now a global industry and aquaculture has become a significant threat to coastal ecosystems. About 20 percent of the world's mangrove forests have been destroyed since 1980, partly due to shrimp farming. Over four decades, 660,000 acres of Indonesian mangroves were converted to shrimp farms, but most of these farms are abandoned within a decade because of the toxin build-up and damage to the environment.

Industrial-sized monocultures such as these are very susceptible to disease outbreaks and ecological problems. Pressure and criticism from governments and activists led to changes in the industry in the late 1990s including stronger regulations and a program aimed at developing and promoting more sustainable farming practices.

Virtually all farmed shrimp are of the family Penaeidae, and just two species of shrimp, the Pacific white shrimp and the giant tiger prawn, account for about 80 percent of all farmed shrimp. Most of us have eaten farmed shrimp from Southeast Asia, and find it flavorless and flabby. About 25 percent of farmed shrimp comes from Latin America, where Brazil is the largest producer, and the remaining 75 percent is produced in Asia, in particular in China and Thailand—Thailand being the largest exporter of shrimp in the world.

• Farmed Salmon

The environmental impact of salmon farming is increasing as global production continues to rise. Most salmon are farmed in open pens and cages in coastal waters so waste from these farms, often containing antibiotics and pesticides, is released directly into the ocean. Parasites and diseases from farmed salmon can spread to wild fish swimming near the farms and escaping farmed salmon can harm wild populations.

Salmon farms are typically sited in pristine coastal ecosystems which they then pollute. A farm with 200,000 fish discharges more fecal waste than a city of 60,000 people. There is also an accumulation of heavy metals on the sea floor near salmon farms, particularly copper and zinc. However, some salmon farmers are making changes to improve their practices, including raising U.S. freshwater coho in inland tank-based closed systems. Closed systems reduce environmental risks by containing pollution, disease, and parasites, and reducing fish escapes into the wild.

One of the biggest concerns about farmed salmon is that they require large amounts of protein which is often supplied to them in the form of forage fish. It can take three pounds of wild fish to grow one pound of farmed salmon. Consequently, farmed salmon consume more wild fish than they generate as a final product, and as the salmon farming industry expands, it requires more wild forage fish for feed. The extraction of wild fish from the ocean to feed farmed salmon impacts the survivability of the wild predator fish who rely on them for food.

Another concern is the amount of fish oil fed to farmed salmon. Fish do not actually produce omega-3 fatty acids, but instead accumulate them from either consuming microalgae that produce these fatty acids, as is the case with smaller fish, or by eating prey fish that have accumulated these acids from their food source. To satisfy this requirement, more than 50 percent of the world fish oil production is fed to farmed salmon.

Recently, salmon has been genetically modified for faster growth and there is much concern about the impact these GM fish might have on wild salmon stocks if they escape into the ocean, not to mention the negative effects of eating genetically-modified foods on the human body.

Comparative Vibrational Levels of Health and Disease States	Level	Comparative Nutritional Levels of **Fish and Seafood**
10,000 = Level of Optimal Health e.g. a healthy newborn baby / hunter/gatherer tribes	10,000	Fresh and frozen wild fish and seafood and products (eggs, oil etc) • Organic farmed fish • Canned anchovies • Canned Brunswick sardines, King Oscar sardines & kipper snacks • Bacalau/dried cod
	9,500	Canned: Bumble Bee pink salmon • Starkist tuna • Chicken of The Sea mackerel • Bumble Bee whole oysters, whole baby clams • Beach Cliff sardines in water • Giovanni's anchovy paste
	9,000	Non-organic farmed salmon (from UK) • Bumble Bee albacore tuna • Beach Cliff sardines, mustard sauce
	8,500	Romanoff whitefish caviar
	8,000	Farmed tilapia (from US and South America) • Farmed salmon & trout (US) fresh, frozen, smoked
	7,500	
	7,000	
	6,500	Farmed Tilapia from South East Asia, e.g. China, Taiwan
AVERAGE LEVEL OF HEALTH IN USA Inflammation	6,000	Farmed shrimp from South East Asia
Arthritis starts to manifest	5,500	
Heart Disease starts to manifest	5,000	Bumble Bee Chopped Clams (US) • Beach Cliff sardines in soybean oil • Acme Nova smoked salmon
Cancer cells form: Breast, Prostate, Lung, Colon, Pancreas	4,500	Chicken of The Sea crab meat (Vietnam) • Bumble Bee shrimp & crab (Indonesia)
Diabetes • Osteoporosis	4,000	Ace of Diamonds canned tiny shrimp (Indonesia) • Bumble Bee smoked oysters • Imitation crab meat
Lymphoma • Leukemia • Dementia	3,500	
Congestive heart disease Brain cancer • Multiple sclerosis	3,000	
Breast cancer metastasizes	2,500	
Prostate cancer metastasizes • Common cold/ flu	2,000	
Melanoma	1,500	
Metastatic bone and lung cancer	1,000	
	500	
	50	
Decay and Death	0	

BETTER HEALTH ↑ / WORSENING HEALTH ↓

Measured in Bovis Units of Life Force Energy

Wild Atlantic salmon is commercially extinct, so by definition all Atlantic salmon is farmed. On the other hand, the wild Pacific salmon fishery is well managed by public agencies who control the amount of salmon that is caught, making it a sustainable resource. Seafood Watch recommends wild-caught salmon from Alaska, California, Oregon, and Washington as these are ocean-friendly choices. They advise avoiding purchasing salmon farmed in open net pens, but salmon farmed on land in "closed" or "contained" farms is a viable alternative; this includes clearly labeled U.S. farmed freshwater coho salmon.

Despite all these concerns, recent research has found that the health benefits of both farmed and wild salmon exceed any potential risks from environmental toxins, says Eric Rimm, associate professor of epidemiology and nutrition at the Harvard School of Public Health.

• Farmed Shellfish

Farming shellfish has been especially successful in frigid northern waters, such as in Scotland, Scandinavia, Canada, and the North West and North East coasts of the U.S. The aquaculture of bivalves, such as oysters, clams, mussels and scallops, is a process that is relatively benign to the environment, and in some cases beneficial. Mollusks are filter-feeders and can filter pollutants as well as nutrients from the water, improving water quality in the estuaries and coastal regions where the farming takes place.

Essential Fatty Acids in Fish

Fish oil, derived from the tissues of oily fish, contain the omega-3 fatty acids eicosapentaenoic acid (EPA), and docosahexaenoic acid (DHA), oils that are known to reduce inflammation throughout the body, and are thought to have many health benefits. Fish oil has been studied in a wide variety of other conditions, such as clinical depression, anxiety, cancer, and macular degeneration, and although a benefit is thought to occur in these conditions, the results remain to be scientifically proven.

The American Heart Association recommends the consumption of one gram of fish oil daily, preferably by eating fish, for patients with coronary heart disease, although pregnant and nursing women are advised to avoiding eating fish with high potential for mercury contaminants including mackerel, shark, or swordfish. The U.S. National Institutes of Health recommends fish oil and other omega-3 sources for cardiovascular disease prevention and reduction of high blood pressure.

Fish oil also seems to have an effect on mental health and studies have suggested that EPA may reduce the risk of depression and suicide. One study compared blood samples of 100 suicide-attempt patients to those of controls and found that levels of eicosapentaenoic acid were significantly lower in the washed red blood cells of the suicide-attempt patients. Studies on prisoners in England showed that when the inmates were fed seafood which contains omega-3 fatty acids, there was a drop in rates of assault, and a Finnish study found that prisoners who were convicted of violence had lower levels of omega–3 fatty acids than prisoners convicted of nonviolent offenses. A study from the Orygen Research Centre in Melbourne, Australia, suggests that omega-3 fatty acids could help delay or prevent the onset of schizophrenia, while another study conducted at Sheffield University in England also reported positive results with fish oil on patients suffering from schizophrenia. Participants of the study had previously taken anti-psychotic prescription drugs that were no longer effective. After taking fish oil supplements, participants in the study experienced progress compared to others who were given a placebo.

As already noted, the omega-3 fatty acids in fish originate from algae and smaller forage fish, so in terms of taking a supplement, many nutritional experts are advising us to take krill oil than oil from the livers of larger fish such as cod and salmon that may be contaminated with environmental toxins.

Predatory fish such as shark, sword fish, tilefish, and albacore tuna may be high in omega-3 fatty acids, but due to their position at the top of the food chain, these species can also accumulate toxic substances. For this reason, the FDA recommends limiting consumption of these species due to high levels of toxic contaminants such as mercury, dioxin, PCBs, and chlordane.

Food Poisoning from Fish

Seafood represents the number one cause of food poisoning in the U.S. Seafood poisoning can result in extreme discomfort, kidney damage, nervous system damage, and even death.

There are two ways a person can get food poisoning from consuming fish. The first is called ciguatera poisoning and generally occurs when a person consumes fish from tropical waters that has eaten some sort of poisonous food and whose flesh is contaminated with toxins. Predator species near the top of the food chain in tropical and subtropical waters, such as barracuda, snapper, moray eel, parrotfish, grouper, triggerfish, and amberjack, are most likely to cause ciguatera poisoning, although many other species cause occasional outbreaks. Ciguatoxin is very heat-resistant, so contaminated fish cannot be detoxified by conventional cooking.

The second type of food poisoning which occurs from eating fish is scombroid poisoning. Histamine, sometimes present in fish that hasn't been kept chilled after being caught, or in spoiled fish (especially tuna and mackerel), can cause this condition, which is similar to a fish allergy. The histamine triggers the immune system to attack a possible foreign body or infection. But unlike an allergy, scombroid poisoning would affect anyone who consumed the fish. Just because a person gets scombroid poisoning, it does not necessarily mean they are allergic to the fish they have eaten.

Shellfish sometimes absorb poisons from toxic algal blooms (red tide) which appear in the waters at certain times of year. This can cause various types of neurotoxic shellfish poisonings, and again, everyone who eats the shellfish will be susceptible.

It's best to buy fish from a trusted source, and, of course, fish should smell right—a "fishy" smell tells us that fish is not fresh, so don't buy it.

Allergies to Fish

Fish is included in the list of the eight most common allergens in the U.S. and, according to the Asthma and Allergy Foundation of America, an allergy to fish and seafood is the most common food-related allergic reaction. It is covered under the Food Allergy Labeling and Consumer Protection Act (FALCPA) which requires that manufacturers label the presence of fish in clear language on food labels, either in the list of ingredients or following the word "contains" after the ingredient list. Allergies to fish, crustaceans, and shellfish are usually lifelong conditions.

An allergy to fish and seafood is caused by a malfunction of the immune system where the body does not recognize the protein (parvalbumin) that is present in many fish species and begins to defend itself. The immune system attacks the fish proteins with antibodies and histamine, two chemicals that cause inflammation and swelling in soft tissue in the body. Fish allergies are commonly linked to anaphylactic shock and can cause significant complications if not properly treated. Fish and shellfish are biologically distinct, so people who find they are allergic to shellfish most probably can eat fin fish and vice versa, unless they have allergies to both. People who are allergic to one type of shellfish are often advised to avoid all shellfish.

People with allergies to one type of fish are likely to have (or to develop) allergies to others, so most people with an allergy to one kind of fish are advised to avoid all fish. Pollock, salmon, cod, tuna, snapper, eel, and tilapia are among the fish that commonly trigger fish allergies, while some fish—specifically tuna and mackerel—seem to be less allergenic than others. On the other hand, allergies to shellfish mostly affect adults and are rare among young children. Both shellfish and fish allergies are more likely than many food allergies to start during adulthood and less likely than other allergies to be outgrown.

A fish allergy is linked to an increased risk of severe asthma in adults, and fish has also been linked with oral allergy syndrome (OAS), in which the mouth itches or tingles after eating an allergen, and is often seen in people with occupational contact with fish.

People who are allergic to fish or other seafoods may not need to avoid fish oil, as most fish oils on the market tend to be refined enough to remove all of the proteins that can trigger allergic reactions. Some people may experience allergy symptoms after eating fish by-products, such as gelatin or fish oil capsules.

The fish parasite Anisakis simplex, or cod worm, is a parasite considered to be a major allergen and, like fish allergies, can cause severe allergic reactions including anaphylactic shock. If you have a severe allergic reaction after eating fish but tests to fish allergies come up negative, consider further investigation. Note that while Anisakis larvae can be killed by freezing or cooking, they can still trigger allergies after being killed, so people with Anisakis allergies should avoid fish and shellfish altogether.

Fish & Seafood

The Bottom Line

THE GOOD: Wild fish and seafood from unpolluted waters, fresh or frozen • some farmed shellfish

THE BAD: Most farmed fish

THE DOWNRIGHT DANGEROUS: Fish and shellfish farmed in South East Asia • larger fin fish with high mercury and PCB content • fish that is not fresh

CHAPTER 13

Milk, Dairy Products & Eggs

"Most people believe they need to consume large, daily quantities of milk to achieve good health. NOTHING could be further from the truth."

——*Dr. Joseph Mercola, founder of the World's No. 1 Natural Health Website www.mercola.com*

MILK, LIKE BREAD, USED TO BE one of the healthiest staples of our diet—hearty, wholesome, and nutritious. But something happened to milk on the road to "progress" in the 20th century, and now our grocery stores are full of processed dairy products that have little nutritional value and can actually be detrimental to our health. We continue to be told that we need milk in our diet because it provides calcium, that it's "good for our bones, but scientific research has shown that the opposite is true.

The problem with dairy products arise from three misconceptions:

- One is the mistaken idea that pasteurized and homogenized milk has the same benefits as raw milk
- The second is that cows kept in concentrated animal feeding operations (CAFOs) and fed soy and corn will produce milk that is as nutritious as cows fed on grass in an open field
- The third is the crusade against saturated fat, which has convinced many people that animal fats are bad for us and cause heart disease, and that consuming skimmed milk and low-fat dairy products is actually healthier for us than whole milk dairy products.

In fact, there are so many issues with including dairy products made from commercially-processed milk in our diet that it's hard to know where to begin, but when we see that generic "supermarket" milk calibrates at 5,000, at the level of heart disease, and raw organic milk calibrates at 10,000, the level of perfect health, you really have to wonder what happened to milk to make it so dangerous to our health.

Dairy products are ubiquitous in the American diet, but it must be realized that milk products—butter, cheese, cream, sour cream, and yogurt—are inferior products if they are made from inferior milk, and most commercially-produced pasteurized and homogenized milk is inferior milk. Cows are ruminants and naturally feed on grass for most of the year and on silage, hay, and root vegetables in the winter. Dairy cows in concentrated animal feeding operations are not allowed to roam and graze on grass, but are given food made from soy, corn, cottonseed meal and other commercial feeds. This feed, which is laden with antibiotics, pesticides and herbicides, is not their natural diet and it not only changes the nature of the milk but causes health problems for the cows. The raw milk that comes from these cows contains steroids, antibiotics, pesticides from treated grains, bacteria from infected animals, and genetically engineered growth hormones. Organic milk can also come from cows held in CAFOs, though the grain they are fed must by law be free of antibiotics, hormones and pesticides.

Most people eat these products without question, whether it's milk on a bowl of cereal, cheese melted on an enchilada, or sour cream on a baked potato. All can be healthy foods, but not after they have been through the punishing processing system that produces the average supermarket dairy product.

Another issue with including dairy products in our diets is that many people cannot digest milk or are allergic or sensitive to its proteins, though this is more true for pasteurized milk than for raw milk. Dr. Peter D'Adamo in his book, *Eat Right For Your Type*, maintains that only people with type B blood have evolved to be able to digest dairy products. People with O-type blood and those of African descent seem to have a particularly hard time with dairy products.

Comparative Vibrational Levels of Health and Disease States		Comparative Nutritional Levels of **Dairy Products & Eggs**
10,000 = Level of Optimal Health e.g. a healthy newborn baby / hunter/gatherer tribes	10,000	Organic milk, butter, cream, cheese & yogurt (cow, sheep, goat), preferably raw • organic eggs
	9,500	Kerry Gold Irish Butter • Organic Valley eggs • Pete & Gerry's organic eggs
	9,000	
	8,500	Kate's Pure Butter
	8,000	Horizon organic milk and butter • Stonyfield organic fat-free milk • Breakstone's reduced-fat sour cream • Siggi's Icelandic-style yogurt • Chobani Greek yogurt • Fage Greek yogurt
	7,500	The Organic Cow whole milk • Stonyfield low-fat organic milk • Breakstone's sour cream • Earth Balance spread • Average supermarket eggs
	7,000	Stonyfield Farms Organic Strawberry Yogurt
	6,500	Land O'Lakes butter • Sorrento ricotta cheese • Breakstone's cottage cheese • Lactaid milk
AVERAGE LEVEL OF HEALTH IN USA		
Inflammation	6,000	Garelick whole milk • Land O'Lakes light butter • Smart Balance butter spread • Promise spread • Hood light cream/sour cream • Generic fat-free milk & sour cream • Cracker Barrel cheese
Arthritis starts to manifest	5,500	Land O' Lakes butter • Philadelphia cream cheese • Sorrento Stringsters cheese • Kraft shredded cheese • Generic 1% milk • Hood milk, whipping cream, half & half and cottage cheese
Heart Disease starts to manifest	5,000	Supermarket whole milk and 2% milk • Kraft Singles fat-free processed cheese • Weight-Watchers string cheese • Kraft Polly-O string cheese
Cancer cells form: Breast, Prostate, Lung, Colon, Pancreas	4,500	Kraft Singles processed cheese • Yoplait Plus • Activia Yogurt
Diabetes • Osteoporosis	4,000	Land O'Lakes & Fleichmann's margarine • I Can't Believe It's Not Butter spread • Yoplait Trix & Yoplait Kids yogurt • Weight-Watchers strawberry yogurt • Danimals Smoothie (Danone yogurt)
Lymphoma • Leukemia • Dementia	3,500	Egg Beaters® Original
Congestive heart disease Brain cancer • Multiple sclerosis	3,000	Egg Beaters® 100% Egg Whites
Breast cancer metastasizes	2,500	MacDonald's milk shake • Sara Lee cheesecake • Chocolate milk
Prostate cancer metastasizes • Common cold/ flu	2,000	Carnation Evaporated Milk • Cadbury's milk chocolate
Melanoma	1,500	Carnation Condensed Milk • Lindt milk chocolate
Metastatic bone and lung cancer	1,000	Cool Whip • Butter Buds Sprinkles • Molly McButter Butter Flavor Sprinkles • Godiva milk chocolate
	500	Hershey's milk chocolate
	50	
Decay and Death	0	

BETTER HEALTH (levels 6,500–10,000) · WORSENING HEALTH (levels 6,000 and below)

Measured in Bovis Units of Life Force Energy

Do We Need to Include Dairy Products in Our Diet at All?

The answer to this question may be NO. Many nutritional experts believe that dairy products should not be part of our diets because they are hard for humans to digest, especially when made from pasteurized milk. In fact, many cultures around the world have historically consumed little, if any, dairy products at all.

Frank A. Oski, MD, former director of the Department of Pediatrics at Johns Hopkins University, wrote in his book *Don't Drink Your Milk*: "In no mammalian species, except for the human, is milk consumption continued after the weaning period. Calves thrive on cow milk. Cow milk is for calves. In many other parts of the world, most particularly in East Asia, Africa, and South America, people regard cow milk as unfit for consumption by adult human beings."

We are given the message repeatedly in ads and in the press that "milk does a body good." Starlets pose with "milk moustaches," a glass of milk supposedly makes a bowlful of sugary cereal "a nutritious breakfast," and the calcium in milk is touted as being a prevention for osteoporosis. But evidence is growing that consumption of pasteurized dairy products is bad for our health. As Dr. Oski says in his book: "The drinking of cow milk has been linked to iron-deficiency anemia in infants and children; it has been named as the cause of cramps and diarrhea in much of the world's population, and the cause of multiple forms of allergy as well; and the possibility has been raised that it may play a central role in the origins of atherosclerosis and heart attacks."

The Physician's Committee for Responsible Medicine has reported: "Milk's main selling point is calcium, and milk-drinking is touted for building strong bones in children and preventing osteoporosis in older persons. However, clinical research shows that dairy products have little or no benefit for bones . . . Prostate and breast cancers have been linked to consumption of dairy products, presumably related to increases in a compound called insulin-like growth factor (IGF-I) . . . Milk and dairy products are not necessary in the diet and can, in fact, be harmful to health." And it's not just bad for humans—one study showed that even calves fed pasteurized milk do poorly and many die before maturity.

Most of these studies were done on the effects of pasteurized milk, and new research has demonstrated the enormous benefits of raw milk. For many people, raw dairy products made from grass-fed cows, including milk, butter, cheese, cream, and yogurt, are a healthy choice. But, according to Dr. Peter J. D'Adamo in his book *Eat Right for Your Type*, people who do best on the so-called Paleolithic or Caveman Diet, typically people with type-O blood, may find they need to stay away from dairy products altogether. Those with type A blood do best with fermented dairy products, while those with type B blood are the only group that seems to be able to digest dairy products without problems.

There is more bad news about drinking milk from CAFO cows—a report from the Harvard School of Public Health suggests that milk from factory farms may be associated with hormone-related cancers because of the industrial agricultural practice of milking a cow throughout her pregnancy. An increasing amount of hormones appear in the milk of cows at the later stages of pregnancy, and can contain up to 33 times as much of an estrogen compound (estrone sulfate) as milk from a cow following pregnancy, as well as much higher levels of other hormones. The healthiest milk would therefore be raw, grass-fed, organic, and from a cow that is only milked for the first six months after giving birth, which would include the first four months of a new pregnancy.

Raw Milk vs. Pasteurized Milk

The biggest problem with milk is the way it is processed, and all the evidence points to the fact that organic raw milk is better for us than pasteurized, homogenized milk. Many adults as well as children have difficulty digesting pasteurized milk, and allergies to pasteurized milk products are common.

Pasteurization destroys many nutritious components of raw milk, including enzymes, vitamins and "good" bacteria. These bacteria, or probiotics, include lactobacillus and acidophilus which are healthy bacteria that live naturally in the intestines and have a beneficial impact on overall immune function. Raw milk also contains phosphatase, an enzyme that aids in the absorption of calcium in the bones, and the enzyme lipase, which helps to hydrolyze and absorb fats. These enzymes are deactivated when the milk is heated above 120 degrees F and are completely destroyed at a temperature of 150 or 160 degrees F, so, in essence, there are no health benefits to be derived from pasteurized dairy products.

The consumption of raw organic pasture-raised milk has many health benefits and medicinal qualities. These benefits are being rediscovered and some physicians today are treating illnesses with raw milk with spectacular results. According to Mark McAfee, founder of The Raw Milk Institute, increasing numbers of doctors are now prescribing raw organic dairy products for children with asthma, hay fever, recurrent ear infections, and chronic inflammation. Two important studies from Europe—the PARSIFAL study in 2006, involving 15,000 children, and the more recent GABRIELA study—showed that the whey protein in raw milk stabilizes mast cells, improving asthma in children and in some cases completely curing it.

McAfee explains that pasteurized milk contains a large number of dead bacteria which cause histamines to be released, creating inflammation in the body, which is the underlying cause of such conditions as asthma, increased mucus, and ear infections. "Raw milk does exactly the opposite," he says. "Milk is alive [with beneficial] bacteria and your body recognizes it . . . [These beneficial bacteria] colonize and become part of your immune system."

We are taught through the media to fear raw milk, that it's unhygienic and a health hazard; but in fact, there was not a single death in the U.S. due to raw milk for the decade from 1998 to 2008. And it's important to note that the largest recorded outbreak of Salmonella in the U.S. resulted from *pasteurized* milk. The incident, which occurred between June 1984 and April 1985, resulted in 200,000 illnesses and 18 deaths. Yet the CDC never issued a specific Morbidity and Mortality report for this outbreak. McAfee believes that the CDC has an ongoing bias against raw dairy products, and says that this and other outbreaks of illness resulting from the consumption of pasteurized milk are kept from public knowledge, so we don't hear about any warnings from the CDC and FDA. "We haven't seen any deaths from raw milk since the data started being collected in 1973," he states.

Currently, 25 states have laws banning the sale of raw milk for human consumption, and it is a violation of federal law to sell raw milk packaged for consumer use across state lines. But states around the country are starting to introduce bills to legalize the sale of raw milk for human consumption. You may be able to find a local supplier for raw milk at RawMilkInstitute.org and the Campaign for Real Milk at www.realmilk.com

The Pasteurization Process

Pasteurization of milk is required by State and Federal Laws. Pasteurization's main purpose is to extend the shelf life of milk and to kill certain pathogens, especially *Mycobacterium Bovis*, which causes tuberculosis. The pasteurization process was named after French chemist and microbiologist Louis Pasteur who developed the process in 1862 with the original intent of preventing wine and beer from souring. However, pasteurization should not be confused with sterilization, which is used to kill *all* micro-organisms in food. Sterilization of food is known to adversely affect the taste and quality of the product, while pasteurization aims to reduce the number of pathogens so they are unlikely to cause disease.

The pasteurization process heats milk to temperatures below boiling, since at very high temperatures the protein particles in milk aggregate, or curdle. There are two basic methods of pasteurization in the U.S: High Temperature Short Time (HTST) pasteurization process, in which milk is heated to 161° F for 15–20 seconds. This temperature kills virtually all of the viable micro-organisms, and is considered adequate for destroying almost all yeasts, molds, and common bacteria. HTST milk has a refrigerated shelf life of two to three weeks. The second method is Ultra-pasteurized (UHT) milk, which is heated to 275° F for a minimum of one second and can last for up to two or three months on the shelf. When ultra-heat treatment of milk is combined with sterile handling, the result is sterilized milk which can be stored unrefrigerated for six to nine months.

Most bigger dairies use UHT pasteurization to pasteurize their milk, but this kills all bacteria, both good and bad, as well as any healthy enzymes. This process is used because it is faster and more milk can be processed in a day. But some smaller dairies prefer to use a third method, called Low Temperature Pasteurization, which is healthier because the milk is only heated up to the minimum temperature required by law and held there for 30 minutes. By heating milk only to the minimum required temperature, more of the good bacteria and enzymes are preserved. The same process is used for home pasteurization, where milk is heated at 145° F for 30 minutes.

Proponents for raw milk point out that milk only needs to be pasteurized if it comes from large herds of cows fed in confined feedlots, where sanitation is a big concern. Raw milk from inspected herds of dairy cows at smaller farms is perfectly safe. Many farmers are now changing to direct sales of raw milk because of the increased income—farmers selling their milk to dairy companies in the conventional system receive about $1 per gallon for their product, about the same price that dairy farmers received during World War II, while farmers selling raw milk can receive between $4 and $13 per gallon, according to www.realmilk.com.

The Homogenization Process

Homogenization, unlike pasteurization, is not mandated by law, and you can purchase non-homogenized milk from small dairies. Homogenization was introduced so that milk of various qualities and from many different milking herds and dairies could be mixed together for the sake of greater consistency and sold for one uniform price.

Cow's milk is 88 percent water with globules of butterfat and proteins, including casein and whey, suspended in it. The butterfat globules naturally rise to the top as cream. Many people will remember the days before homogenization when milk was delivered every day by the milkman. There was a choice of three types of milk: regular, silver top and gold top. Each represented a different quality of milk with gold-top having the most cream. The more valuable milk had the highest butterfat content and could be sold at a premium. In the

U.S., there are federal standards for minimum legal amounts of butterfat in dairy products—for instance, whole milk must contain at least 3.25 percent fat, and heavy cream must contain a minimum of 36 percent fat. The irony is that skim milk is sold in the U.S. as a healthier food, but in fact, butter-fat is in milk for a reason—without it, the body cannot absorb and utilize the fat-soluble vitamins and minerals in the milk. Butterfat contains valuable trace minerals and short chain fatty acids, and is the best source of vitamin A in our diet.

Homogenization is the mechanical process of breaking down the fat globules in milk so they become the same size as other particles of the milk solids. The milk will then stay integrated rather than separating as cream. Milk is homogenized by passing it through a fine filter at high pressure so the fat globules are reduced in size, from 1-10 micrometers to 0.80 micrometers or smaller.

But there are serious issues with homogenization, the main one being that the tiny homogenized fat globules and smaller particles of milk proteins are able to survive digestion. These particles, that would normally be digested in the stomach or gut, are not broken down and are absorbed directly into the bloodstream, creating an allergic response. And as the much smaller fat globules begin to reassemble, they include fragments of the milk proteins whey and casein in their walls. It is these new, chemically altered protein-heavy fat globules that some researchers think can cause allergic reactions.

According to Dr. Frank Lipman, an internationally recognized expert in the field of integrative medicine, this process makes homogenized milk much harder to digest. "Proteins that would normally be digested in the stomach are not broken down and instead are absorbed into the bloodstream. Often the body reacts to these 'foreign proteins' by triggering the immune system, causing inflammation. It can even trigger auto-immune problems. Homogenized milk has also been linked to heart disease probably because of the fat globules that are dispersed by the process."

Some People Have Allergies to Pasteurized Dairy Products

Cow's milk is the number one food allergen in this country. It is the most common food allergy in American children and it is believed that about 2.5 percent of children are allergic to the proteins in dairy products, though most grow out of it by the time they are teenagers. True cow's milk allergy is rare in adults. Symptoms of true milk allergy are severe, with rashes, vomiting, and breathing difficulties occurring within the first 15 minutes to hour after ingestion.

Many people are lactose intolerant—a common sensitivity to the sugar found in milk. It is caused by a lack of the enzymes needed to digest the sugar lactose, a condition that is common in people from an Asian background. About one in 20 Caucasians and 95 percent of African-Americans are also thought to be lactose intolerant. Symptoms include bloating, gassiness, intestinal cramping, and diarrhea, and may occur within an hour of eating dairy products, or reactions may be delayed for up to 12 hours. Raw grass-fed milk may be tolerated by those who are lactose intolerant.

There are two main types of proteins in milk: casein and whey. Casein is a highly digestible form of milk protein, but whey protein is less easily digested. When whey protein is not digested fully in the intestine, some of the intact protein may stimulate a localized intestinal or a systemic immune response.

Milk protein is 80 percent casein, and the casein in dairy products can promote the formation of mucous. It can also make existing mucous thicker in the nose and sinuses, leaving a person with the feeling of being completely congested, and may also cause a runny nose or post-nasal drip. Many singers have learned to avoid dairy products before a performance because they tend to produce phlegm and thickened mucous in the airways. Casein is used in the manufacture of adhesives such as glue, bottle labels, and wood glue for furniture, so that makes you think about the affect casein might have on the narrow passages of the sinus.

Pasteurized milk has been shown to be the primary cause of recurrent ear infections in children, and has also been linked to the development of such conditions as insulin dependent diabetes, rheumatoid arthritis, and infertility. According to Robert Cohen, author of the book *Milk The Deadly Poison*, milk and refined sugar make two of the largest contributions to food-induced ill health in the U.S. Cohen founded and is executive director of America's Dairy Education Board, a group of nationally prominent doctors dedicated to dispelling the myth that milk is nature's perfect food, and says that milk has been well documented as a cause in diarrhea, cramps, bloating, gas, gastrointestinal bleeding, iron-deficiency anemia, skin rashes, atherosclerosis, and acne.

According to the Organic Consumers Association, a recent Dutch study suggests that children are one third less likely to suffer from allergies before age two if they're raised on organic dairy products. In the study, children and breast-feeding mothers ate organic milk, cheese, and yogurt and found that the risk for eczema, asthma, and other allergies decreased. Researchers believe it may, in part, be due to the higher concentrations of conjugated linoleic acids that are found in organic milk, and also the fact that organic milk contains 71 percent more omega-3 fatty acids than conventional milk.

Saturated Fat is Good for Us

> ". . . There is no significant evidence for concluding that dietary saturated fat is associated with an increased risk of coronary heart disease or stroke and cardiovascular disease."
>
> —*from a study published in* **The American Journal of Clinical Nutrition,** *2010*

Saturated fats provide a concentrated source of energy in our diets and form the building blocks for the cell membranes of the body. They also provide a variety of hormones and hormone-like substances that are essential to our health.

As described more fully in the chapter on Meat & Poultry, there has been a trend in this country over the past 50 years to blame saturated fats as a cause of heart disease. However, despite countless studies and nearly a billion dollars spent on research, there has been no conclusive evidence that a diet high in animal fats has a significant effect on heart disease. Yet the notion that a healthy diet is one with minimal fat has persisted. Americans dutifully reduced their intake of animal fats, butter, and eggs, but rates of obesity and degenerative diseases, and especially diabetes, sky-rocketed.

Eating low-fat and skimmed dairy products was a part of these dietary recommendations. But full-fat dairy products contain a substance called conjugated linolenic acid (CLA), which has been shown to have strong anti-carcinogenic properties and helps reduce body fat. When milk is skimmed, the CLA is discarded with the butter fat, and without butterfat, it is difficult for the body to assimilate the vitamins and minerals in the rest of the milk. Without a doubt, full-fat milk is healthier than low-fat or skimmed milk, and research shows that consuming full-fat dairy may help reduce a person's risk of diabetes, cancer, and heart disease. Butter is a very healthy food with a host of beneficial nutrients, including an "anti-stiffness" factor which protects against calcification of the joints. But to consider butterfat a healthy food, it needs to come from unprocessed, organic milk.

Two European studies link a diet high in CLA with a lower risk of breast cancer—in Finland, researchers measured CLA levels in the serum of women with and without breast cancer. Those women with the most CLA had a significantly lower risk of the disease. Meanwhile, French researchers measured CLA levels in the breast tissues of 360 women and found that women with the most CLA had the lowest risk of cancer—in fact, the women with the highest levels of CLA had a staggering 74 percent lower risk of breast cancer than the women with the lowest levels.

Eating food containing CLA also helps us to lose weight as well as reducing the risk of cancer and diabetes. The Organic Center, an organization promoting organic farming, states the following: "Milk, most dairy products, beef, lamb, and pork are the major dietary sources of CLA. The 'magical properties' of CLA include reducing the propensity to store fat (especially abdominal fat), inhibiting tumor development, promoting sensitivity to insulin in cells, increasing immune response against viral antigens, and modulating inflammatory processes . . . Milk from dairy cows on organic farms, particularly pasture-based operations, contains significantly higher CLA levels."

The most effective way to increase intake of CLA is to eat the meat and dairy products of grass-fed animals. It's worth noting that milk from grass-fed Irish cows is two to three times higher in CLA than milk from grain-fed American cows.

Eggs—The Perfect Food

The common practice of including eggs in our diet has taken a particularly bad rap over the past couple of decades. Eaten by people all over the world for eons, suddenly 30 years ago they were demonized as not being "heart healthy," as if people who'd eaten eggs all their lives suddenly had "unhealthy hearts." But eggs are one of the most nutritious foods we can eat, and they have been shown to be protective against diseases, including heart disease.

Cutting back on egg consumption was widely recommended by doctors as a way to supposedly lower blood cholesterol levels and prevent heart disease; the advice was to eat no more than two eggs per week. However, a recent study where researchers took a close look at the egg-eating habits and heart health of 118,000 men and women found "no evidence of an overall significant association between egg consumption and risk of CHD [coronary heart disease] in either men or women." In fact, they found that people who ate from five to six eggs per week had a lower risk of heart disease than those who ate less than one egg per week.

Of course, free-range organic eggs are far superior when it comes to nutrient content. An egg is considered organic if the chicken was fed organic food, which means it will not have accumulated high levels of pesticides from the grains, mostly GM corn, fed to typical chickens. The best source for high quality eggs is to buy them locally from an organic farm or farmers' market, or from individuals who keep chickens and sell their eggs.

Some people are allergic to eggs, but often this allergy is to egg whites and they do fine with the egg yolks, which is in fact the most nutritious part of the egg. Be aware that the product EggBeaters is one of the worst foods you can eat. How hard is it to crack and whisk up a couple of eggs? Pour them into a saute pan with a knob of butter, and in a minute you've whipped up an omelette—nothing can be simpler or more nutritious than that.

Milk Products: Butter, Cheese and Yogurt

Most of these products were originally developed as a way of preserving milk, since fresh raw milk goes sour (curdles) very quickly if not kept chilled at 40 degrees F. Milk contains naturally-occurring bacteria and these feed on the lactose, or milk sugar, changing the lactose into lactose acid, which tastes sour. When this happens, the milk has curdled. Milk can be made to last longer by separating it into butter, cream, water, and milk solids (powdered milk). Powdered milk lasts a long time, and even butter if kept cool can have a long storage time.

All dairy products start with milk, so the higher the quality of the milk, the better the products. Milk products made from low-grade milk are low-grade products. All cow's milk products sold in stores in America are made from pasteurized milk. Smaller local dairies, however, may sell products made from raw milk, especially cheese, in areas where it is legal to do so. Some cheeses imported from Europe are made from raw milk, most often sheep and goat cheese.

For millennia, people around the globe have prized butter for its health benefits. The origins of butter go back thousands of years to when our ancestors first started domesticating animals; the first written reference to butter was found on a 4,500-year old limestone tablet illustrating how butter was made. In India, ghee (clarified butter) has been a staple food for more than 3000 years, and is also used as an offering to the gods in religious ceremonies. But the crusade over the past 40 years against saturated fats has meant that we were advised against eating butter and told to eat margarine instead. Because of butter's obvious health benefits, it is a tragedy that it was turned into such a villain in our diet.

Despite what the ads from the food industry lead us to believe, margarine is NOT better for us than butter, far from it. Margarine is a processed food made from refined polyunsaturated oils treated to make them solid at room temperature. This process is called hydrogenation, and margarine and similar hydrogenated or processed polyunsaturated oils are more detrimental to our health than any saturated fat. As you can see from the chart, Kerry Gold Irish butter calibrates at 9,500 while Land O' Lakes margarine calibrates at 4,000, the level of diabetes.

The best butter is raw, organic butter because pasteurization destroys nutrients, but unfortunately, the sale of raw butter is prohibited in most of our 50 states. You can, however, make your own healthy butter—Body Ecology (bodyecology.com) sells a culture starter kit which you simply add to organic cream. Cultured butter is full of good bacteria such as *lactobacillus planterum* and *lactococcus lactis*, microflora which are essential for a healthy inner ecosystem.

Making cheese is another way of preserving milk. To make cheese, milk is left to stand overnight allowing the cream to rise to the surface. This cream is skimmed off and churned to make butter, while the milk underneath is used to make cheese. Milk needs to be curdled first so that the solids separate from the liquid, resulting in curds and whey, usually by adding rennet, made from enzymes removed from the fourth stomach of a calf. Certain bacteria and molds convert the milk to cheese and in doing so create acids that kill the microbes that would spoil the milk or cheese, including lactic acid. Molds also have the function of breaking down fats and proteins thereby reducing the amount of fat in the cheese which enables it to be stored longer.

Yogurt contains a special kind of bacteria, the probiotic acidophilus, which promotes good digestion and a healthy body. But not all yogurts contain good bacteria—most are highly processed and are combined with fruit and sugar, so their nutritional value is virtually useless. It's therefore important to purchase yogurt that contains live culture or live microorganisms, for instance Greek-style yogurt. Yogurt with live culture is especially useful after taking a course of antibiotics. The problem with antibiotics is that they destroy the good bacteria along with the bad, so that yeasts and other naturally-occurring bacteria have the opportunity to outnumber and overwhelm the probiotics, which can lead to yeast infections and digestive issues.

Yogurt can be made at home with a "starter" from a little

> "The greatest cause of death in America . . . is heart and blood vessel disease. The greatest cause of pain and disability is the nation's crumbling skeletons, associated with osteoporosis, arthritis and joint disease. The single vitamin complex that is the most anti-plaque, as well as the most bone-building and bone-healing, is vitamin K2. The main source of K2 for humans is butter oil—that is, butter from cows that eat newly sprouted and fast-growing green grass. The more fake oils, margarines and 'heart-healthy' fake foods you eat, the worse your deficiency of vitamin K2 will become."
>
> — *Dr. Bruce West in his newsletter "Health Alert"*

plain yogurt with active cultures, or by using freeze-dried yogurt starter cultures. Obviously the best yogurt is made from the best milk, so make sure it's organic milk from pasture-raised cows, and raw if possible. Some people who cannot tolerate dairy products have no problem digesting yogurt.

Essential Fatty Acids in Milk

As stated before in this book, but it's an important point worth repeating, our modern diets are highly unbalanced in their omega-3 to omega-6 fatty acid ratio, being too low in beneficial omega-3s and too high in inflammatory omega-6s, which leads to a host of degenerative conditions.

Raw milk from grass-fed cows has a high omega-3 essential fatty acid (EFA) content, while CAFO-raised cows fed on grains have a high omega-6 EFA content. Several sources of information suggest that human beings evolved on a diet with a ratio of omega-3 to omega-6 of approximately 1:1 or 1:2, whereas in Western diets the ratio now is more like 1:15 or even 1:20. It has been shown that a healthy ratio of fatty acids will dramatically reduce the risk of many chronic diseases such as arthritis, diabetes, cancer, heart disease, and Alzheimer's. In published studies, a higher level of omega-3 EFAs in women was associated with a decreased risk of breast cancer, patients with rheumatoid arthritis who had a higher level of omega-3s had less inflammation, and it also had a beneficial effect on patients with asthma.

Organic Milk Can Come from Cows in Confined Feedlots

How nutritious is organic milk? In some cases, it may not be much better than regular milk. The Organic Consumers Association has revealed conflicting ties between industry giants, organic products and politicians which make it highly improbable that we can depend on the purity and safety of organic milk products.

The newest GM crop to be approved for use by the Federal Government is alfalfa, and most of it will be used to feed dairy cows producing milk for Dean Foods. Dean Foods, the largest processor and distributor of milk in the U.S., owns Horizon, the leading brand of organic milk. Though one might assume that organic milk comes from small family farms where cows contentedly munch on fresh grass, in fact much of Horizon's organic milk is produced in huge factory farms where the animals are fed corn and soy, albeit organic corn and soy—but it still is not the cow's natural food. It is strongly believed that the new GM alfalfa represents a major threat to the integrity of organic milk, as GM alfalfa will inevitably contaminate organic alfalfa fields.

Land O' Lakes is also a Dean Foods brand, along with Silk and International Delight. Representatives from Kraft, Dole, and Dean Foods sit on the board of the Organic Trade Association, the board that makes the regulations for organic products. They have recently voted to allow synthetic hormones to be added to organic products in amounts so small they do not have to be included in the list of ingredients.

The Organic Consumers Association states on their website: "As you know, Genetically Modified Organisms, factory farms, and deceptively labeled consumer products pose a mortal threat to public health, climate stability, and all living things . . . consumers are inadvertently ingesting genetically engineered organisms and pesticide-tainted foods, organic farms are being contaminated with Monsanto's GMOs, climate-destabilizing chemical fertilizers are being massively applied to crops, and small farmers and farm workers are being exploited."

The Organic Consumers Association is calling for a boycott of Dean Foods and all of its brands, including Horizon and Silk, to protest GM alfalfa and all of the other crimes against human health, worker safety, animal rights, and the environment caused by Dean's factory-farmed dairies.

However, there is hope: Dean Foods' CEO Gregg Engles recently blamed "soft" milk sales partly on "a weak cereal category, which drives roughly 30 percent of milk use." Which means that consumption of pasteurized milk is going down along with reduced breakfast cereal consumption. The message seems to be getting out that cornflakes and milk do NOT make a healthy breakfast.

Safe Brands of Dairy

Public health officials and the National Dairy Council have worked together to make it difficult for us to obtain wholesome, fresh, raw dairy products. But they can be found with a little effort. In some states, you can buy raw milk and cream directly from farmers, and whole, pasteurized, non-homogenized milk from cows raised on non-grain organic feed is now available in many gourmet shops and health food stores. This high-quality milk can be cultured to restore enzyme content, at least partially, and cultured buttermilk is often more easily digested than regular milk, and is an excellent product to use in baking. Many shops now carry whole cream that is merely pasteurized (not ultra pasteurized like most commercial cream); diluted with water, it is delicious on cereal and a good substitute for those allergic to milk.

Reputable brands of organic and naturally-produced dairy products include Organic Valley, Kerry Gold butter and cheese from Ireland, Kate's butter, and Eden Foods, which was selected as the best food company in the world in 2009 by *The Better World Shopping Guide.*

Milk Alternatives

Some people with allergies to pasteurized cow's milk can tolerate raw cow's milk, or they can try goat's milk. They may also be able to eat goat and sheep's cheese. Other alternatives are almond milk, coconut milk, rice milk, and organic unsweetened soy milk (but it's best to consume soy in moderation.) Hemp milk is a new product on the market which is easy to make at home by blending hemp seeds and water in a high-speed blender; almond milk can be made by the same method.

Many people who are lactose intolerant find that their symptoms disappear if they consume raw dairy products made from grass-fed cows. They should also be able to tolerate milk that has had the lactose removed, such as Lactaid milk, but be warned that Lactaid is highly pasteurized and homogenized and not organic, so is not a healthful alternative.

Ice Cream

ICE CREAM, AS AMERICAN AS APPLE PIE AND BASEBALL, was once a treat for a special occasion, but has now pretty much become an everyday food. And, judging by the numbers, some people *are* eating it every day. Americans now consume about 48 pints per person per year, more than any other country in the world, and ice cream is now a $21 billion a year industry.

Ice cream may be a treat for the taste buds, but certainly not for the rest of the body, especially now that many flavors and varieties of ice cream contain high-carb "chunky" ingredients, such as cookie dough and broken-up candy bars, not to mention extravagant toppings of sprinkles, candy, and syrups.

Historic records tell us that different types of frozen desserts have been eaten for thousands of year. But they remained an expensive treat until the middle of the 19th century when rail could be used to transport ice from the north to warmer areas. After refrigeration became common, ice cream became popular throughout the world, and with it came an explosion of ice cream stores and vendors. They sold all all types and flavours of ice cream, expanding on the basic vanilla/chocolate/strawberry flavors to compete with each other to invent the most exotic and appealing products. Howard Johnson's restaurants advertised "a world of 28 flavors," and Baskin-Robbins out-did them, producing 31 flavors. Ben & Jerry's upped the ante when it developed its now famous range of "chunky" ice cream flavors, adding ingredients such as nuts, candy, and fruit, and other manufacturers followed suit. But, despite all their efforts, the most popular flavours today remain vanilla and chocolate.

The original recipe for ice cream was simple and nourishing: cream, honey to sweeten it, and flavorings such as fruit, vanilla, coffee, and chocolate. But today's commercial ice creams are laced with artificial ingredients making them almost unrecognizable from the healthy treat enjoyed for centuries, to the extent that ice cream is now a dangerous food. And these frozen treats are being eaten in increasingly larger and larger individual servings, especially by children. Ben & Jerry's has introduced the Vermonster, a large ice cream sundae consisting of 20 scoops of ice cream, four bananas, four ladles of hot fudge sauce, three chocolate chip cookies, a chocolate fudge brownie, ten scoops of walnuts, two scoops each of four different toppings, and whipped cream. Let's hope this is intended for more than one person!

Ice cream is made by stirring the ingredients slowly while cooling them, which incorporates air and prevents large ice crystals from forming. The result is a smoothly textured semi-solid foam that can be scooped when frozen. This basic ice cream isn't so bad for us—as the chart shows, it's the extras that create the problems. The cone, made of refined wheat, is often dipped in chocolate, and the chunky ingredients that are blended into the ice cream, like cookie dough or candy bars, and the various toppings add an additional load of sugar to an already sugary food.

Soft ice cream was developed in the 1930s and is made by using a method that doubles the amount of air in the ice cream, meaning that manufacturers use less of the ingredients, thereby reducing costs. Cones can be filled on order from a point-of-sale machine with a spigot, and such companies as Dairy Queen, Carvel, and Tastee-Freez established chains of soft-serve ice cream outlets. Sherbert, actually an incorrect usage for the word "sherbet," is a frozen dessert containing

Comparative Vibrational Levels of Health and Disease States		Comparative Nutritional Levels of **Ice Cream**
10,000 = Level of Optimal Health e.g. a healthy newborn baby / hunter/gatherer tribes	10,000	Ice cream made with organic cream, organic fruit, natural sweeteners, and natural flavorings
	9,500	
	9,000	
	8,500	
	8,000	
	7,500	Ben & Jerry's Vanilla
	7,000	Ben & Jerry's Chocolate, Strawberry, Coffee, Banana, White Russian
	6,500	Ben & Jerry's pistachio
AVERAGE LEVEL OF HEALTH IN USA Inflammation	6,000	Haagen-Dazs Vanilla, Vanilla Swiss Almond
Arthritis starts to manifest	5,500	Haagen-Dazs Dulce de Leche • Dreyer's Vanilla
Heart Disease starts to manifest	5,000	Ben & Jerry's Chunky Monkey, Banana Split • Dreyer's Chocolate, Strawberry, Coffee • Breyer's Vanilla, Chocolate • Tofutti Soy Ice Cream
Cancer cells form: Breast, Prostate, Lung, Colon, Pancreas	4,500	Dreyer's Rocky Road
Diabetes • Osteoporosis	4,000	Ben & Jerry's Cherry Garcia, Mint Chocolate Chunk • Breyer's Butter Pecan • Haagen-Dazs Mint Chip
Lymphoma • Leukemia • Dementia	3,500	Ben & Jerry's Cheesecake Brownie, Creme Brulee • Breyer's Cherry Vanilla • Haagen-Dazs Chocolate Chip Cookie
Congestive heart disease Brain cancer • Multiple sclerosis	3,000	Ben & Jerry's Peanut Brittle, Mud Pie, Mint Chocolate Cookie, Milk & Cookies • Baskin Robbins Vanilla
Breast cancer metastasizes	2,500	Ben & Jerry's Cinnamon Buns • Baskin Robbins Chocolate, Butter Pecan, Rum Raisin, Egg Nog
Prostate cancer metastasizes • Common cold/ flu	2,000	Baskin Robbins—most other flavors • Haagen-Dazs Cookies & Cream • Friendly's Cookies & Cream
Melanoma	1,500	
Metastatic bone and lung cancer	1,000	
	500	Soft Serve Ice Cream: Carvel, Dairy Queen, Mr. Softie, and Tastee-Freez
	50	All sherberts and sorbets: Baskin Robbins, Dreyer's, Edy's, Haagen Dazs etc.
Decay and Death	0	

BETTER HEALTH

WORSENING HEALTH

Measured in Bovis Units of Life Force Energy

both fruit juice and between one and two percent butterfat, and sometimes egg-white or gelatin, while sorbet is a frozen dessert made from sweetened water flavored with fruit juice or puree. Sorbet is marketed as being a non-fat or low-fat alternative to ice cream, but of course, as we now know, sugar is much more dangerous than the fat found in cream or milk.

To enjoy ice cream, choose a small portion of high quality ice cream and savor every mouthful. As we can see from the chart, most commercial ice cream calibrates really low on the scale, at the level of heart disease and diabetes, and the more "stuff" that's added, the lower the level gets and the more unhealthy it becomes. Even Haagen Dazs, which promotes itself as being a premium ice cream, calibrates "below the line." The best quality of the commercial ice cream varieties is Ben & Jerry's, but be aware that the more ingredients that are added, the less healthy it becomes. Ben & Jerry's plain vanilla ice cream, for instance, calibrates at a reasonably healthy 7,500, while their Mint Chocolate Cookie calibrates at 3,000—not due to the quality of the basic ice cream, but because of the added ingredients.

As a matter of interest, all the better-known ice cream brands that you find in your supermarket freezer cases are owned by major food corporations: Ben & Jerry's and Breyer's are owned by Unilever, Drayer's and Edy's by Nestle, Baskin Robbins by Dunkin' Donuts, and Haagen Dazs by Pillsbury.

Dairy Products

The Bottom Line

THE GOOD: Raw organic milk and dairy products made from pasture-raised cows • certain brands of low-heat pasteurized, non-homogenized organic dairy products • eggs from chickens fed organic feed • Ben & Jerry's non-chunky varieties of ice cream

THE BAD: Homogenized organic milk • organic milk and dairy products from CAFO grain-fed cows • Supermarket eggs from battery-raised hens

THE DOWNRIGHT DANGEROUS: All pasteurized, homogenized non-organic milk and dairy products, especially when sugar is added (yogurt, ice cream, puddings, ice cream and creamy desserts)

CHAPTER 14

Beans and Legumes

NUTRITIONISTS URGE US TO EAT BEANS as an important part of our diet, but many of us do not seem to like them very much—unless they are disguised in a highly-flavored sauce, as in baked beans or chili. It seems, despite their much touted benefits, that beans are not everyone's favorite food. Maybe it's because they cause digestive disturbances—gas!—or because they also contain toxins, called lectins, and the body may have a natural aversion to eating them.

Beans as we know them today derived from a common ancestor that originated in Peru. Migrating Indian traders took kidney beans with them on their travels to other countries throughout South and Central America, and Spanish explorers introduced beans into Europe in the 15th century, bringing them back from their voyages to the New World, along with potatoes and tobacco. Subsequently, European traders introduced kidney beans into Africa and Asia, and beans are now popular in many cultures throughout the world. Today, the largest commercial producers of dried common beans are India, China, Indonesia, Brazil, and the United States.

Beans and peas, also called pulses, are annual leguminous crops which are used both for human and animal food. The term "bean" originally referred to the seed of the broad bean, or fava bean, but was later expanded to include members of the genus Phaseolus, such as the common bean and the runner bean. Other beans such as the azuki bean and mung bean were originally classified as Phaseolus and later reclassified, and the use of word "bean" can refer to different species of pulses around the world. The word bean is also sometimes used to refer to the seeds or pods of plants that are not in the family *leguminosae*, but which bear a resemblance to true beans—for example coffee beans, castor beans, cocoa beans, and vanilla beans, which superficially resemble bean pods. The term "bean" is now applied generally to many related plants such as peas, lentils, chickpeas (garbanzos), vetches, lupins, and soy beans. However, soy has its own issues as a food for humans, which are covered in the next chapter.

Green beans and green peas are considered vegetable crops, while the term "pulse" is generally reserved for crops grown for their dry seed. Soy beans and peanuts (or ground nuts), which are a legumes and not true nuts, are grown both for human and animal consumption, as well as for their oil. Some legumes are eaten young while still in their pods and cooked whole, such as sugar-snap peas and green beans, or runner beans. Dried beans come from both Old World varieties of broad beans (fava beans) and New World varieties (kidney, black, cranberry, pinto, navy/haricot).

Beans are a summer crop and need warm temperatures to grow. As the bean pods mature, they turn yellow and dry up, and the beans inside change from green to their mature color. Bean plants are vines that need external support, which may be provided by frames or poles. Native Americans customarily grew beans along with corn and squash, the so-called "three sisters," with the tall cornstalks acting as support for the beans. However, nowadays the so-called bush bean has been developed which does not require support and is more practical for commercial production and harvesting.

Peas and beans are about 20 to 25 percent protein by weight, which is double the protein content of wheat and three times that of rice, but it is not a "complete" protein, meaning they do not contain the full range of essential amino acids required by the body. Pulses are often relatively poor in the essential amino acid methionine while grains tend to be deficient in lysine, and for this reason beans and grains are often combined in a meal to form a complete protein, as in beans and rice. Though combining beans with grains does make a complete protein, it is still deficient in B vitamins compared to animal protein. Soy beans are also not a complete protein, though they are often described as such—they are deficient in the sulfur-containing amino acids methionine and cystine, and lysine is adversely affected during processing. Beans are high in purines, which are metabolized to uric acid. Uric acid is known to promote the development or exacerbation of gout and for this reason, people with gout are advised to limit their consumption of beans.

Beans and Digestive Disturbances

Many people avoid eating beans because of their unfortunate side effects—gas, bloating, and digestive disturbances. Beans have this effect because they contain a type of fibre called oligosaccharides, composed of three to five sugar molecules linked together in such a way that the body cannot digest or absorb it. This fiber passes intact into the large intestine where bacteria breaks it down and gas is produced. Haricot and lima beans are generally major culprits, while peanuts are the least offensive because they have lower levels of oligosaccharides.

Soaking beans before cooking helps, and by discarding the soaking water prior to cooking, you will get rid of up to 80 percent of the oligosaccharides that cause flatulence. They can be soaked at room temperature for eight hours or overnight, or boiled briskly for two or three minutes, covered and set aside for one hour, and then drained well. Cooking times will vary with the variety, age, and size of beans, but generally cook them for one to two hours, or until the beans are tender when mashed or pierced with a fork. The U.S. Food and Drug Administration recommends an initial soak of at least five hours in water, which should then be discarded.

If you don't eat beans often, your body will not have the chance to fully adapt to digesting them, so the more often you eat them, the more your digestive system will adjust to them. Adding certain ingredients to the beans when they are cooking, such as a few bay leaves or a pinch of cumin, can have gas-reducing properties. But note that beans cooked with added sweeteners, such as sugar or maple syrup, may be even more difficult for some people to digest.

When all else fails, there's always Beano. Beano and similar products contain digestive enzymes that help break down the oligosaccharides before they reach the large intestine, specifically alpha galactosidase, derived from the fungus *Aspergillus niger.* This enzyme breaks down the complex sugars into simple sugars, making beans and peas more digestible, and reducing intestinal gas. Beano also works on a variety of "problem" foods, including cabbage, broccoli, cauliflower, grains, cereals, nuts, and seeds.

Beans Contain Natural Toxins

Plant poisonings are the most common cause of calls to the Poison Control Center. It is thought that all plants contain a small amount of toxin which acts as a natural defense against being eaten by insects and animals, but it is not usually a problem due to the small amounts involved.

Beans contain a toxin called phytohaemagglutinin (PHA), a member of a very common class of proteins called lectins. Lectins are glycoproteins that are present in a wide variety of edible plants, particularly in the seeds. In most cases, they are not harmful and possibly beneficial, but some lectins are known to be toxic. One of the most dangerous poisons known, ricin, is a lectin derived from the seeds of the castor bean *Ricinus communis*—but it is not a true bean, so this is not the same lectin found in edible beans and other legumes. Foods with high concentrations of lectins, such as beans, cereal grains, seeds, and nuts, may be harmful if consumed in excess. Adverse effects include allergic reactions, nutritional deficiencies, and immune reactions. It is thought that the susceptibility to the lectins in beans is hereditary.

Different beans may have different effects on the body depending on a person's blood type. Many people with type O blood, for instance, do not tolerate kidney beans, navy beans, and lentils very well as they contain lectins that deposit in muscle tissues, according to Dr. D'Adamo in his book *Eat Right for Your Type.* His research has led him to believe that those with type A blood can also have problems with kidney beans and navy beans, and they should also avoid lima beans and chickpeas. It seems prudent for each person to identify through trial and error which beans they can digest and which cause problems.

The PHA lectin is found in many species of beans, but the highest concentration is found in red kidney beans. The unit of toxin measured is the hemagglutinating unit (hau). Raw kidney beans contain from 20,000 to 70,000 hau, but this number is reduced to as low as 200 to 400 hau when the beans are fully cooked. White kidney beans contain only about one-third the amount of toxin as the red variety, and broad beans, or fava beans, contain five to ten percent of the amount that red kidney beans contain. But in fact most beans contain a little PHA.

PHA causes red blood cells to clump together, resulting in nausea, vomiting, and diarrhoea. Symptoms develop from between one to three hours after consumption, usually as extreme nausea followed by vomiting, which may be severe. Some people have been hospitalized, but recovery is usually rapid and spontaneous. The syndrome is usually caused by the ingestion of raw, soaked kidney beans, either alone or in salads or casseroles. As few as four or five raw beans can trigger symptoms. Several outbreaks have been associated with "slow cookers" or crock pots, or in casseroles which had not reached a high enough internal temperature to destroy the lectin. It has been shown that heating the beans to 176 degrees F may increase the toxicity five-fold, so these beans are actually more toxic when partially-cooked than if eaten raw. PHA in beans is deactivated and reduced to safe levels by as little as ten minutes of boiling, which is sufficient to degrade the toxin, but not to cook the beans.

Obviously, cooking beans properly is very important. All

Comparative Vibrational Levels of Health and Disease States		Comparative Nutritional Levels of **Beans, Peas and Legumes**
10,000 = Level of Optimal Health e.g. a healthy newborn baby / hunter/gatherer tribes	10,000	Organic beans, peas & legumes—fresh, dried, canned, cooked • Organic peanut butter
	9,500	Antonio's Lupini Beans, bottled
B	9,000	Bird's Eye and Green Giant frozen green beans
E T	8,500	Average supermarket fresh green beans and peas
T E R	8,000	Organic canned beans and peas (kidney, black, pinto, navy, white, butter, cannellini, lentils, etc.)
H E	7,500	Average supermarket dried beans, peas and lentils • Goya & Gouveia dried beans, peas and lentils
A L	7,000	Le Sueur Canned Peas
T H	6,500	Average store-bought hummus (made from chick peas)
AVERAGE LEVEL OF HEALTH IN USA Inflammation	6,000	Planter's Dry Roasted Peanuts • Progresso Fava Beans, canned
Arthritis starts to manifest	5,500	
Heart Disease starts to manifest	5,000	Canned kidney, black, pinto, navy, white, butter, cannellini, lentils, etc by Goya, Progresso, Rienzi
Cancer cells form: Breast, Prostate, Lung, Colon, Pancreas	4,500	Old El Paso Refried Beans, canned • Peanut oil
Diabetes • Osteoporosis	4,000	Goya canned beans in sauce • Goya Black Bean Soup
Lymphoma • Leukemia • Dementia	3,500	
Congestive heart disease Brain cancer • Multiple sclerosis	3,000	Heinz Baked Beans • Progresso Pea Soup, and Lentil Soup
Breast cancer metastasizes	2,500	Campbell's Beef & Bean Chili, Split Pea & Ham Soup, Hearty Bean & Ham Soup
Prostate cancer metastasizes • Common cold/ flu	2,000	Campell's Pork & Beans • Planter's Cocktail Peanuts (roasted in peanut and/or cottonseed oil)
Melanoma	1,500	Campbell's Baked Beans
Metastatic bone and lung cancer	1,000	Skippy® & Jif® Peanut Butter • Bush's Baked Beans
	500	Bush's Grillin' Beans, all flavors
	50	Planter's Honey-Roasted Peanuts • Beer Nuts
Decay and Death	0	

(Arrow labels: BETTER HEALTH ↑ / WORSENING HEALTH ↓)

Measured in Bovis Units of Life Force Energy

dried beans should be soaked overnight, and then boiled for 10 or 15 minutes before being cooked since under-cooked beans may be more toxic than raw beans. Kidney beans should never be sprouted for use in salads, such as three-bean salad, and it is not likely that stir-frying kidney bean sprouts is safe, either. The presence of PHA has also been found in significant levels in fava beans, or broad beans, while lima beans, or butter beans, can also be quite dangerous when consumed raw, but in this case the culprit is a different toxin altogether: linamarin, a cyanogenic glucoside, which is the same toxic substance found in cassava root.

Toxins in String Beans

String beans, though technically a bean, are usually classified as a vegetable; however, it's worth mentioning here that, in common with other beans, the raw mature green bean, also called the string bean or runner bean, is poisonous, containing varying amounts of prussic (hydrocyanic) acid or cyanogenic aminoglycoside. It was only as recently as 1957 that prussic acid was discovered in green beans. If eaten raw in moderation when young and tender, these beans probably won't cause a problem. But to be safe, green beans should be thoroughly cooked to neutralize any harmful poison. Mature beans are usually toxic when they have turned purple and the outer casing is "stringy." Some individuals have become sick with vomiting, stomach ache, circulation problems, convulsions, or heart palpitations a few hours after eating raw runner beans, so don't put them in a veggie smoothie and eat them raw—it's safer to cook them.

Beans and Legumes

The Bottom Line

THE GOOD: Organic beans, peas, and legumes, properly cooked • canned organic beans • organic peanut butter (no sugar added) • baked beans made with organic beans and honey, molasses or maple syrup • hummus prepared from organic garbanzo beans

THE NOT-SO-BAD: Store-bought hummus

THE BAD: Non-organic canned beans

THE DOWNRIGHT DANGEROUS: Baked beans made with sugar or HFCS • most canned soups containing peas and beans, including Progresso and Campbell's • peanut butter with added sugar, such as Skippy and Jif • sugar-coated peanuts, such as Beer Nuts

CHAPTER 15

Soy and Soy Products

BEAN CURD. TOFU. TEXTURED SOY PROTEIN. Soy by any other name doesn't sound any sweeter. Tofu not only looks unappetizing, even its name sounds sinister. Does anyone actually *like* tofu, or have we been obediently eating it because we've been told we will save the planet by doing so?

In the 1980s, when "they" told us we should avoid animal fats full of "artery clogging cholesterol" and embrace soy, I bought a book called *The Joy of Tofu.* As a young child growing up in Hong Kong, soy, then called bean curd, seemed pretty off-putting to me. The look, the taste, the texture, and the name were all a big turn-off to a five-year-old. But I thought I should give it a try as an adult, and try it I did. I may have found joy in cooking and joy in sex, but I never found joy in eating tofu. And now, having done the research for this chapter, I know why. Plainly, we should not be eating it—at least, not in its unfermented form, and certainly not if it's genetically-modified (GM), which is true of most of the soy grown in this country. Organic, properly fermented soy products do have some health benefits, but unfermented soy foods, which include soy milk, tofu and soy protein, are not healthy choices.

The stats on soy are that the soybean is a species of legume native to East Asia and is actually classed as an oil seed rather than a pulse by the Food and Agricultural Organization of the United Nations, as the bulk of the soybean crop is grown for oil production. Most of the remainder is used as livestock feed, with a small percentage used for human consumption. Soybeans are now grown on more than 72 million acres of U.S. farmland, all heavily subsidized by the government. Soy consumption in the U.S. has skyrocketed since the early 1990s, with soy food sales climbing from $300 million in 1992 to over $4 billion in 2008. It is the second-most valuable agricultural export in the U.S., behind corn, and it's interesting, if not ironic, to note that soy and corn are also two foods that we could readily remove from our diets and we'd be the healthier for it. Soy also has many industrial applications including diesel fuel, waterproof cement, anti-corrosion agents, and soy-based printing inks.

Since it is estimated that more than 90 percent of soybeans grown in this country are genetically-modified (GM), we are probably consuming GM substances when we eat any foods with soy in them, especially as soy is used extensively in processed foods in various forms such as soybean oil, soy lecithin, and textured soy protein isolate. Soybean meal is a low-cost source of protein for animal feeds and prepackaged meals for humans, often added to processed foods containing meat and dairy products and labelled as "textured vegetable protein."

According to the United Soybean Board, soybean oil represents approximately 79 percent of all edible oil consumed in the United States, and if it's not labeled organic, remember that there's a 90 percent chance it's made from GM soy.

Allergy to soy is common, and soy is high on the list of the main foods that can cause allergies, including milk, wheat, corn, eggs, peanuts, tree nuts, and shellfish. This can be a problem for people with a soy allergy since it is hidden in so many different foods.

> "The meteoric rise of soy as a 'health food' is a perfect example of how a brilliant marketing strategy can fool millions. But make no mistake about it, unfermented soy products are NOT healthful additions to your diet."
>
> — *Nutritional Expert Dr. Joseph Mercola*

Unfermented Soy should not be Included in the Human Diet

For many years, soy has been promoted as being a healthy alternative to meat and dairy products by the food industry who, through the media and advertising, have led us to believe that Asians have lower rates of cancer and heart disease because they eat soy products. But according to an article by The Weston A. Price Foundation, "Dangers of Eating Soy: It Could be Slowly and Silently Killing You," it is a myth that Asians consume large amounts of soy foods. In fact, average daily consumption of soy foods in Japan and China is 10 grams, about two teaspoons per day. Asians consume fermented soy foods, such as soy sauce, fermented bean paste, natto, and tempeh, in small amounts as a condiment, and not as a replacement for animal protein. It is also myth, they say, that modern unfermented soy products confer the same health benefits as traditionally fermented soy foods.

Kaayla T. Daniel, PhD, explains in her book, *The Whole Soy Story: The Dark Side of America's Favorite Health Food*, that the Chinese first started eating soybeans about 2,500 years ago, after they learned how to ferment it. They knew that soybeans contained many toxins after cooking and they learned to neutralize those toxins through fermentation. She also explains how tofu was first used in monasteries in China about 2,000 years ago, in part to promote sexual abstinence, since the phytoestrogens in soy can lower testosterone levels. Only very recently has soy been eaten the way we typically eat it, consuming large amounts in an unfermented and often highly processed form.

It is now known that problems resulting from eating unfermented soy include:

- Malnutrition and digestive problems
- Thyroid dysfunction
- Cognitive decline
- Reproductive disorders
- Immune system breakdowns
- Heart disease and cancer

Eating unfermented soy depletes the body of vitamin B12 and increases the body's need for vitamin D. The phytates in soy bind to metal ions, preventing the absorption of certain minerals, including calcium, magnesium, iron, and zinc, which is particularly problematic for vegetarians. The soybean has one of the highest phytate levels of any grain or legume, and these phytates are highly resistant to normal phytate-reducing techniques such as long, slow cooking. The traditional way of preparing soybeans for human consumption—a long period of fermentation—significantly reduces the phytate content of soybeans, but modern soy foods are not fermented and are processed in a way that denatures the protein and increases the levels of carcinogens.

The isoflavones in soy act as goitrogens, substances that suppress thyroid function, causing a range of health problems including anxiety and mood swings, insomnia, weight gain, infertility, digestive problems, and food allergies.

Soy milk has been shown to be a significant contributor to thyroid dysfunction or hypothyroidism in women in the U.S. A recent study found that women with the highest levels of estrogen in their blood had the lowest levels of cognitive function, and in Japanese-Americans, tofu consumption in mid-life is associated with the occurrence of Alzheimer's disease in later life. Studies have shown that as little as four tablespoons a day can result in hypothyroidism with symptoms of lethargy, constipation, weight gain, and fatigue.

There is also the notion that modern soy foods protect against many types of cancer, but a report by the British government concluded that there is little evidence that soy foods protect against breast cancer or any other forms of cancer, and in fact, soy foods may result in an *increased* risk of cancer. The high temperature needed to process soybeans to make textured vegetable protein and soy protein isolate results in the formation of toxic lysinoalanine and highly carcinogenic nitrosamines. And neither do soy foods protect against heart disease—there are hundreds of studies linking unfermented soy consumption to heart and other diseases.

Soy also contains natural toxins known as "anti-nutrients," such as saponins, soyatoxin, protease inhibitors, and oxalates, some of which can interfere with the enzymes needed to digest protein. While a small amount of these anti-nutrients

> "Our bodies are simply not designed or adapted to safely use and metabolize more than very small quantities of any food, including soy, which is not part of the original human diet . . . for the best long-term health, we should consume soy and soy products sparingly, if at all."
>
> — *Dr. Jonathan Wright, author of the "Nutrition & Healing" newsletter*

Comparative Vibrational Levels of Health and Disease States		Comparative Nutritional Levels of **Soy and Soy Products**
10,000 = Level of Optimal Health e.g. a healthy newborn baby / hunter/gatherer tribes	10,000	Organic fermented soy products: tempeh, miso, natto, soy sauce
	9,500	
	9,000	
	8,500	
	8,000	West Soy organic soy milk, unsweetened • Eden organic soy milk, unsweetened
	7,500	Organic soy bean flour
	7,000	Eden organic soy milk, vanilla flavor
	6,500	Generic soy bean flour • West Soy and Eden soy milk, sweetened/vanilla
AVERAGE LEVEL OF HEALTH IN USA Inflammation	6,000	
Arthritis starts to manifest	5,500	Soy protein isolate • Tofu (made from organic soy beans)
Heart Disease starts to manifest	5,000	Tofutti cream cheese and sour cream • Tofutti ice Cream
Cancer cells form: Breast, Prostate, Lung, Colon, Pancreas	4,500	Pacific Ultra soy milk (not organic) • Tofu (from non-organic soy beans)
Diabetes • Osteoporosis	4,000	Crisco soybean oil • Kikkoman soy sauce
Lymphoma • Leukemia • Dementia	3,500	Soy protein concentrate
Congestive heart disease Brain cancer • Multiple sclerosis	3,000	
Breast cancer metastasizes	2,500	
Prostate cancer metastasizes • Common cold/ flu	2,000	
Melanoma	1,500	
Metastatic bone and lung cancer	1,000	Aurora roasted soy beans • Nature's Promise soy crisps
	500	Nature's Promise soy crisps, Creamy Ranch flavor
	50	Monosodium glutamate made from soy • Soy lecithin • Soy Slender soy milk with Splenda
Decay and Death	0	

BETTER HEALTH (6,500–10,000) · WORSENING HEALTH (below 6,500)

Measured in Bovis Units of Life Force Energy

would probably not be harmful, the high levels of soy that many Americans are now unknowingly consuming could be problematic.

Yet, according to a 2008 survey by the United Soybean Board, 85 percent of consumers in the U.S. perceive soy products as healthful, 70 percent of consumers believe soybean oil is good for them, 33 percent eat soy foods or beverages at least once a month, and 84 percent of consumers agree with the FDA's claim that consuming 25 grams of soy protein daily reduces your risk of heart disease.

Nutritional expert Dr. Joseph Mercola, who publishes the most widely-read healthcare website in the U.S., says, "Unfortunately, many Americans who are committed to healthy lifestyles have been misled and grossly manipulated into believing that unfermented and processed soy products like soy milk, soy cheese, soy burgers and soy ice cream are health foods."

Soy Protein is Not a Complete Protein

Soybeans are also touted by many agencies as a source of complete protein, one that contains all the essential amino acids needed by the body, but in fact this is a myth: in common with all legumes, soybeans are deficient in the sulfur-containing amino acids methionine and cystine, and the processing of soybeans also adversely affects the amino acid lysine.

Soy protein isolate is a dry powder that has been separated or isolated from the other components of the soybean, making it 90 to 95 percent protein and nearly carbohydrate- and fat-free. This soy product can be found in all kinds of food items, from protein bars, protein shakes, soups and sauces to meat substitutes, baked goods, and breakfast cereals. There are many different names for this processed soy, some of which hide in ingredient lists under the title of "bouillon," "natural flavor" and "textured plant protein." Others names given to soy protein isolate are mono-diglyceride, TSF (textured soy flour) or TSP (textured soy protein), TVP (textured vegetable protein), lecithin, and MSG (monosodium glutamate). Not all textured vegetable protein is made from soy, but a great deal of it is. Lecithin can also be made from eggs, sunflower seeds, and corn.

The processing of soybeans to make soy protein isolate requires acid washing in aluminum tanks, which is designed to remove some of the anti-nutrients. But this process also leaches aluminum into the final product. Aluminum can have adverse effects on brain development and cause symptoms such as antisocial behavior, learning disabilities, and Alzheimer's disease and dementia.

The Phytoestrogens in Soy are a Danger for Humans of all Ages

Isoflavones are a type of phytoestrogen, a plant compound resembling human estrogen. They are found in small amounts in a number of grains, vegetables, and legumes, but soybeans represent by far the most concentrated source in the human diet. Studies show that the phytoestrogens genistein and daidzein in soy are powerful endocrine disrupters in animals and humans. Studies have shown that consuming phytoestrogens during pregnancy, even at moderate levels, can have adverse affects on the developing fetus and the timing of puberty later in life.

Premature sexual development of girls has been linked to the use of soy formula and exposure to environmental estrogen-mimickers such as PCBs and DDE. Almost 15 percent of white girls and 50 percent of African-American girls in the U.S. show signs of puberty before the age of eight, and some are showing sexual development before the age of three. Studies show that babies fed soy-based formula have 13,000 to 22,000 times more estrogen compounds in their blood than babies fed milk-based formula, meaning that some infants are receiving the estrogenic equivalent of four birth control pills per day. When babies are fed formula containing soy, it floods the bloodstream with female hormones that inhibit testosterone, which is a possible cause of disrupted development patterns in boys, including learning disabilities and ADD.

Male babies normally have a testosterone surge during the first few months of life which establishes a program that will express male characteristics after puberty, not only in the development of their sexual organs and other masculinity traits, but also in setting patterns in the brain characteristic of male behavior. Feeding them soy formula can have a devastating effect on these hormonal changes. The natural isoflavones found in soy mimic estrogen so well that they have been known to cause a variety of alarming side effects in men such as breast enlargement (gynecomastia), decreased facial and body hair growth, decreased libido, mood swings, erectile dysfunction, and lowered sperm count.

Numerous studies show that soy foods cause infertility in animals and can prevent ovulation. Consuming soy foods can also stimulate the growth of estrogen-dependent tumors, and stimulate the growth of cancer cells.

Archer Daniels Midland, a major U.S. soy producer, recently withdrew its application to the FDA for "generally recognized as safe" (GRAS) status for soy isoflavones following an outpouring of protest from the scientific community. The FDA never approved GRAS status for soy protein isolate because of concern regarding the presence of toxins and carcinogens in processed soy.

Genetically-Modified (GM) Soy

Probably the biggest danger from eating soy and soy products in the U.S. is that most of it is genetically-modified. It's true that 98 percent of the U.S. soybean crop is used for animal feed and is not for human consumption, but when we eat animals, we are eating what they eat too.

In 1997, about eight percent of soybeans grown for the commercial market in the U.S. were GM; by 2010, the figure had risen to 93 percent. But the reluctance of the agritech business to allow research to be done on GM products means that there are only a handful of studies on the safety of GM soybeans.

In 1995, Monsanto Company introduced Roundup Ready soybeans that were genetically modified to be resistant to Monsanto's herbicide Roundup, meaning they were chemically engineered to withstand heavy doses of herbicides. Roundup's active ingredient, glyphosate, is the most used herbicide in the U.S. and there is considerable evidence that it is dangerous to humans, affecting the endocrine and reproductive systems and altering fertility by throwing off the delicate hormonal balance that governs the reproductive cycle. It has been shown to interfere with aromatase, which produces estrogen, and is highly toxic to the placenta in pregnant women. In a 2009 French study, scientists discovered that glyphosate can kill the cells in the outer layer of the human placenta which in turn can kill the placenta. To learn more about GM food, refer to the GM chapter at the beginning of the book.

Soy as Animal Feed

Raw soybeans, including the immature green form, are toxic to humans and to all monogastric animals (those with single stomachs). To make soy palatable to animals, the bulk of the U.S. soy crop is solvent-extracted with hexane to create a "toasted" defatted soy meal that is 50 percent protein. Producing animal feed on this scale has made it possible to raise farm animals such as chicken, turkeys, and pigs on huge factory farms. Over 30 million tons of soybean meal are consumed by livestock in a year; even the hulls are used as a component of cattle feed. Environmental groups have reported that soybean cultivation in Brazil has destroyed huge areas of Amazon rainforest, and predict further deforestation in the future.

The natural food for cattle is grass, which is rich in beneficial omega-3 fatty acids. But when cattle eat soy, which is high in omega-6 fatty acids, their meat is also rich in omega-6 fatty acids, which are already too abundant in the modern American diet. Consumption of soy-fed meat by humans directly contributes to the imbalance between levels of omega-3 and omega-6 fatty acids in the diet, which has an inflammatory effect on the body and contributes greatly to degenerative disease. Soybean meal is also used in lower-end dog foods, hardly their natural food, and has the same issue of creating a serious omega fatty acid imbalance leading to inflammation and disease.

Soy Products

The Bottom Line

THE GOOD: Organic, naturally-fermented soy products such as tempeh, miso, and soy sauce

THE BAD: All unfermented soy products, even if organic

THE DOWNRIGHT DANGEROUS: All non-organic soy products and meat from animals fed GM soy feed

CHAPTER 16

Vegetables

YOU REALLY CAN'T SAY ANYTHING BAD about vegetables, they are an essential part of a healthy diet—until you consider the fact that many of the edible plants we cultivate are toxic. Whoever would have thought that a stick of celery or a runner bean could be life-threatening? But for some people, they are. Most plant toxins, though, are not directed at humans—they are manufactured by the plant to deter herbivores and pests from nibbling them to death, but it does mean we have to be careful and know how to prepare and cook vegetables properly.

A plant is termed a vegetable when part of it is customarily consumed by humans, usually the stem (celery), root (carrot), flower (artichoke), leaf (lettuce), and fruit (tomato, zucchini, peppers). Generally, vegetables are savory but not sweet, though new hybrids are being developed that are much sweeter than in the past, such as sweet potatoes and sugar-snap peas. In past centuries, the staple vegetables in northern climes were cabbage, carrots, onions, and root vegetables such as rutabaga, parsnips, radishes, and turnips (though later potatoes took their place). Many of the vegetables we now eat, such as bell peppers, eggplant, and avocados, were then virtually unknown.

A primary difference between plants and animals is a plant's ability to manufacture its own food. Most people are familiar with basic plant chemistry, that miracle of self-sufficiency called photosynthesis, where the chloroplasts in green leaves make food from carbon dioxide from the air and hydrogen from water combined with light from the sun. Photosynthesis literally means to "put together with light." Plants utilize the carbon dioxide animals and humans give off when they breathe, and in return give off oxygen as a by-product of photosynthesis. Without this carbon dioxide/oxygen exchange, life on earth could not exist. But this plant chemistry also enables plants to manufacture all kinds of chemical compounds that are designed to be toxic to the animals and insects who want to eat them, including us.

In the diet, vegetables can be eaten freely, and are healthiest if grown organically. It's best to eat them as fresh as possible, either by growing them yourself in season, or purchasing them from a local farmers' market. Most supermarkets these days have organic produce sections, often at very little more than the price of regular vegetables, and specialty stores such as Trader Joe's and Whole Foods Market offer excellent quality at reasonable prices. But even basic supermarket vegetables are not so bad. Yes, organic is best, but when you look at the range of foodstuffs that the average person consumes in a day, non-organic veggies are the least of their problems.

The charts in this book demonstrate that an unhealthy diet is not caused by eating too few vegetables—it's all the "other stuff" we eat that creates the problems. But as with other foods that are processed, vegetables, too, calibrate much lower when canned or pre-cooked and frozen. Fresh is important: freshly-picked romaine lettuce, for instance, has a total nutritional level of 10,000, but after three to five days of being stored in a cool place it drops to 9,000. After one week, it's down to 7,000, and after 10 days it drops to 4,000. But at that point it's wilted, and we can see quite clearly that it's not edible, nor nutritious. There's also much concern about the impact of pesticides, insecticides, and artificial fertilizers on vegetables and the declining fertility of soil in America. But the truth is, fresh vegetables, no matter how they have been grown, are still more healthy to eat compared with the packaged and processed foods that fill so many grocery carts.

Comparative Vibrational Levels of Health and Disease States		Comparative Nutritional Levels of **Vegetables**
10,000 = Level of Optimal Health e.g. a healthy newborn baby / hunter/gatherer tribes	10,000	Most vegetables grown in fertile soil untreated with artificial fertilizers, herbicides, and pesticides, fresh or frozen • cooked organic root vegetables • cooked spinach • most edible mushrooms
	9,500	Supermarket red and yellow onions • supermarket tomatoes • most canned tomatoes • most frozen vegetables (no sauce) • Green Giant bottled whole mushrooms
	9,000	Most supermarket vegetables • Del Monte canned potatoes • Most frozen vegetables with sauce
	8,500	Supermarket Iceberg lettuce, leaf lettuce, scallions
	8,000	Supermarket avocados, cucumbers • Bird's Eye frozen butternut squash and yellow turnips
	7,500	Supermarket green peppers, red peppers, celery
	7,000	
	6,500	
AVERAGE LEVEL OF HEALTH IN USA Inflammation	6,000	Raw organic root vegetables: potatoes, carrots, beets, parsnips, turnips, rutabaga, yams • Raw spinach
Arthritis starts to manifest	5,500	Raw non-organic potatoes and root vegetables
Heart Disease starts to manifest	5,000	Aunt Nellie's bottled white onions • Del Monte canned sliced beets
Cancer cells form: Breast, Prostate, Lung, Colon, Pancreas	4,500	Del Monte: canned lima beans, green beans, sweet peas, spinach • Lesueur canned peas • Cento canned artichoke hearts
Diabetes • Osteoporosis	4,000	Del Monte canned vegetables: carrots, Italian beans, spinach, zucchini in tomato sauce • Shurfine canned asparagus
Lymphoma • Leukemia • Dementia	3,500	Del Monte canned wax beans
Congestive heart disease Brain cancer • Multiple sclerosis	3,000	Ore Ida frozen French fries, Shoestrings, and Tater Tots
Breast cancer metastasizes	2,500	
Prostate cancer metastasizes • Common cold/ flu	2,000	Generic deli cole-slaw and three-bean salad
Melanoma	1,500	Claussen dill pickle (cucumber) • French's French Fried Onions
Metastatic bone and lung cancer	1,000	
	500	Mancini Ready To Serve Sweet Fried Peppers
	50	Hanover frozen candied sweet yams • Vlasic Polish dill spears and sweet gherkins (cucumber)
Decay and Death	0	

BETTER HEALTH ↑ / WORSENING HEALTH ↓

Measured in Bovis Units of Life Force Energy

Why Doesn't Everyone Like Vegetables?

"I do not like broccoli, and I haven't liked it since I was a little kid and my mother made me eat it. And I'm President of the United States, and I'm not going to eat any more broccoli!"
—*President George H. W. Bush*

"Eat your veggies!" parents urge their children. But why is it such a battle to get some children to eat vegetables? And it's not only children—remember President George Bush and his dislike of broccoli? One reason is that a large sector of the population (about 45 percent in the U.S.) has type O blood, and type Os can exhibit a natural aversion to vegetables in the brassica group and to the sulphur smell they emit when being cooked. This is a genus of plants in the mustard family, and includes cabbage, cauliflower, broccoli, kale, mustard greens, and Brussels sprouts. There's a reason for this: type Os tend towards low levels of thyroid hormone and these vegetables contain goitrogens, which suppress thyroid function, and can induce hypothyroidism and goiter. This is a good example of a human body instinctively knowing what is right for it. And yes, President Bush has type O blood. Kelp, a sea vegetable, is useful for supplying the thyroid with iodine.

On the other hand, leafy greens such as collard greens, romaine lettuce, and spinach have been found to be particularly beneficial for type Os because they contain Vitamin K which helps with blood clotting factors, a process that can be deficient in people with type O blood.

Those who do well on a vegetarian diet are most likely to have type A blood, explains Dr. D'Adamo in his book *Eat Right For Your Type*. His research has shown that most people with type A blood need about four times as many vegetables as type Os, while type Os typically need more animal protein. So those people who identify themselves as "steak-and-potatoes" eaters are most likely to have type O blood.

Vegetarian and Vegan Diets

"I joke that a big juicy steak is my beauty secret. But seriously, I love red meat. I was a vegan for a long time, and it nearly killed me. I found I was not getting enough nutrition."
—*Angelina Jolie, film actress*

People who follow vegetarian and vegan diets do so for two main reasons: ethics, and better nutritional health. There can be no argument with the first—there are few things on this planet more shameful than how animals are treated in factory farms, and many people simply feel that killing animals to eat them is just plain wrong. But the second reason, that a vegetarian or vegan diet is healthier, is now thought by many nutritional experts to be misguided. Many people have based their decision to avoid meat due to reports that animal protein and fat (cholesterol) are bad for our health. But in fact, that is not true.

Dr. Joseph Mercola has said: "A largely vegetarian diet may be appropriate for some, but to promote it as the only, or even the best, way to improve health is foolhardy at best, because some two-thirds of people simply cannot and will not thrive on a meatless diet."

Vegetarians often cite *The China Study* by T. Colin Campbell, PhD, as being proof that such a diet is healthy. But this "study" has been found to have fundamental flaws since it is not actually a study but a theory built around a comprehensive set of observations, and Dr. Campbell's assertion that animal protein should be avoided has never been tested on live patients. Dr. Campbell's findings have been found to be untrue by many nutritionally oriented physicians, including Dr. Mercola, who have collectively treated tens of thousands of patients and found that promoting a diet free of animal protein for everyone invariably causes harm and suffering in those whose nutritional type requires large amounts of fat and protein. Dr. Mercola relates that he was initially inspired by Dr. Campbell's research and believed that his patients should improve on his recommended dietary regimen. But he found that large numbers of his sick patients failed to improve on this diet, and in fact many significantly worsened and nearly died. Some left his practice because they lost faith in his ability to use diet as a tool to help them regain their health.

Another nutritional physician who took a hard look at Dr. Campbell's book and the studies that form the basis of his conclusions is Michael R. Eades, M.D., who has been in the full-time practice of nutritional and metabolic medicine since 1986. He points out that Dr. Campbell is not a practicing physician and had no real-world experience to support his nutritional recommendations. As Dr. Eades writes in his blog, "In my studied opinion, *The China Study* is a masterpiece of obfuscation. It would be difficult for a mere mortal to pen so much confusion, ambiguity, distortion and misunderstanding in what is basically a book-length argument for a personal opinion masquerading as hard science."

But our goal needs to be good health through a nutritious diet, not a battle over what people should or should not eat. The unavoidable truth is that different kinds of people need to eat different kinds of foods. I do not think that people who are meat-eaters enjoy the idea that animals have to be killed to feed them, but there are many animal lovers who eat meat. Growing up on a farm was one way people learned to understand how domesticated animals fit into the circle of life. Perhaps the Native Americans, 98 percent of whom have type O blood, learned best to deal with this unavoidable truth by honoring the animals they hunted by performing sacred ceremonies for their spirits.

Toxins in Plants

Plants are armed with an arsenal of weapons to protect them from "enemies" such as humans, insects, and herbivores. These deterrents include thorns, stinging leaves, and toxins. "Plants are by far the biggest manufacturers of chemical weapons on earth," writes Dr. Sharon Moalem in his book, *Survival of the Sickest.*

The fruits of plants contain seeds which need to be dispersed so that new plants can grow. One of the ways this happens is when animals eat the fruit and deposit the seeds via excretion far from the original plant. That's why fruit looks so tempting and tastes so good—the plant wants it to be eaten! But the plant does not want its leaves, stems or roots to be eaten—it needs those to survive, and that is where the toxins are to be found.

In medicine, it is said that there are no toxins, only toxic doses (the Arndt-Schultz law). It is thought that all plants might contain a small amount of toxin, most often cyanide, which acts as a natural defense against foraging animals, but it is not usually a problem due to the small amounts involved. Plants also produce alkaloids primarily designed to help protect them from insects. There are many edible plants that are known to contain toxins, including raw runner beans, broad beans, and unripe (green) potatoes and tomatoes. Even asparagus is a poisonous plant. Some people are very sensitive to the sulphur compounds in raw asparagus shoots. After peeling asparagus or coming into contact with the plant, they may suffer from allergic reactions, asthma, inflammation of the skin and eyes, and allergic rhinitis. The red berries of asparagus are also slightly toxic—people have experience vomiting and abdominal pain after ingesting more than five of the ripe berries.

Some people are very sensitive to hot peppers which contain capsaicin, a sticky poison that adheres to mucous membranes. If you eat a very hot pepper, drink milk or eat something with fat in it which will help peel the capsaicin away from the mucous membrane. Capsaicin can also cause degeneration of some types of neurons, so, in large quantities, hot peppers can be very harmful. In populations in some tropical countries such as Sri Lanka, where hot peppers are eaten regularly, there is a high rate of stomach cancer.

Celery, celery root, parsley, and parsnips contain toxins called psoralens, also known as furocoumarin. Psoralens can damage DNA and cause phytophotodermatitis, which is sensitivity to sunlight caused by contact with a plant. Phytophotodermatitis from celery has been seen among grocery store workers. Handling these plants and then sunbathing can lead to bad sunburn, rashes, blisters, and skin discoloration; photosensitivity from eating these vegetables can occur, but it is quite unusual. This may be the reason why celery is traditionally grown in the dark, the stem mounded up with soil so the stalk stays white.

Poisonous Edible Plants

Some people have allergic reactions to the nightshade family of plants, which includes tomato, potato, eggplant, sweet bell peppers, and tobacco. Tomatillos, tamarios, pepinos, pimentos, paprika, cayenne, and Tabasco sauce are also classified as nightshade foods. The active alkaloid in nightshades, solanine, is more familiar to us as nicotine. The leaves of all these nightshades foods contain some level of nicotine, but it is called solanine in potatoes, tomatine in tomatoes, alpha-solanine in eggplants, and solanadine in chillies and capsicums. This drug-like alkaloid may affect sensitive individuals, especially the nervous system or joints, and it seems that certain people notice that their symptoms of a variety of mental, emotional and physical conditions subside when they remove nightshades from their diet.

Alkaloids may affect the metabolism of calcium in a way that is not yet understood. It seems that nightshade vegetables may cause the removal of calcium from the bones, depositing it in soft tissue which might be the start of arthritis. For these reasons, medical professionals often recommend that people with osteoarthritis, rheumatoid arthritis or other joint problems like gout eliminate nightshade vegetables from their diet. One in three people with arthritis, studies have shown, will react badly to nightshades, and some researchers believe that arthritis is often misdiagnosed in people who may in fact only be experiencing the effects of consumption of vegetables from the nightshade family. In 1980, The Arthritis Nightshades Research Foundation was established to study the nightshade/arthritis connection. Their determination was, "If nightshades can be eaten or used sparingly, arthritis can be slowed in developing."

Like many other plants of the nightshade family, tomato leaves and stems contain atropine and other tropane alkaloids that are toxic if ingested, causing digestive upset and nervous excitement. The ripened fruit does not contain these compounds, but the green unripe fruit of the tomato plant contains small amounts of the poisonous alkaloid tomatine. Use of tomato leaves in tea (tisane) has been responsible for at least one death. However, levels of tomatine are generally too small to be dangerous. Tomato plants can be toxic to dogs if they eat large amounts of the fruit, or chew plant material.

The seemingly innocuous zucchini can also cause problems as members of the cucumber family (Cucurbitacea) are able to produce a group of highly potent toxins (cucurbitacins) that have insecticidal and/or fungicidal properties, though the amount of cucurbitacin is normally present in such low concentrations that it cannot be tasted. The production of cucurbitacins is controlled by the plant so that they are only made when they are needed, such as when climate conditions seem to be right for a possible insect infestation or fungal infection. In 2001, several New Zealanders complained of stomach cramps after they had eaten zucchini. Over the period of a few weeks, more and more cases were reported, which led the health authorities to investigate. Many of the people who became ill remembered that the zucchini tasted very bitter. And that was the culprit. Cucurbitacins are intensely toxic and taste very bitter—in fact, they have such a bitter taste that it is very unlikely that anyone could stand to eat enough zucchini-containing cucurbitacins to cause significant harm. Cucumbers that taste bitter will also have a higher level of cucurbitacins, and some varieties have higher levels than others.

• Toxins in String Beans

While beans and peas, also called pulses, are annual leguminous crops, the green bean, broad bean, lima bean, and garden pea are considered vegetable crops. These beans and peas are eaten young when still in their pods, or cooked whole, for example, green beans and sugar-snap peas. The mature green bean, also called the string bean or runner bean, is poisonous, containing varying amounts of prussic (hydrocyanic) acid or cyanogenic aminoglycoside. It was only as recently as 1957 that prussic acid was discovered in green beans. When eaten in moderation when young and tender, raw runner beans should not be a problem. But to be safe, green beans eaten in quantity should be thoroughly cooked to neutralise the harmful poison. As mentioned in the chapter on Beans, some individuals have become sick with vomiting, stomach ache, circulation problems, convulsions, and heart palpitations a few hours after eating raw green beans, so, to be safe, always eat green beans cooked or steamed.

• Oxalic Acid in Vegetables

Spinach, chard, beet greens, and rhubarb contain significant amounts of oxalic acid which can interfere with absorption of some minerals, especially calcium. It imparts a sharp taste to these leafy vegetables, especially in older leaves. Levels are so high in rhubarb leaves that we don't eat them—they're poisonous. However, the oxalic acid in vegetables is broken down during cooking and so doesn't interfere with the absorption of calcium present in other foods which might be eaten at the same time.

Interestingly, raw spinach calibrates at the level of 6,000 but reaches 10,000 when cooked, so it actually becomes more nutritious when it's cooked. Anyone who has chewed their way through a plate of spinach salad appreciates how much easier and quicker it is to eat the same amount of spinach when steamed!

Root Vegetables

Root vegetables include potatoes, carrots, beets, parsnips, turnips, rutabagas, jicama, yams, and other roots such as cassava. Because they grow underground devoid of sunlight, root vegetables calibrate low when raw, around 5,500 to 6,000, but reach the high nutritional level of 10,000 when they are cooked. They can be baked, boiled, steamed, fried and sauteed, but be aware that cooking them in a microwave oven actually reduces their nutritional level, whereas cooking by gas, electricity or fire increases it. A microwaved baked potato, for instance, is far less nutritious than one baked in a conventional oven. I was led to believe that it was best to eat beets raw and would religiously grate them into my salad, but I now realize that my grandmother was right all along—beets *are* more nutritious when cooked. However, carrots calibrate at 5,000 when raw, but the digestion process raises their level to 10,000 in the body, but this is not true of other root vegetables, so it's best not to eat them raw.

Cassava, or manioc, is a starchy thick-skinned tuber which is a dietary staple in many tropical countries. Raw cassava contains toxic cyanogenic glucosides, and can be classified as sweet or bitter, depending on the level of toxins present. Improper preparation of cassava can leave enough residual cyanide to cause acute cyanide intoxication and goiters, and has been linked to partial paralysis. Cassava must be cooked properly to detoxify it before it is ready for human or animal consumption. It is made into a flour that we call tapioca, which is a useful alternative to wheat in gluten-free bakery products.

Sometimes carrots may have an off-flavor such as a bitter or petroleum-like taste, usually the result of being exposed to ethylene, a normal fruit-ripening hormone that may react with natural chemical compounds found in carrots. Carrots, therefore, should not be stored with ethylene-producing fruit and vegetables such as apples, avocados, bananas, pears, peaches, plums, cantaloupes, honeydew melons and tomatoes. Carrots stored in perforated plastic bags at a low temperature retain the best taste.

Potatoes

Potatoes are America's most popular vegetable, according to the USDA's Economic Research Service. The typical American consumes more than 140 pounds of them every year, which is 50 pounds more than the per-capita consumption of tomatoes, the potato's closest competitor. Although they do get a bad rap, potatoes can be part of a healthy diet, being one of the few common starches we eat that is not a grain.

Potato registers high on the glycemic index and plain mashed potato is thought to elevate blood sugar levels, but in fact we rarely eat plain cooked potatoes—we usually eat them with butter, sour cream or gravy, which slows their absorption into the

Comparative Vibrational Levels of Health and Disease States	Measured in Bovis Units of Life Force Energy	Comparative Nutritional Levels of **Potatoes**
10,000 = Level of Optimal Health e.g. a healthy newborn baby / hunter/gatherer tribes	10,000	Cooked organic potatoes: boiled, steamed, mashed, baked, roasted, or sauteed in olive oil
	9,500	Organic potatoes fried in olive oil, coconut oil, or lard from grass-fed cattle
BETTER HEALTH	9,000	Average supermarket potatoes fried in lard from grass-fed cattle • Shurfine canned new potatoes
	8,500	
	8,000	Supermarket potatoes fried in lard from corn-fed cattle
	7,500	
	7,000	
	6,500	Raw organic potatoes
AVERAGE LEVEL OF HEALTH IN USA		
Inflammation	6,000	Raw supermarket potatoes • Generic dried "mashed" potatoes in packets
Arthritis starts to manifest	5,500	Supermarket potato baked in microwave oven
Heart Disease starts to manifest	5,000	
Cancer cells form: Breast, Prostate, Lung, Colon, Pancreas	4,500	
Diabetes • Osteoporosis	4,000	Supermarket potatoes fried in canola or soy bean oil
Lymphoma • Leukemia • Dementia	3,500	Cape Cod potato chips • Utz reduced fat potato chips
Congestive heart disease Brain cancer • Multiple sclerosis	3,000	Lay's & Utz potato chips • Ore Ida & generic frozen French fries, Hash Browns, Steak Fries
Breast cancer metastasizes	2,500	McDonald's fries • Burger King fries • Utz Medley potato chips • Kettle Krinkle Cut potato chips
Prostate cancer metastasizes • Common cold/ flu	2,000	Wendy's fries • Average supermarket potatoes fried in cottonseed oil or corn oil
Melanoma	1,500	
Metastatic bone and lung cancer	1,000	
WORSENING HEALTH	500	Pringles potato chips, all flavors
	50	
Decay and Death	0	

blood stream. In fact, potatoes are beneficial in the diet because a small but significant portion of the starch in potato is resistant to digestion by enzymes in the stomach and small intestine, and so it reaches the large intestine essentially intact. This resistant starch is considered to have similar physiological effects and health benefits as fiber in the gut and improves glucose tolerance and insulin sensitivity—quite the opposite of its reputation.

Most people know not to eat green potatoes because they contain toxins known as glycoalkaloids which are concentrated in the green portions of the plant—its leaves, stems and sprouts. Exposure to light, physical damage, and age can all increase the glycoalkaloid content of a potato, with the highest concentrations occurring just underneath the skin, but this can be peeled away before cooking. The concentration of glycoalkaloid in wild potatoes is enough to produce toxic effects in humans, affecting the nervous system, causing headaches, diarrhea and intense digestive disturbances, cramps, weakness and confusion, and in severe cases coma and death. Happily, cultivated potato varieties contain lower toxin levels, and cooking at high temperatures (over 170°C or 340°F) destroys the toxin. Food safety specialists note that, as far as they are aware, no serious cases of potato poisoning have occurred in the U.S. in the last 50 years.

Sweet potato, which is not related to the white potato, contains an enzyme inhibitor that blocks the action of trypsin, an enzyme that digests proteins. This makes raw sweet potato difficult to digest as the trypsin inhibitor is deactivated by cooking. so it's best to always cook sweet potatoes.

• Our Favorite Form of Potato—French Fries

Everyone loves French fries! They are tasty, filling and nutritious—so long as they are cooked in healthy oil. When I was growing up in England, fast food meant fish and chips, with the chips, or fries, being hefty slices of potatoes fried in lard—and what a flavor they had. And in fact, the taste of a French fry is largely determined by the cooking oil. For decades, McDonald's cooked its French fries in a mix of about 90 percent beef tallow and the balance cottonseed oil. But in 1990, amid fears over high levels of cholesterol in the American diet, McDonald's switched to pure vegetable oil. When McDonald's fries were cooked in beef fat, they calibrated at the healthy level of 9,000, but now their health level has plummeted to 2,500. This switch from frying food in animal fats to vegetable oils has been a major factor in causing the current health crisis in this country. Refined vegetable oils are one of the unhealthiest products we can eat, and heating them to high temperatures makes them all the more dangerous. So make your fries just like your grandmother used to—deep-fried in lard, from pasture-fed cattle if possible.

Pesticides and Herbicides in Vegetables

Three independent studies have found that children whose mothers are exposed to common agricultural pesticides are more likely to experience a range of harmful effects to their cognitive development, including lower IQ, as well as impaired reasoning and memory. A report from *Consumer Reports* has revealed unsafe levels of pesticide residues on certain fresh fruits and vegetables, including many that are grown in the United States. The worst offender was winter squash, followed by spinach, then spinach from Mexico, and then domestically-grown celery and green beans. Others that tested high on the list included sweet bell peppers, potatoes, lettuce, kale, and collard greens. The vegetables that contained the least amounts of pesticides were onions, avocados, sweet corn, sweet peas, asparagus, cabbage, eggplant, sweet potatoes, and red onions. Illegal insecticides found on the produce were not due to current use, but to low levels of chemicals that are attributed to persistent residues in soils or to wind dispersal of pesticides applied legally to nearby fields. It is commonly thought that imported foods from Mexico and South America are more contaminated than U.S. grown foods, but in fact 11 of the 12 highest contaminated foods in the samples tested were U.S. grown.

One chemical, methyl parathion, accounts for more than 90 percent of the total toxicity load of much fruit and green beans and peas. The high toxicity values for winter squash from the U.S. are almost entirely due to residues of dieldrin, a very toxic carcinogenic insecticide that was banned 25 years ago, but is still present in the soil in some areas.

Bud Nip, also called Sprout Nip, or Beet-Kleen, is a chemical called chlorpropham which is sprayed on potatoes to prevent sprouts from growing on them. Chlorpropham is also used as a plant growth regulator used for controlling grass weeds in various crops including blueberries, cane berries, carrots, cranberries, garlic, onions, spinach and tomatoes. Though it is sprayed on the outside of these food items, the chlorpropham is absorbed into the entire plant. The Extension Toxicology Network reports that "Long-term exposure to chlorpropham may cause tumors" and "may cause adverse reproductive effects. Chlorpropham may cross the placenta." If you plan to grow potatoes, buy organic varieties, otherwise the "eyes" will not sprout into new plants.

Bisphenol A Found in Canned Foods

BPA is used to harden plastic and is found in food can linings and polycarbonate plastics for beverage bottles. BPA is a synthetic estrogen, an endocrine disrupter that interferes with the body's hormones and "disrupts" the human endocrine system. It has been linked to serious health problems such as early puberty, brain and heart disorders, infertility, and prostate and breast cancer. In 2007, the Environmental Working Group released the first study showing that BPA can leach from can linings into canned foods. Since then, many other studies have found the same thing. In fact, BPA is so pervasive that scientists have found that 95 percent of people tested have potentially dangerous levels of BPA in their bodies. Many vegetables that we commonly eat, such as tomatoes, artichoke hearts, and beans, are canned for convenience, so this is another reason to eat fresh or frozen when possible.

Make Organic your Choice

There are more reasons to eat organic foods than for nutritional value—purchasing organic produce encourages sustainable agriculture and supports smaller farms that practice healthy soil and crop management without using dangerous chemicals. According to data posted by the USDA, certified organic acreage in the United States expanded to more than four million acres in 2008. California leads with the most certified organic cropland, with over 430,000 acres, largely used for fruit and vegetable production.

The more we demand fresh, healthy, sustainably-grown food, the more our suppliers will provide it for us. According to the Organic Trade Association, the organic foods industry grossed $26.7 billion in 2010, up from $1 billion in 1990, and sales in 2010 increased 7.7 percent over the year before. The highest growth was seen in organic fruits and vegetables, up 11.8 percent over 2009 sales. We are obviously moving slowly but surely in the right direction.

For parents concerned about the effects of pesticides used in conventional food production on their children, buying organic makes sense, according to a study at the University of Washington. Children used to eating non-organic foods were switched for five days to an organic diet and pesticide levels were measured in their urine before and after the change. The study found that some pesticides disappeared from the children's urine after eating the organic food. Previously published results showed that children consuming produce and juice grown using conventional farming practices had urine levels of some pesticide types that were five to seven times higher than for children with a 75 percent organic diet.

Research Has Shown that Plants are Alchemists

New research has shown that plants are able to extract minerals from the earth and transmute them into other substances. Albrecht von Herzeele, author of *The Origin of Inorganic Substances*, proved that, far from simply absorbing matter from the soil and the air, and in contradiction to the law of the conservation of matter, living plants are continuously creating matter. Researchers at the Agricultural Research Institute at Rothamsted in England, in experiments that spanned 17 years, found the same thing—plants were shown to be able to extract from soil samples more elements than they originally contained. Similarly, there is evidence that we too are able to transmute certain nutrients from the foods we eat into other substances that our body needs.

Vegetables

The Bottom Line

THE GOOD: Most fresh vegetables • cooked root vegetables • cooked spinach and green beans • fresh, dried and canned tomatoes • vegetables fried in good quality animal fat (lard), coconut oil or olive oil

THE NOT-SO-GOOD: Raw root vegetables, raw spinach, raw green beans

THE BAD: Most canned vegetables • some raw vegetables that might contain natural toxins

THE DOWNRIGHT DANGEROUS: Vegetables deep-fried in refined vegetable oil • most processed and frozen French fries • vegetables combined with sugar, such as candied yams and glazed carrots

CHAPTER 17

Fruit & Berries

LUSCIOUS FRESH FRUITS AND BERRIES ARE THE GLORIES of the vegetable kingdom. Who hasn't believed they were in heaven when biting into a sun-ripened peach or munching on strawberries straight from the garden? But so often, purchasing fruit can be a severe disappointment. Just think about how much money we have wasted on woolly peaches, nectarines like bullets, mushy blueberries and tasteless apples. These disgraces are usually due to the fruit being grown thousands of miles away, harvested while unripe, and transported great distances to their final destination. Fruits and berries are definitely one food category that is best consumed locally, in season.

In terms of food, rather than botany, fruits are the sweet-tasting seed-bearing parts of plants, or occasionally sweet parts of plants which do not bear seeds, such as the banana. Some foods technically considered to be fruits in botany are not considered fruits in cuisine because they lack the characteristic sweet taste, such as tomatoes and avocados.

Fruits are touted as essential for a healthy diet. The American Cancer Society recommends eating five or more servings of fruit and vegetables each day, but that is a bit vague, and could be interpreted by some people to mean five bananas per day! Other dietary guidelines call for five to thirteen servings of fruit and vegetables daily, a whopping amount. Lumping fruit and vegetables together as one category in this way is clearly not a good idea.

Back in the hunter-gatherer days, humans ate fruits when they were in season, usually for only a few weeks in a year. But now that there is plenty of fruit available in food markets all year long, much of it imported from warmer climes, we feel that we have *carte blanche* to eat them freely. Fruit tastes yummier than vegetables so it's easy to overdose. But it's a mistake to think that fruit and vegetables have the same nutritional values. Vegetables can be eaten liberally, but fruit should be eaten in moderation as they contain a high level of fructose. Fructose, or fruit sugar, can be a problem in the diet because it is metabolized in the liver, not in the bloodstream like glucose, and then circulates in the blood as triglycerides. When these triglycerides reach a high enough level in the blood, they are deposited as fat in the body. So, despite what we have been led to believe, fruit is high in carbohydrates that can be stored as fat, and many nutritionists now suggest that we eat no more than three servings of fruit per day. For some people, moderation in fruit-eating may be even more important, because over-indulging can cause allergic reactions that lead to hives, hay fever, and digestive disturbances, and for some with severe allergies, anaphylactic shock. And others can have a fructose-malabsorption issue, which can cause digestive disturbances after eating certain fruits.

That said, fruits and berries contain some of the most powerful healing compounds known to man, and in certain cases act as important medicinal plants. For example, blueberries are rich in polyphenols, a type of antioxident that is anti-inflammatory and has been shown to be protective against Alzheimer's and other age-related changes in the brain. Cherries, cranberries, blackberries and goji berries also contain healing polyphenols. And papaya and pineapple contain proteolytic enzymes, meaning that they digest proteins, and thus provide a wide variety of health benefits. Note that conventional wisdom tells us that bananas are high in potassium, but in fact they contain only half the potassium that is found in an equivalent amount of green vegetables.

The old Welsh proverb, "an apple a day keeps the doctor away," is, like much of the wisdom passed down to us from earlier generations, actually grounded in fact, and is probably one of the best things you can do for your health—but make sure it's organic.

Comparative Vibrational Levels of Health and Disease States	Bovis Units	Comparative Nutritional Levels of **Fruits and Berries**
10,000 = Level of Optimal Health e.g. a healthy newborn baby / hunter/gatherer tribes	10,000	Organically-grown fresh fruit, dried fruit and frozen fruit • Wyman's canned wild blueberries
	9,500	Conventionally-grown fresh pineapple, grapefruit, tangerines, mangoes • Oregon tart red cherries, canned in water
	9,000	Conventionally-grown cantaloupe melon, pineapple • Batth Farms raisins • Sun-Maid currants
	8,500	Conventionally-grown pomegranates, Kiwi fruit, red grapes, honeydew melon, oranges, dates • Dole raisins • Sun-Maid raisins
	8,000	Conventionally-grown bananas, apples, raspberries, plums, prunes, green grapes, apricots, lemons, limes
	7,500	Conventionally-grown pears, blueberries, blackberries, cranberries, cherries, watermelon, peaches
	7,000	Conventionally-grown strawberries, nectarines • Musselman's apple sauce
	6,500	
AVERAGE LEVEL OF HEALTH IN USA		
Inflammation	6,000	
Arthritis starts to manifest	5,500	
Heart Disease starts to manifest	5,000	Mott's apple sauce • Sun-Maid Dried Fruit Bits, Mixed Fruit
Cancer cells form: Breast, Prostate, Lung, Colon, Pancreas	4,500	
Diabetes • Osteoporosis	4,000	Del Monte canned peaches, pineapple, mandarin oranges, grapefruit (in fruit juice)
Lymphoma • Leukemia • Dementia	3,500	
Congestive heart disease Brain cancer • Multiple sclerosis	3,000	
Breast cancer metastasizes	2,500	Mariani Banana Chips
Prostate cancer metastasizes • Common cold/ flu	2,000	
Melanoma	1,500	
Metastatic bone and lung cancer	1,000	Sun-Maid Yogurt Raisins
	500	Libby's Canned Fruit Mix in light syrup • Del Monte Canned Pear Halves & Fruit Cocktail in light syrup
	50	Del Monte Canned Peaches, Pineapple, Mandarin Oranges in light syrup • Ocean Spray Craisins Aurora dried cranberries • Glace cherries • Crystallized and candied fruit
Decay and Death	0	

BETTER HEALTH (arrow up) / WORSENING HEALTH (arrow down)

Measured in Bovis Units of Life Force Energy

Pesticides in Fruit & Berries

Fruit crops have the dubious distinction of having the highest amounts of herbicides and pesticides sprayed on them. The worst culprits, in order of danger, are peaches, apples, blueberries, nectarines, strawberries, cherries, grapes, pears, raspberries, plums and oranges. One chemical, methyl parathion, accounts for more than 90 percent of the total toxicity load of peaches, apples, and pears. The fruits that were found to have the lowest levels of herbicides and therefore can be eaten without too much worry are pineapples, mangos, Kiwi fruit, cantaloupe, tangerines, and grapefruit. All fruit should be washed before eating, since it does reduce toxin levels to some degree, but other pesticides are absorbed into the plant and cannot be washed off.

Bananas are typically grown with one of the highest pesticide loads of any tropical crop, but they actually present little risk of pesticide ingestion to the consumer. But the environment where they are grown is heavily contaminated, so, in order to protect the environment, choose organic bananas—they cost only a small amount more than those that are conventionally-grown, and taste better too. Surprisingly, domestically-grown cherries were found to be three times more contaminated than their imported counterparts, which were among the cleanest fruits and vegetables analyzed.

Three independent studies found that children whose mothers were exposed to common agricultural pesticides were more likely to experience a range of harmful effects to their cognitive development, including lower IQ, as well as impaired reasoning and memory. The peer-reviewed studies, all funded by the National Institutes of Health, found links between delayed cognitive development and both dietary and environmental exposure to some of the most widely used agricultural pesticides. Many other studies have raised additional concerns about pesticides, and recently, the President's Cancer Panel issued a report highlighting the link between exposure to environmental contaminants, including pesticides, and increased risks of cancer. Shortly thereafter, a study published in the journal *Pediatrics* concluded that exposure to organophosphate pesticides at levels common among U.S. children may contribute to the prevalence of attention deficit hyperactivity disorder (ADHD) in these children. All the more reason to choose fruit and berries that have been organically-grown.

Natural Poisons Exist in Fruit

All plants seem to contain a small amount of toxin, most often cyanide, as a natural defense against insects and animals that might eat them. Plants also produce toxic alkaloids primarily designed to help protect them from insects, which are usually found in the leaves, stem and roots—the parts of the plant that it does NOT want to get eaten. Ripe fruit is generally free of toxins, and is also why fruit tastes so good and looks so tempting—the plant wants them to be eaten! The fruits of plants contain seeds which need to be dispersed so that new plants can grow, and one of the ways this can happen is when animals eat the fruit and deposit the seeds via excretion far from the original plant.

Cherries, plums, apricots, and peaches contain highly poisonous compounds in their leaves and seeds. When the seeds of cherries are crushed or chewed, they produce prussic acid (hydrogen cyanide), so don't suck on or chew cherry pips. Apple seeds also contain cyanide but in much smaller doses—you would need to chew and consume a lot to get sick. But never give apple cores containing seeds to dogs.

Rhubarb stalks and leaves contain notable quantities of oxalic acid, which is a nephrotoxic and corrosive acid that is present in many plants, but the stems are edible and non-toxic. Symptoms of poisoning include kidney disorders, convulsions and coma, but it is rarely fatal. Rhubarb needs to be cooked with a sweetener added, and is commonly combined with strawberries to make strawberry-rhubarb pie in early summer.

Elderberry trees are covered in spring with thousands of fragrant white flowers which are used for making elder flower champagne and for flavoring soda. But the berries are poisonous and will cause severe stomach problems. A good wine can be made from elderberries as the fermentation process neutralizes the toxins, but NEVER eat raw elderberries or drink raw elderberry juice—the result can be catastrophic.

Allergies to Fruit

Some people have the great misfortune to be allergic to fruit, mostly berries such as strawberries. There are many different reactions but the most severe is pseudoanaphylaxis, similar to allergic anaphylaxis except that it does not involve a true allergic response. But in susceptible people, strawberries act as a histamine liberator and this reaction is very serious. A more common reaction to strawberries is called oral allergy syndrome (OAS), tingling and swelling in the mouth, which usually develops in individuals who already suffer from hay fever allergies. People with an allergy to red strawberries might be able to tolerate the new white or yellow varieties. Allergists estimate that 70 percent of people with allergic rhinitis, or hay fever, have some form of OAS. Other reactions can mimic hay fever, causing dermatitis or hives, and breathing difficulties. Some people break out in an itchy rash after over-indulging, which is very easy to do in strawberry season. All the more reason to eat fruit only when it's in season, as you are far less likely to build up a sensitivity to foods if you only eat them for a few weeks each year.

Salicylates are chemicals that naturally occur in various plants and are chemically similar to aspirin. Although salicylates are a natural substance, some people experience an allergic reaction when exposed to even a small amount. Salicylates are found in blackberries and other common fruits including cherries, oranges, prunes, pineapple, dates, grapes, raspberries, plums, and blueberries. Symptoms can develop immediately after ingesting the fruit, causing itchy skin, hives, or eczema. Sinuses can become congested, and itchy, watery and red eyes are a common symptom of a salicylate intolerance, as well as shortness of breath and wheezing. In rare instances, anaphylaxis may develop, a life-threatening reaction that could cause death.

With mild allergies, sometimes just peeling the fruit is enough to solve the problem, as most of the allergy-inducing proteins are found in the peel or skin. You can also place the fruit in a microwave oven for around 30 seconds, which will denature the proteins but not cook the fruit. Or cut the fruit open and let it sit so that oxidation will cause digestive enzymes to be released and break down the proteins.

Fructose Malabsorption

Fructose malabsorption, formerly named "dietary fructose intolerance," is a digestive disorder in which absorption of fructose is impaired by deficient fructose carriers in the small intestine. It is found in more than 30 percent of the population of Western countries and Africa, and in about 10 percent of the population of Asia. About 50 percent of people with Type O blood are thought to suffer from fructose malabsorption. This condition is common in people with irritable bowel syndrome. Symptoms include bloating (from fermentation in the small and large intestine), diarrhea and/or constipation, flatulence, stomach pain (as a result of muscle spasms, the intensity of which can vary from mild and chronic to acute but erratic), vomiting (if great quantities are consumed), and early signs of mental depression. Other symptoms include aching eyes, "fuzzy head" or "brain fog," and fatigue.

A small proportion of people with both fructose malabsorption and lactose intolerance also suffer from celiac disease. Sufferers may benefit by avoiding foods containing sorbitol. Sorbitol is present in some diet drinks and foods, and occurs naturally in some stone fruits and berries. They should also avoid xylitol and other sugar alcohols, such as erythritol, mannitol, and other ingredients that end with -tol, commonly added as sweeteners in commercial foods.

People with fructose malabsorption should avoid fruits and foods that contain more fructose than glucose. These include apple, pear, guava, honeydew melon, papaya, quince, star fruit, watermelon, dried fruit (apple, currant, date, fig, pear, raisin, sultana), fortified wines, and foods containing added sugars, such as agave nectar, some corn syrups, and fruit juice concentrates. Fructose levels in grapes varies depending on ripeness and variety.

Fruits with fructose level equal to or less than glucose includes stone fruits (apricot, nectarine, peach, and plum—but be careful as these fruits also contain sorbitol), berry fruits, citrus fruits, and other fruit such as ripe banana, kiwi fruit, passion fruit, pineapple, and rhubarb.

Canned Fruit

As with all foods, when they are sweetened with sugar they lose much of their nutritional value, though fruit canned in fruit juice is marginally healthier. Frozen fruit fares better, though the process is most successful for berries, such as blueberries.

Fruit & Berries

The Bottom Line

THE GOOD: All organically-grown fruit and berries, fresh or dried, eaten in moderation • fruit desserts made with organic ingredients and sweetened with honey or maple syrup

THE BAD: Fruit canned in fruit juice

THE DOWNRIGHT DANGEROUS: Fruit canned in sugar syrup • dried cranberries with added sugar • fruit pies and desserts made with sugar added as a sweetener

CHAPTER 18

Fruit Juice

THE QUESTION WE NEED TO ASK ABOUT FRUIT JUICE is not what kind of juice is good for us, but whether it's good for us at all. "There are not many things in life I am sure of, but one of them is that juice is harmful to nearly everyone, ESPECIALLY children," writes Dr. Joseph Mercola in an article on his website www.mercola.com.

People think of fruit juice as a healthy food, but in fact, human beings are not meant to drink their calories. It turns out that fruit juice has just about as much sugar as soft drinks—an eight-ounce glass of fruit juice contains the equivalent of eight spoonfuls of sugar—and the fact that the sugar comes from fruit doesn't make it any better for us. Sweet liquids like fruit juice, high in sugar and with no material substance, enter the blood stream rapidly and cause problems with blood sugar levels which can lead to diabetes and obesity. With obesity reaching epidemic proportions in the U.S., taking a hard look at whether fruit juice is just adding empty calories to our diets is long overdue.

Most fruit contains two sugars, a more-or-less equal balance between glucose and fructose. When you eat a whole fruit, it takes longer for the sugar to break down in the body because the fruit contains natural enzymes, nutrients, and fiber. But the fructose in fruit juice, when separated from other nutrients in the whole fruit, becomes a refined unnatural product which is difficult for the body to deal with. Fructose is metabolized in the body through very specific pathways that differ from those of glucose, and heavy fructose consumption can result in obesity due to the proliferation of fat cells around vital organs, and can trigger the early stages of diabetes, heart disease, and liver disease. Under normal circumstances, when a person eats 120 calories of fructose, 40 calories are stored as fat. But if they eat the same number of calories from glucose, only 6 calories get stored as fat. This huge difference in how much extra fat is stored from fructose is why consuming large amounts can be even more dangerous than sugar.

Fructose is now the number one source of calories in the American diet and, besides causing obesity and diabetes, it can be a factor in the development of a number of other common diseases, including high blood pressure, inflammation, oxidative stress, endothelial dysfunction, microvascular disease, kidney injury, and fatty liver disease. But the delusion that fructose is an acceptable form of sugar is prevalent in many nutritional circles, and it has been promoted as being healthier than glucose because it registers lower on the glycemic index—in other words, it enters the blood stream more slowly than glucose. But its effects on the body are far more serious.

A study from 2008 showed that drinking just one glass of orange juice a day can significantly increase a person's risk of diabetes. The researchers followed the long-term health of 70,000 female nurses over an 18-year period and found that women who had one glass of fruit juice a day increased their odds of developing type 2 diabetes by 18 percent. Many nutritionists and the new U.S. dietary guidelines both agree on the same recommendation: it is better to eat whole fresh fruit than to consume fruit juice. Of course, a small amount of fruit juice occasionally does not present a problem, but drinking juice regularly on a daily basis is not a good idea, nor is allowing children to drink juice. And starting the day with a glass of processed orange juice is one of the worse things a person can do for their waistline, no matter what the ads tell us.

> "The inconvenient truth, many experts say, is that 100% fruit juice poses the same obesity-related health risks as Coke, Pepsi and other widely vilified beverages. 'It's pretty much the same as sugar water,' said Dr. Charles Billington, an appetite researcher at the University of Minnesota. 'In the modern diet, there's no need for any juice at all.' "
>
> —*Karen Kaplan, writing in the* **Los Angeles Times**

Comparative Vibrational Levels of Health and Disease States		Comparative Nutritional Levels of **Fruit Juice, Fruit Drinks & Fruit Cocktails**
10,000 = Level of Optimal Health e.g. a healthy newborn baby / hunter/gatherer tribes	10,000	Fresh-squeezed organic fruit and vegetable juices, unpasteurized
	9,500	Mountain Sun Pure Cranberry, unsweetened • Mott's Garden Blend vegetable • Lakewood pomegranate • Walnut Acres Organic Harvest Apple • Welch's Black Cherry/Concord Grape
BETTER HEALTH	9,000	Knudsen Organic Grape • Lakewood Organic Black Cherry Juice • Welch's Concord Grape • V-8
	8,500	Tropicana Grapefruit Juice
	8,000	Tropicana Orange Juice • V-8 Juice "Hot & Spicy" • Campbell's Tomato Juice
	7,500	V-8 Tomato Juice • Hood Orange Juice
	7,000	Cumberland Farms Orange Juice • Hood Apple Juice • Hood Fruit Punch
	6,500	Nantucket Nectars Apple Juice
AVERAGE LEVEL OF HEALTH IN USA Inflammation	6,000	Cumberland Farms Apple • Mott's Apple • Sunsweet Plum Smart • Apple & Eve Apple, Cranberry
WORSENING HEALTH Arthritis starts to manifest	5,500	Sunsweet Prune Juice • Ocean Spray Ruby/Tangerine • Mott's Plus for Kids' Health & Immune Support
Heart Disease starts to manifest	5,000	Tropicana Lemonade • Snapple Apple • Mott's Tots apple/white grape • Ocean Spray cranberry blend
Cancer cells form: Breast, Prostate, Lung, Colon, Pancreas	4,500	Ocean Spray orange juice • Minute Maid orange juice
Diabetes • Osteoporosis	4,000	Snapple grapeade • Snapple kiwi & strawberry • Hood lemonade • Juicy Juice & Minute Maid apple
Lymphoma • Leukemia • Dementia	3,500	Juicy Juice: Berry, Cherry, Grape
Congestive heart disease Brain cancer • Multiple sclerosis	3,000	Juicy Juice: Apple-Raspberry, Mango, Orange-Tangerine, Strawberry-Banana, Sparkling Apple Ocean Spray Cranberry Juice Cocktail & Apple • Hawaiian Punch, all flavors • Capri Sun, all flavors
Breast cancer metastasizes	2,500	Ocean Spray Cranberry-Blueberry-Blackberry • Ocean Spray Blueberry-Lemonade
Prostate cancer metastasizes • Common cold/ flu	2,000	Ocean Spray Light Cranberry Juice Cocktail • Ocean Spray Diet Cranberry Juice Drink
Melanoma	1,500	
Metastatic bone and lung cancer	1,000	
	500	Koolaid, all flavors • Crystal Light, all flavors
	50	
Decay and Death	0	

Measured in Bovis Units of Life Force Energy

Fruit Juice Leads to Obesity and Other Problems, Starting in Childhood

"People incorrectly think juice is natural and healthy simply because it's extracted from fruit. But there's nothing natural about extracting juice from fruit. It's the fruit in its entirety that's good for you. Drinking juice—even if it says '100% natural'—is no better than drinking soda."

—Dr. Robert H. Lustig, professor of pediatric endocrinology at UCSF and director of the Weight Assessment for Teen and Child Health Clinic

Children are the largest consumers of fruit juice in the United States and, experts say, juice is undoubtedly contributing to the rise in childhood obesity. But the high-glycemic nature of these beverages can cause other problems, such as hyperactivity.

Cautions food expert Dr. Joseph Mercola, "The high sugar content [of fruit juice] will play havoc with their neurotransmitters and is one of the main contributing factors to ADHD (hyperactivity). It will also contribute to colds, dental decay and chronic ill health."

Elizabeth Ward, registered dietitian and author of *Healthy Food, Healthy Families: Feeding Your Child from Birth to Six Years Old*, says parents often view juice as healthy and think that if a little is good, a lot is better. The American Academy of Pediatrics recommends limiting preschoolers to four or six ounces of juice per day, and are telling parents that infants who drink too much fruit juice may become malnourished if the beverage replaces human milk or formula. And babies may be at risk for digestive problems from certain types of juice. The study found that sensitive infants were more likely to suffer from gas and sleep problems after drinking apple juice, which contains high concentrations of the sugars sorbitol and fructose. They also found that infants with digestive symptoms were more likely to have tried fruit juice at an earlier age than other babies. The results of the study, which supports the American Academy of Pediatrics' recommendation to avoid giving babies fruit juice until they are at least six months of age, may help those parents who suffer from sleepless nights due to their child's colic. These children may well have fructose malabsorption (read more about it in the chapter on Fruit & Berries.) There is nothing wrong with giving children plain water to drink—in fact, they need it.

Gout is Caused by Fructose Consumption

Gout used to be regarded as a kind of joke, something that 18th century kings suffered from. But it's no joke to those who suffer from it, and sadly it's enjoying a revival. Gout is an extremely painful form of arthritis caused by uric acid crystals that arise from consuming too much fructose. Fructose is the ONLY sugar that raises uric acid levels, and drinking too much fruit juice, or soda sweetened with HFCS, will increase a person's risk of developing gout. If left untreated, gout can become increasingly painful and lead to joint damage.

One study found that women who drank 12 ounces or more of processed orange juice a day, or two or more cans of soda sweetened with HFCS, were more than twice as likely to develop gout. Women who drank just one six-ounce glass of juice per day or one can of soda were at 41 percent and 74 percent greater risk, respectively. The study concluded that: "The culprit appears to be fructose . . . fructose increases levels of the chemical uric acid, which causes gout. When uric acid levels in the body get too high, the acid hardens into sharp crystals that are deposited in joints."

The Truth about Orange Juice

Real fresh-squeezed orange juice lasts only a few days, as most of us know from experience. So if orange juice purchased in a store lasts for weeks, or even months, it is by definition a processed food.

You would think that the flavor of orange juice would vary from batch to batch, because not every orange tastes exactly the same. But the truth is, the uniform orange flavor of commercially-produced orange juice comes from a formulated additive that gives each carton of juice the same taste.

When oranges are squeezed to make commercial fruit juice, the juice is stored in giant holding tanks and the oxygen is removed, which allows the liquid to keep for up to a year without spoiling. But this process makes the juice completely flavorless, so "flavor" has to be added back into the juice. Juice companies hire flavoring experts to engineer flavor packs to give the orange juice its familiar flavor and make it taste "fresh."

According to the Food Renegade website: "Flavor packs aren't listed as an ingredient on the label because technically they are derived from orange essence and oil. Yet those in the industry will tell you that the flavor packs, whether made for reconstituted or pasteurized orange juice, resemble nothing found in nature." One of the substances used is a chemical called ethyl butyrate, a compound that's added to perfume as well as orange juice in order to make it taste and smell like oranges.

Another issue is that many commercial producers of orange juice use fruit that is substandard and may be contaminated with mold from bruising and other damage, and some people are very sensitive to these mold toxins.

Alissa Hamilton J.D., PhD, a Food and Society Policy Fellow with the Institute for Agriculture and Trade Policy, reveals the truth about mass-produced orange juice in her book, *Squeezed:*

What You Don't Know About Orange Juice. One review of this book says, "It's a potent reminder of just how important it is to really understand how your food is manufactured and processed because the label tells neither the whole story nor the whole truth."

If you would like to wean yourself or your children off orange juice, start by diluting it with water, and slowly keep diluting it every day until it's almost plain water, which can be flavored with a slice of lemon. Or switch to a healthier juice, such as organic black cherry or pomegranate, and dilute it half and half with sparkling water. And remember that there is far more healthy nourishment in a whole orange than in a glass of processed orange juice.

However, though not a perfect food, a glass of processed orange juice is still a better choice than a can of soda—it's the quantity consumed that is the real issue here.

The Truth about Apple Juice

Apples and apple juice have a very high sugar content, with a higher percentage of fructose than glucose. Apples also contain sorbitol, a naturally occurring but indigestible sugar. Many people have a sensitivity to sorbitol—even drinking small amounts of apple juice may cause problems, and especially with young children. A study on rats published in the December 2006 issue of the *World Journal of Gastroenterology* revealed that diarrhea triggered by sorbitol is the result of the intestine's inability to absorb this compound. Some artificially sweetened apple juice may contain added chemical sorbitol.

Apple juice also contains oxalates, so it should be avoided by those with a tendency towards kidney stones. An article published in the *American Journal of Epidemiology* indicates that study participants who consumed 240 mL of apple juice each day demonstrated a 35 percent increase in their risk of forming kidney stones.

Apple juice can also contain mold from the skins, to which some people are very sensitive, especially the mycotoxin patulin, a toxin produced by the *P. expansum, Aspergillus, Penicillium,* and *Paecilomyces* fungal species. *P. expansum* is especially associated with a range of moldy fruits and vegetables, in particular rotting apples and figs. It is destroyed by the fermentation process and so is not found in hard cider. Patulin has been reported to damage the immune system in animals, and in 2004, the European Community set limits to the concentrations of patulin in food products.

"I strongly suggest not drinking apple juice," says food expert David Lawrence Dewey. "Even though juices are pasteurized, heated to kill bacteria and most fungus, apple juice has the highest capability of breeding more of the fungus as it sits on the shelf." Juices that contain the least amount of fungus after sitting on a shelf are cranberry, papaya, white or red grape, and pineapple.

• Arsenic-Laced Apple Juice from China

In the last 10 years, the amount of food the U.S. imports from the People's Republic of China has grown enormously. According to the group Food & Water Watch (F&WW), more than 70 percent of the apple juice consumed in the United States now comes from China, where the government has acknowledged problems enforcing new food safety laws. Sometimes juice companies like Mott's and Nestle's Juicy-Juice will have the countries of origin (including China) stamped or listed on the back of the packages, and Veryfine brand, which claims to be an American classic, uses Washington apples . . . from China. "Veryfine Juices are a great way to start any day. Apple juice concentrate product of Germany, Italy, Argentina, and China," says their website.

F&WW reports that China still uses arsenic-based pesticides in farming, and it has called on the FDA to test more imported foods. The FDA tests less than two percent of imported food and have never set tolerance levels for arsenic and heavy metals. The request for FDA action came after F&WW and its partner, the Empire State Consumer Project, announced the results of tests by Paradigm Environmental Services showing that samples of Mott's Apple Juice had arsenic levels of 55 parts per billion. The U.S. Environmental Protection Agency limits arsenic in public drinking water to 10 parts per billion, so some apple juice drinkers may have unknowingly been consuming unsafe levels of arsenic for years.

It has been found that exposure to arsenic is related to poor scores in language, memory, and other brain functions. Michael Harbut, M.D., chief of the environmental cancer program at Karmanos Institute in Detroit, says, "Given what we know about the wide range of arsenic exposure sources we have in this country,

"PepsiCo Inc. is returning to using only oranges from Florida in its Tropicana Pure Premium orange juices, a decision made several months ago, before low levels of fungicide were found in oranges from Brazil, the company confirmed on Monday. Tropicana Pure Premium had used 100 percent Florida oranges until 2007, when problems with the Florida crop caused the company to look at alternative sources."

—*featured article in the* **Chicago Tribune,** *January 16, 2012*

I suspect there is an awful lot of chronic, low-level arsenic poisoning going on that's never properly diagnosed."

And Joshua Hamilton, Ph.D., a toxicologist specializing in arsenic research and the chief academic and scientific officer at the Marine Biological Laboratory in Woods Hole, Massachusetts, says, "People sometimes say, 'If arsenic exposure is so bad, why don't you see more people sick or dying from it?' But the many diseases likely to be increased by exposure even at relatively low levels are so common already that its effects are overlooked simply because no one has looked carefully for the connection."

Symptoms of chronic exposure to arsenic can initially cause gastrointestinal problems and skin discoloration or lesions. Exposure over time, which the World Health Organization says could be five to twenty years, could increase the risk of various cancers, high blood pressure, diabetes, and reproductive problems. Signs of chronic low-level arsenic exposure can be mistaken for other ailments such as chronic fatigue syndrome.

In the U.S., apple juice is considered an appropriate drink for toddlers and children, but the evidence indicates that this attitude needs to change.

Yes, There are Healthy Fruit Juices!

Of course, the best juice is freshly-made from organic fruit, but several companies make excellent juices, including Walnut Acres, Mountain Sun, Knudsen, and Lakewood, available at health food stores and some grocery stores and supermarkets. Top of the list are black cherry, pomegranate, grape, and blueberry. Pomegranate juice is wonderful to make at home if you have a juicer—it's a difficult fruit to eat without juicing it, and it doesn't need a sweetener. Cranberry juice is also good to make at home, but it does need to be sweetened and is good blended with other fresh fruit, such as Concord grape, which usually can be harvested from the vine or bought in stores at the same time of year that cranberries are in season.

Fruit Juice

The Bottom Line

THE GOOD: Fresh squeezed juice made from organic or home-grown fruit • bottled organic juices not made from concentrate such as Walnut Acres, Welch's, Mountain Sun, Knudsen and Lakewood

THE NOT-SO-BAD: Some processed orange, grapefruit, and apple juice, including Tropicana and Snapple

THE BAD: Certain brands of processed and pasteurized juice, such as Juicy Juice, Minute Maid, Mott's and Ocean Spray

THE DOWNRIGHT DANGEROUS: Processed and pasteurized fruit juice with added sugar or high fructose corn syrup • any fruit juice imported from China and certain other countries • some brands of blended fruit juice and fruit cocktails, such as Hawaiian Punch and Capri Sun • Koolaid • Crystal Light • commercial processed lemonade

CHAPTER 19

Beverages: Water, Tea, Coffee and Soft Drinks

WHEN WE LOOK AT THE LIST OF BEVERAGES on the charts opposite we become aware of the wide range of substances we imbibe, from water, coffee and tea to alcohol, fruit juice, sodas and milk-based drinks such as shakes and ice cream sodas—a lot of choices when all the body really needs is water. The main problem with many of these beverages is that they contain extra calories, most of them "empty" calories, and in fact, statistics show that we now consume nearly twice as many calories from beverages as we did 30 years ago.

We live on a planet where more than 70 percent of the earth's surface is covered with water. Without water, life would never have developed on earth. Water is essential for life and is the major constituent of almost all life forms, accounting for 50 to 75 percent of the weight of plants and about 70 percent of the weight of the human body. Water content is highest in a newborn infant but it progressively decreases from birth to old age. We can exist without food for about a month, but without water we can only survive for a few days. Water performs many functions in the body—it is essential for digestion, nutrient absorption and elimination; aids circulation; controls the body's temperature; lubricates and cushions joints; keeps the skin healthy; and helps remove toxins from the body.

Every civilization throughout time has valued water and many celebrated its source, usually a spring in the mountains that fed a mighty river. Many of these springs and fountains were attributed magical properties and some sites used in ancient worship were built atop scared springs, including medieval cathedrals in Europe. Water from the sacred spring at Lourdes is still venerated and continues to provide healing properties. Native Americans also worshipped springs where they believed nature spirits dwelled.

Water forms the base of most of the beverages we drink, so it follows that the higher the quality of the water used, the healthier the beverage. Coffee and tea made from spring water calibrate higher than if made from city tap water, for instance, and the same is true for milk-based drinks—a milk shake made with organic milk, fresh fruit and honey would calibrate a lot higher than one from McDonald's, for instance. As for soft drinks, they are simply sweetened water, carbonated to add fizz, and flavored with a variety of fruit and edible roots, such as in ginger ale and root beer, not to mention the substance that originally gave Coca-Cola its oomph—kola leaves. In fact, some people call soda "liquid candy. But everyone must know by now that drinking soda is not healthy, and especially not for children—an estimated 56 percent of eight-year-old children drink soda daily, and once the teenage years come, some kids drink three cans of soda each day or more. So just say no, for you AND your kids. Drinking soda on a regular basis is one of the worst things anyone can do for their health.

"The essence of a human being is water . . . All that lives must vibrate . . . each cell must vibrate . . . No vibration means death . . . vibration cannot continue forever without something causing it. Water carries vibration, the source of energy. We must pay respect to water, feel love and gratitude, and receive vibrations with a positive attitude. Then, water changes, you change, and I change. Because both you and I are water."

— *Masaru Emoto, author of* **The True Power of Water**

The Physical Properties of Water

Water is actually formed from two gases, oxygen and hydrogen, and is the only substance on earth that exists in all the three physical states: solid, liquid and gas. Water has historically been viewed as an inert solvent, but in fact it always contains different elements or particles in solution or in suspension. So there is actually no such thing as pure water.

Unadulterated water has a neutral pH, so it is neither acidic nor alkaline. But since it is an excellent solvent, its pH changes according to what it has recently absorbed, so that rain water, for example, is acidic because it contains some carbon dioxide and other substances, while mineral water tends to be alkaline because of the particles of basic minerals it contains.

Water at first glance seems to have a simple atomic structure, consisting of two atoms of hydrogen bonded to one atom of oxygen—the familiar formula of H_2O, or more correctly, dihydogen monoxide. But recently, is has been found that water is a much more complex element than originally thought. The nature of the structure of water causes its molecules to have unique electrochemical properties; the hydrogen side of the water molecule has a slight positive charge, while the other side has a negative charge. This polarity means that water is a powerful solvent, and also has a high surface tension, making it adhesive and elastic, so it tends to form drops rather than spread out over a surface as a thin film. It is water's high surface tension that allows for the formation of water droplets and waves.

Any wave can carry information in the form of energy. Waves transmit energy through a material, often called a medium. Water waves carry energy through liquid water, sound waves carry energy through air (and many other media), and seismic waves carry energy through the earth. The latest research shows that water carries information, and it is believed that this is how homeopathic remedies work, by absorbing and transmitting the healing "energy" or information of a substance in the water with which the substances are mixed.

Water also has a high specific heat and can absorb large amounts of heat energy before it begins to get hot. This helps moderate the earth's climate and enables organisms to regulate their body temperature more efficiently.

How Much Water Do We Need?

Though no one can say exactly how much water we need on a daily basis, getting enough water is important. Every day we lose water from the body through urine and sweat, and this fluid needs to be replenished. An important bodily mechanism—thirst—tells us when to replenish our supply. When our body begins to lose from one to two percent of its total water, our thirst mechanism lets us know that it's time to take in some water. The thirst mechanism works better when we are young. As we age, we can confuse the urge to drink with the urge to eat so older adults should make sure they drink water regularly—when older people feel hunger, it's good a idea for them to drink a glass of water before eating something. Of course, people will require more water when the weather is hot or they are engaged in exercise or other vigorous activity.

Various recommendations of how much water we need range from eight glasses a day to one quart for every 50 pounds of body weight. But an article in *Family Practice Newspaper* by an Institute of Medicine Panel states that on a daily basis people get enough water from normal drinking behavior, such as drinking beverages at meals and in other social situations, and by letting their thirst guide them. If you are healthy, drinking whenever you feel thirsty should be an adequate guide of how much water you need. Some physicians advise people to determine if they are drinking enough from the color of their urine. Urine should be a very light-colored yellow, if it is a deeper color, then it's likely they are not drinking enough water.

There is no recommended upper limit to how much water we can take in because healthy individuals have the ability to excrete excess water and maintain an adequate water balance. However, acute water toxicity has been reported due to the rapid consumption of large quantities of fluids that greatly exceeded the kidney's ability to excrete it, which is at the rate of approximately 0.7 to 1.0 liter per hour. Exercise scientist Dr. Tim Noakes, the author of *Waterlogged: The Serious Problem of Overhydration in Endurance Sports*, reports that at least a dozen deaths have occurred in endurance events due to drinking too much fluid. He believes that athletes have been encouraged to drink too much water while participating in strenuous events, and cites research that has found that overhydrating actually worsens athletic performance, not improves it.

What Kind of Water is Best?

Obviously, it's best to drink fresh, pure water from a natural source. Rural well water is good, but it's not an option for people who live in the suburbs, as well water in built-up areas can be contaminated with nitrates and other groundwater pollutants. Municipal tap water is disinfected with chlorine, often laced with fluoride, and contains residues of toxins, chemicals and pharmaceutical drugs.

Bottled water is often no better than tap water. Dasani, for instance, is not spring water but filtered tap water bottled and distributed by Coca-Cola. Bottled water can cost anywhere between $0.89 to $8.26 per gallon while the price of tap water at the average house costs about $0.002 per gallon. The bottling process has also turned out to be a huge strain on the environment which is one reason why filtering our own water is so important. A reverse-osmosis filtering system can be a very

Comparative Vibrational Levels of Health and Disease States	Bovis Units	Comparative Nutritional Levels of **Water & Soft Drinks**
10,000 = Level of Optimal Health e.g. a healthy newborn baby / hunter/gatherer tribes	10,000	Spring water from source • unpolluted river water and sea water • rain water • some well water
	9,500	Poland Spring • Fiji • Volvic • Evian • Gerolstein • Acadia • San Pellegrino in glass bottle
	9,000	Poland Spring sparkling • O-Water • Aquafina • Acadia flavored sparkling
	8,500	Most rural municipal tap water • Dasani • Sobe Life Energy • San Pellegrino in plastic bottle • Vitamin Water • Nestle Pure Life • Schweppes Club Soda
	8,000	Most municipal city tap water
	7,500	Perrier • Propel • Skinny Water • Polar Seltzer • Distilled water
	7,000	
	6,500	Clear Splash • Powerade Zero
AVERAGE LEVEL OF HEALTH IN USA Inflammation	6,000	Powerade Sports Drink
Arthritis starts to manifest	5,500	Gatorade Perform
Heart Disease starts to manifest	5,000	
Cancer cells form: Breast, Prostate, Lung, Colon, Pancreas	4,500	
Diabetes • Osteoporosis	4,000	
Lymphoma • Leukemia • Dementia	3,500	Pepsi • Schweppes Ginger Ale • Schweppes Tonic Water
Congestive heart disease Brain cancer • Multiple sclerosis	3,000	Schweppes Diet Ginger Ale • Schweppes Diet Tonic Water
Breast cancer metastasizes	2,500	Canada Dry Ginger Ale
Prostate cancer metastasizes • Common cold/ flu	2,000	Coca Cola • Diet Pepsi
Melanoma	1,500	Sprite • Fresca • Fanta • 7-Up • Minute Maid Lemonade • Waist Watcher's Diet Sod • Generic supermarket sodas
Metastatic bone and lung cancer	1,000	Diet Coke • Sprite Zero • Generic supermarket diet sodas
	500	
	50	
Decay and Death	0	

BETTER HEALTH (arrow up, 6,500–10,000)

WORSENING HEALTH (arrow down, 6,000–0)

Measured in Bovis Units of Life Force Energy

cost-effective device to install under the sink. But remember that plastic water containers can leach unsafe chemicals into water, especially Bisphenol A (BPA), an endocrine disrupter which alters the function of the endocrine system by mimicking the role of the body's natural hormones. So use a glass or metal bottle to store filtered water at home or when you go on trips.

Soda and Soft Drinks

It is estimated that the average American drinks around 50 gallons of sweetened soda drinks per year. The sweeteners used in sodas are highly refined sugars, unnatural substances which give the body a huge jolt, especially when combined with caffeine and phosphoric acid, which gives soda its fizz and is highly acidic to the body. Research has shown that drinking just one can of soda per day increases a person's risk of diabetes by 85 percent over time, and the effect on children is more severe than in adults.

Americans spend more than $66 billion a year on carbonated drinks and many have no idea what a negative affect on their health this habit can have. Manufacturing, distributing and advertising soft drinks is BIG business. Coca-Cola, for instance, spends more than $2.9 billion a year on advertising, much of it aimed at children. Again, it's greed-driven, with the goal of using the cheapest ingredients—in this case, water, sweetener and flavorings—to realize the greatest profits. And if the ingredients are addictive, so much the better for business.

According to Dr. Robert Lustig in his lecture "The Real Truth About Sugar," which has had over two million views on YouTube, Coca-Cola is specially formulated to cause addiction and thirst. The main ingredients of Coke are caffeine, which is a mild stimulant and diuretic, and salt, about 55 mg per can. A hefty dose of sugar, or high fructose corn syrup, is added to mask the taste of the salt, and phosphoric acid is pumped in which adds fizz to help the concoction go down. (Ever tried drinking a warm, flat Coke? It's undrinkable.) But when ingested together, claims Dr. Lustig, this mixture actually makes you *more thirsty,* not less, and so people drink more of it. He calls this the "Coca-Cola Conspiracy" because he believes "they knew what they were doing."

It has been proven again and again that a diet high in sugar exacts a toll on emotional health as well as physical health. A study published in the journal *Psychology Today* found a strong link between high sugar consumption and the risk of both depression and schizophrenia. A diet high in sugar, fructose, and sweetened beverages like soda also causes excessive insulin release, which can lead to falling blood sugar levels, or hypoglycemia. Hypoglycemia, in turn, causes the brain to secrete glutamate in levels that can cause agitation, depression, anger, anxiety, and panic attacks.

Drinking soda is linked to numerous health problems among children and adults, including obesity, liver disease and even violent behavior—new research shows that frequent soft drink consumption is associated with a 9 to 15 percent increase in aggressive behavior. Schools that have taken soda machines out of their cafeterias have reported a lower level of disruptive behavior in the schools and higher test scores. The Fizzy Drink Study in Christchurch, England, explored the effects on obesity when soda machines were removed from schools for one year. Obesity stayed constant in the schools where the machines were removed, but in schools where soda machines remained, obesity rates continued to rise. However, the soft drink industry disagrees with the most obvious of facts, that sugar and high fructose corn syrup cause obesity. Says Richard Adamson, a scientist from the National Soft Drink Association, "There is no association between sugar consumption and obesity."

Diet Soda

Diet soda is actually worse than regular soda. Diet soda contains artificial sweeteners, such as aspartame and sucralose (Splenda), instead of sugar and high fructose corn syrup. These artificial sweeteners are toxic chemicals that have been silently damaging people's health for the past 30 years. Regular consumption of aspartame and Splenda have been suspected of causing such symptoms and diseases as lymphoma, leukemia, brain cancer, asthma, headaches, depressed and anxious mood, seizures, memory loss, hallucinations, dizziness, visual changes, weakness and fatigue, joint pain, sleep disorders, weight gain and diabetes, abdominal cramps, nausea, vomiting and diarrhea, rashes and hives.

And there is no evidence that these chemicals help with weight loss—in fact, it has been found that the sweet taste from artificial sweeteners stimulates the same surge of insulin that real sugar causes, so there is no benefit in that respect. Many scientists now agree that artificial sweeteners may interact with our body's sense of sugar satisfaction, believing that artificial sweeteners confuse our taste buds. Sharon P. Fowler, MPH, and colleagues at the University of Texas Health Science Center in San Antonio, studied more than 1500 people between the ages of 25 and 64, looking at whether each consumed regular or diet soft drinks. They found a correlation between the daily consumption of multiple cans of all soft drinks and obesity, which was expected, but they also found that the risk of obesity was *even higher* with the consumption of diet soda. The researchers found that for each can of diet soft drink consumed per day, the risk of obesity went up by 41 percent.

Researchers at the American Stroke Association's International Stroke Conference in 2011 reported that drinking diet soda may also cause stroke, heart attacks, and other lethal vascular events. The researchers concluded that: "This study suggests that diet soda is not an optimal substitute for sugar-sweetened beverages, and may be associated with a greater risk of stroke, myocardial

Comparative Vibrational Levels of Health and Disease States		Comparative Nutritional Levels of **Coffee, Tea and Related Drinks**
10,000 = Level of Optimal Health e.g. a healthy newborn baby / hunter/gatherer tribes	10,000	Herbal teas • Green and white tea • Fresh unpasteurized cow and goat milk • Any of these sweetened with a natural sweetener such as raw honey, maple syrup or stevia
	9,500	Organic black tea made with spring water
	9,000	Organic coffee made with spring water • Organic hot chocolate made with organic milk & raw honey
	8,500	Regular black tea made with well water, no milk
	8,000	Horizon organic milk • Average local dairy milk
	7,500	Regular black tea made with city tap water, no milk
	7,000	Nescafe made with city tap water
	6,500	Coffee from Starbucks, Dunkin' Donuts, McDonald's, no cream or sugar • Black tea w/milk & sugar
AVERAGE LEVEL OF HEALTH IN USA Inflammation	6,000	
Arthritis starts to manifest	5,500	
Heart Disease starts to manifest	5,000	Average supermarket milk
Cancer cells form: Breast, Prostate, Lung, Colon, Pancreas	4,500	
Diabetes • Osteoporosis	4,000	Starbucks coffee with cream, no sugar • Dunkin' Donuts hot chocolate • Lipton iced tea
Lymphoma • Leukemia • Dementia	3,500	Dunkin Donuts coffee with cream, no sugar • Burger King fat-free milk
Congestive heart disease Brain cancer • Multiple sclerosis	3,000	Starbucks coffee with cream and sugar • Lipton diet green tea
Breast cancer metastasizes	2,500	Dunkin' Donuts coffee with cream and sugar • McDonald's milkshake • Nestea • Ensure "Immune Health" shake
Prostate cancer metastasizes • Common cold/ flu	2,000	Generic coffee-shop coffee with cream and sugar • Dunkin' Donuts iced latte, mocha • Burger King vanilla shake • Nestle's hot chocolate • Ensure "Nutrition Shake"
Melanoma	1,500	Dunkin' Donuts iced latte, caramel • Starbucks Coffee Frappuccino, Chai Latte • Yoohoo chocolate drink
Metastatic bone and lung cancer	1,000	Starbucks Caramel Frappuccino • Wendy's Frosty milkshake • Arizona iced tea
	500	Wendy's caramel apple frosty parfait • Burger King Oreo® sundae shake, chocolate • Arizona sweet tea
	50	Flavoring syrups such as Chocolate, Caramel, Butterscotch, and Strawberry
Decay and Death	0	

BETTER HEALTH ↑ / WORSENING HEALTH ↓

Measured in Bovis Units of Life Force Energy

infarction, or vascular death than regular soda."

If you are the type of person who keeps your intake of sugar and high fructose corn syrup under control, then as a treat, it's fine to drink the occasional Coke—and sometimes there's nothing better on a hot summer's day, or if you have an upset stomach. But stay away from diet sodas altogether. Diet soda is NOT healthier than regular soda.

Coffee and Tea

Compared with the evils of soda, there's not much negative press about our favorite hot beverages, coffee and tea. Yes, people who are sensitive to caffeine would be advised to minimize their caffeine intake, but there are many good quality decaffeinated versions of coffee and tea to choose from.

In the tea category, herbal teas and green and white tea are the healthiest choices; black tea calibrates a little lower on the scale as it is smoked, as does coffee, due to the roasting and grinding process. Beyond that, the health level of the beverage depends upon the quality of the water used to make it, and its additives, such as sugar and milk. As has been stated before in this book, when you add sugar to any food item, its health level plummets, and it's the same with coffee and tea. For instance, a cup of Starbucks coffee with cream and sugar calibrates at 3,000, the level of heart disease, while a cup of organic coffee made from spring water with organic raw milk added and honey as sweetener would calibrate at 9,000, a very healthy level.

One way we can vote with our wallet to protect the environment as well as our health is to purchase organic, shade-grown, free-trade coffee, and to patronize coffee shops that sell these products and support these principles. And start asking your favorite cafe to provide organic milk or cream, and honey as a sweetener.

How to Revitalize Water

Well water or tap water can be revitalized at home by this method: fill a glass pitcher with filtered water and swish it around vigorously with a metal spoon. This will allow the water molecules to reorganize, in the same way as water cascading over a waterfall reinvigorates the molecules. It represents the difference between the molecular structure of stagnant water and a rushing stream, or when you take a bath and when you take a shower—the water in the shower is much more invigorating. Tap water can also be revitalized by the sun's energy by leaving it outdoors in sunlight in a glass container for a day, or about eight hours of daylight.

Water, Tea, Coffee and Soft Drinks

The Bottom Line

THE GOOD: Spring water from an unpolluted source • vitalized well water • some brands of imported mineral water in glass bottles • coffee, black tea, and herbal tea made with spring water, organic dairy products and honey

THE NOT-SO-GOOD: Municipal tap water and beverages made with it • filtered tap water in plastic containers • carbonated water, which is very acidic

THE BAD: Sports drinks • tea and coffee sweetened with sugar and conventional dairy products

THE DOWNRIGHT DANGEROUS: Sodas and soft drinks sweetened with sugar, high fructose corn syrup or artificial sweeteners • diet sodas • sweetened milk-based drinks such as milkshakes and ice cream sodas

CHAPTER 20

Beverages: Beer, Wine & Spirits

"Fermented dietary beverage . . . was so common an element in the various cultures that it was takenfor granted as one of the basic elements of survival and self-preservation . . . thus, while alcohol has always been misused by a minority of drinkers, it has proved to be beneficial to most."

— David J. Hanson, Ph.D., Professor Emeritus of Sociology at the State University of New York and an expert on alcohol

THROUGHOUT HISTORY, ALCOHOL HAS BEEN HIGHLY VALUED and has been used since the earliest days of our civilization for a variety of purposes, including pleasure, nutrition, medicine, ritual, and a source of currency.

Alcohol, or ethyl alcohol (ethanol), refers to the intoxicating ingredient found in wine, beer and hard liquor. Alcohol arises naturally from carbohydrates when certain micro-organisms metabolize them in the absence of oxygen, a process known as fermentation. The first use of alcohol by humans was probably the result of an accident, a fortuitous contamination of fruit juice or other rustic beverage by wild yeasts. Many of us will remember discovering when we were young that raw apple cider would turn delightfully fizzy after sitting for a few days due to natural yeasts causing it to ferment.

In earlier days, alcoholic beverages were sources of needed nutrients and were also used for their medicinal, antiseptic and analgesic properties. Levels of amino acids and vitamins increase during fermentation so it is possible to achieve nutritional enrichment naturally through fermentation. In ancient Egypt, the phrase "bread and beer" stood for all food and was also a common greeting. Many alcoholic beverages, such as Egyptian bouza and Sudanese merissa, contain high levels of protein, fat and carbohydrates, a fact that helps explain the frequent lack of nutritional deficiencies in some populations whose diets are generally poor but whose populace consumes alcohol.

These days, drinking alcohol is considered normal social behavior for much of the world's population, and is a way of relaxing, especially when in the company of others. Alcohol can serve as a social lubricant, provide pharmacological pleasure, and enhance the flavors of food, and the consumption of alcohol is an important part of American society, considered an appropriate activity when socializing.

Though alcohol has famously been misused by a minority of drinkers, there is much evidence that it plays an important role in enhancing the enjoyment of life for millions of people. In the words of the Founding Director of the National Institute on Alcohol Abuse and Alcoholism: ". . . alcohol has existed longer than all human memory. It has outlived generations, nations, epochs and ages. It is a part of us, and that is fortunate indeed. For although alcohol will always be the master of some, for most of us it will continue to be the servant of man."

Though alcohol should be regarded as a recreational drug with potentially serious adverse effects and should be treated as such, it is evident that the consumption of alcohol has played an important role in generally enhancing the enjoyment and quality of life.

"I believe the intrinsic hado [life force energy] of alcohol is good. It merges with both water and oil. It is a rare substance that can bridge between water, spirituality, and materialism. Alcohol is considered to have a *hado* [energy, or vibration] that we humans need."

— Masaru Emoto, author of **The True Power of Water**

A Brief History of Alcohol Use From Earliest Times

The discovery of late Stone Age beer jugs suggests that intentionally fermented beverages existed at least as early as the Neolithic period, about 10,000 years B.C. The art of wine making was evident in Greece by about 2,000 B.C., though the first alcoholic beverage to obtain widespread popularity in that area was mead, a fermented beverage made from honey and water. By 1,700 B.C., wine making was commonplace, and during the next thousand years wine was used for medicinal purposes, was incorporated into religious rituals, and became important in socializing and an accompaniment to daily meals. As a beverage, it was drunk in many ways: warm or chilled, pure or mixed with water, plain or spiced.

Wine and beer were the common alcoholic beverages consumed up until the Middle Ages when the process of distillation was discovered. Knowledge of this process spread slowly among monks, physicians and alchemists, who were interested in distilled alcohol as a cure for ailments. At that time it was called *aqua vitae*, "water of life," but was later known as brandy. This distilled alcohol, or spirits, were largely used for medicinal purposes throughout most of the 16th century. It has been said of distilled alcohol that "the 16th century created it; the 17th century consolidated it; the 18th century popularized it."

In the 17th century, Dom Perignon, the wine-master of a French abbey, developed the method for making sparkling wine, now known as champagne, but it took another century before the problems of bursting bottles and suitable corks could be solved and champagne would become popular.

The Virginia colonists, who arrived in North America in the 17th century, brought with them the traditional belief that alcoholic beverages were a natural food and were beneficial when used in moderation. These first colonists brought their beer-making skills with them, as they considered it essential to their well-being. The Puritan minister Increase Mather preached in favor of alcohol but against its abuse: "Drink is in itself a good creature of God, and to be received with thankfulness, but the abuse of drink is from Satan; the wine is from God, but the Drunkard is from the Devil."

Early Consumption of Wine

The consumption of wine has been widely noted throughout world literature from the earliest times, including in the Bible. But there is some evidence that this beverage so often referred to—or translated—as "wine" was little more than preserved fruit juice. Wine drinking was initially seen as a way to preserve fruit juice, rich in Vitamin C, so abundant in the summer months but scarce in the winter. The Roman author and philosopher Pliny wrote about wine that was always sweet and was produced with care. Early records suggest that casks of fresh fruit juice were plunged into water and kept there until cold weather set in. Since the juice was kept below 40 degrees F, the yeast settled to the bottom and the wine did not ferment. This juice, or wine, was often given to children, so it would make sense that it had a very low alcohol level. Personally, I find I am able to drink my neighbor's home-made wine in Italy, which is pure fermented grape juice—it gives me no hangover and no headache, and is in fact the only wine I can drink with no side effects. If this is the kind of "wine" that is referred to in our historical documents, reflecting the customs of earlier times, then it bears little resemblance to the tipple that is transported halfway across the world and laced with preservatives, clarifiers, and sweeteners. As the chart on the right shows, home-made wine tops the charts as being healthy, while bottled wine calibrates much lower.

Alcoholic Beverages Were an Antidote to Water Pollution and Food Poisoning

Water pollution plagued citizens in earlier times, and city dwellers had little option but to drink the water from polluted rivers which often served as open sewers. Coffee and tea were not introduced into Europe until the mid 17th century and it would be another hundred years or more before they were commonly consumed on a daily basis, so alcoholic beverages such as wine, beer and mead were drunk freely if potable water was not available.

From early times, it was also considered preferable to drink wine with meals rather than water, since drinking alcohol was believed to guard against food poisoning. And in fact, according to a recent article in the *New York Times*, drinking alcohol with a meal has been proven to lower the risk of food poisoning, or at least reduce its effects. It appears that the higher the alcoholic content or proof of the beverage, the more protective it is against food poisoning. Scientists at Oregon State University have demonstrated the ability of alcohol to kill salmonella, shigella, listeria, and E-coli in the laboratory. In laboratory studies, the wine's combination of ethanol, organic acids, and low pH appeared to scramble the genetic material of bacteria. All wines have some effect, say researchers, but red wines are the most potent.

The Downside

The International Agency for Research on Cancer of the World Health Organization has classified alcohol as a Group 1 carcinogen. Its evaluation states, "There is sufficient evidence for the carcinogenicity of alcoholic beverages in humans [to classify]

Comparative Vibrational Levels of Health and Disease States		Comparative Nutritional Levels of **Beer, Wine & Spirits**
10,000 = Level of Optimal Health e.g. a healthy newborn baby / hunter/gatherer tribes	10,000	Homemade beer • Homemade and local wine, unbottled • Champagne Ayala by Bollinger (no sugar)
	9,500	Moet et Chandon & Bollinger French champagne (sugar added in fermentation)
BETTER HEALTH	9,000	Organic wine, bottled • local wine, bottled • Krug and Taittinger champagne • Beck's lager
	8,500	Italian red wine • All Australian wine • Stella Artois lager • Draft Guinness • Micro-brewed beer
	8,000	Italian white wine • California wine • Korbel sparking wine • Bottled Guinness • Corona beer • Coors beer • Heineken beer • St. Pauli Girl lager
	7,500	French red wine • Molson's beer • Miller beer
	7,000	French white wine • Budweiser beer • Chilean wine
	6,500	Spanish wine • Argentinian wine
AVERAGE LEVEL OF HEALTH IN USA Inflammation	6,000	
WORSENING HEALTH Arthritis starts to manifest	5,500	
Heart Disease starts to manifest	5,000	Bloody Mary (vodka and tomato juice)
Cancer cells form: Breast, Prostate, Lung, Colon, Pancreas	4,500	Irish Whiskey • Grappa (Italian brandy)
Diabetes • Osteoporosis	4,000	French Brandy • Bourbon • Rye Whisky • Meyer's Jamaican Rum • Southern Comfort
Lymphoma • Leukemia • Dementia	3,500	Johnny Walker Red Whisky • Jack Daniels • Absolut Vodka • Creme de Cassis
Congestive heart disease Brain cancer • Multiple sclerosis	3,000	Gordon's Gin • Vodka & tonic • Tia Maria • Crown Royal Reserve Canadian Whisky
Breast cancer metastasizes	2,500	Gordon's Gin & tonic • Pastis
Prostate cancer metastasizes • Common cold/ flu	2,000	Classic Martini • Cape Codder Cocktail • Kahlua • Ouzo
Melanoma	1,500	Manhattan Cocktail • Long Island iced tea • Grand Marnier • Baileys Irish Cream • Curaçao • Absinthe
Metastatic bone and lung cancer	1,000	Liqueurs: Courvoisier, Chartreuse, Amaretto, Drambuie • Godiva Caramel Liqueur
	500	
	50	Margaritaville margarita mix • Master Of Mixes strawberry margarita daiquiri mix, pina colada mix
Decay and Death	0	

Measured in Bovis Units of Life Force Energy

alcoholic beverages as carcinogenic to humans." And the U.S. Department of Health & Human Services' National Toxicology Program listed alcohol as a known carcinogen in 2000.

The long term effects of consuming alcohol range from possible health benefits to severe detrimental effects in cases of chronic alcohol abuse. Long-term use of alcohol in excessive quantities is capable of damaging nearly every organ and system in the body, and the developing adolescent brain is particularly vulnerable to its toxic effects. Heavy alcohol consumption can cause cardiovascular disease, pancreatitis, liver disease, and cancer. Some studies, however, do show a beneficial effect from consuming low amounts of alcohol, due most probably to the relaxing effect of alcohol on the body.

The National Council on Alcoholism and Drug Dependence states that drinking alcohol is associated with a wide range of accidents and injuries resulting from the impaired performance of complex mental and motor functions. The relationship between alcohol and motor vehicle accidents is well known, and alcohol has also been implicated in many railroad, boating, and aircraft accidents. The subtlety and complexity of the skills required to operate these vehicles make them susceptible to impairment by low doses of alcohol. Drinking by U.S. workers in the work place can threaten public safety, impair job performance, and result in costly medical, social, and other problems affecting employees and employers alike. Productivity losses attributed to alcohol on an annual basis can be measured in the billions of dollars.

Heavy alcohol consumption can contribute to malnutrition. At seven calories per gram, alcohol is an energy-rich substance, like pure sugar, and the more calories an individual consumes as alcohol, the less likely it is that they will eat enough food to obtain adequate nutrients. To make matters worse, chronic alcohol abuse also interferes with the body's metabolism of nutrients. Alcohol is absorbed and metabolized very rapidly in the body, unlike solid food, which requires time for digestion. About 20 percent of alcohol is absorbed directly across the walls of an empty stomach and can reach the brain within one minute.

Since drinking alcohol is such an accepted part of modern Western life, learning to drink responsibly is essential. In a *Time* magazine article "Should You Drink with Your Kids?" John Cloud wrote: "Jews, Italians, Greeks, French, Spaniards, Portuguese and many others typically introduce their children to alcoholic beverages at an early age. And they tend to have fewer alcohol-related problems than we do in the U.S. In these groups, people learn how to drink from an early age and do so in the safe and supporting environment of the home. Common sense suggests that it's better to learn how to drink in the parents' house than in the fraternity house."

Beer, Wine & Spirits

The Bottom Line

THE GOOD: Homemade wine and beer • organic bottled wine and beer • artisan-made and imported European beer • naturally fermented champagne (no sugar added)

THE NOT-SO-GOOD: Bottled wine and champagne containing preservatives, clarifiers and added sugars • mass-produced beer

THE BAD: Distilled liquor

THE DOWNRIGHT DANGEROUS: Liqueurs (distilled liquors with added sugar) • cocktails and mixed drinks • distilled liquors mixed with tonic water and soda containing high fructose corn syrup

CHAPTER 21

Oils and Fats

OF ALL THE DIFFERENT FOODS WE EAT, it is probably our choice of fats and oils that has the most profound impact on our health. Fats are the building blocks of our cell membranes, and certain fats are very beneficial to our body, while others, including refined vegetable oils and rancid seed oils, can be seriously bad for our health.

Since the beginning of time, members of the human race have consumed fats and oils in their diet as valuable nutrients for health and energy. Fat is a concentrated source of energy and each tribe or nation that settled in different parts of the world adopted the kind of dietary fat that was readily available from local sources—olive oil in Southern Europe, lard and butter in central and northern Europe, duck fat in South West France, flax oil in Eastern Europe, ghee (clarified butter) in India, sesame oil in Asia, coconut oil in tropical climes, and so on. And for millennia, the world's population remained pretty healthy on that diet, not having been told they should eat otherwise. But in the last 40 years or so, it became the fashion in the U.S. and much of the Western world to view fat, and especially saturated fat, as unhealthy and to be avoided. But in fact, saturated fat is a necessary part of our diet.

Cholesterol is essential for good health and there has been no greater controversy regarding what the "experts" advise us to include or avoid in our diet than the idea that saturated fat causes heart disease. Despite overwhelming evidence to the contrary, the idea still prevails that high levels of serum cholesterol are dangerous and cause arterial disease. In numerous studies performed over four decades, researchers have been unable to prove that patients with heart disease had higher levels of cholesterol in their blood than healthy subjects, nor that the total amount of dietary fats consumed had any effect on cholesterol levels in the blood. Yet these myths have been perpetuated by the health care industry who profits from treating "high" cholesterol levels in the blood.

Fats come in two types: saturated and unsaturated. Saturated fat, such as butter and lard, is hard at room temperature, while unsaturated fat is not. Unsaturated fat can be monounsaturated or polyunsaturated: monounsaturated fats are liquid at room temperature and include olive, sesame, almond, and peanut oils; polyunsaturated fats stay liquid even when refrigerated and include corn, sunflower, and soybean oils, as well as fish oils. Saturated fats have an advantage in that they are more stable when stored at room temperature, and also when used at high temperatures. In fact, many consider the much maligned lard to be the best fat to use for deep-frying, just as our grandmothers did, as vegetable oils when heated to high temperatures for deep-frying are unstable and have been shown to become carcinogenic. Coconut oil, which is a saturated vegetable fat, is also stable at high temperatures and is a good alternative to lard.

Some fats are essential to our diets and these are called essential fatty acids, or EFAs. We need both omega-3 and omega-6 fatty acids in our diets, but it's important to get the balance right—the average American diet has a higher ratio of omega-6 fatty acids compared to omega-3 fatty acids, which causes inflammation in the body leading to a host of degenerative diseases.

One of the most critical issues about fats and oils is how long they can be safely stored. Rancid fats and oils are toxic to the body, causing premature aging, poor skin condition, and compromised cell membrane health. Naturally-occurring oils and fats properly protected from light, heat and oxygen are safe to eat and for this reason butter, lard, olive oil, and coconut oil are especially good because of their stability when stored for long periods, up to a year or more, in a cool, dark place. Unsaturated fats are more delicate and great care must be taken with them to prevent oxygen, heat and light from damaging the molecules, otherwise they quickly go rancid.

The Role of Fats and Oils in Our Diet

Fats and oils are certainly an important part of our diet, but what's crucial is the type and quality of the fats and oils that we consume. Quite simply, good quality oils and fats are beneficial, while highly-refined vegetable oils and fats are incredibly bad for us.

Fats and oils are essential for the building and maintenance of the cells in our bodies. Biologists estimate that the multi-celled organism that is our body has between 60 and 90 trillion individual cells. The health of each cell, and therefore our entire body, is fundamentally dependent on the health of the structure of these cells, especially the cell membrane.

Just as protein is made up of amino acids, so fats are comprised of fatty acids. When we digest the fat in our food, it is broken down into fatty acid molecules of various lengths. These are made up of short, medium, and long chain molecules comprised of many essential fatty acids connected together. Our body then uses these fatty acids as raw materials to assemble the special types of fat it incorporates into its cell membranes. About two-thirds of the substance of our brain is composed of fats, and the membranes of neurons—the specialized brain cells that communicate with each other—are composed of a thin double-layer of fatty acid molecules. Myelin, the protective sheath that covers communicating neurons, is composed of 30 percent protein and 70 percent fat.

In addition, fat carries important fat-soluble vitamins, such as A, D, E, and K, into and around the body. Vitamin K2, which is found in butter, cheese, egg yolks, beef, and fish liver, is the most bone-building and bone-healing of them all and is protective against blood vessel disease and calcification of the aortic valve, which is yet more evidence that limiting healthy animal fats can actually CAUSE heart disease, not prevent it.

Dr. Bruce West, founder of Health Alert/Immune Systems, Inc., has written: "The more fake oils, margarines and 'heart-healthy' fake foods you eat, the worse your deficiency of vitamin K2 will become. The worse your deficiency of vitamin K2 becomes, the faster your arteries will clog with calcium. The faster your arteries clog with calcium, the sooner you will be faced with aortic sclerosis. And the sooner you are diagnosed with aortic sclerosis, the sooner you will get aortic stenosis with its resultant left-side heart disease and bloating, weakness, heart failure and finally death. It is just that simple."

The Importance of Saturated Fat in Our Diet

Saturated fat became the whipping boy of Western diets in the middle of the 20th century when Americans were persuaded by the medical profession that a diet based on meat, butter, and eggs was unhealthy and instead they should eat such "heart healthy" foods as margarine, Egg Beaters, soy, and vegetable oils. But this diet has now been revealed to have been disastrous for the health of the nation—in the 40 years or so since these dietary guidelines were first adopted, rates of cancer, heart disease and diabetes have sky-rocketed, not decreased.

While some plants make cholesterol in very small amounts, all foods comprised of animal protein contain cholesterol to varying degrees. Major dietary sources include cheese, egg yolks, beef, pork, lamb, poultry, fish, and shrimp. Human breast milk also contains significant quantities of cholesterol.

Cholesterol is an essential structural component of cell membranes and is required to establish proper membrane permeability and fluidity. But despite this obvious need for cholesterol, the medical profession, the drug companies and the media still tout the "cholesterol is bad" message, and it's in their financial interest to do so, as blood tests for measuring cholesterol levels in the blood and sales of drugs designed to lower cholesterol levels continue to ring the cash register. And with print media pretty much supported these days by ads from the pharmaceutical industry, who would expect *Time* magazine, for instance, to write a candid article about the value of saturated fat in our diet when on the next page is a three-page ad spread for cholesterol-lowering drugs? The full story of how this travesty came to be foisted on the American public is described in detail by Gary Taubes in his book, *Good Calories, Bad Calories.* It's a fascinating read, even though it is a depressing example of how the public can be manipulated by bad science and successful lobbying, and how severe the consequences can be. It is not an exaggeration to say that this single idea has caused more confusion, suffering, sickness and death than just about any infectious epidemic in the U.S. ever did.

> "From the inception of the diet-heart hypothesis in the early 1950s, those who argued that dietary fat caused heart disease accumulated the evidential equivalent of a mythology to support their belief. These myths are still passed on faithfully to the present day."
>
> — *Gary Taubes, author of* **Good Calories, Bad Calories**

Comparative Vibrational Levels of Health and Disease States		Comparative Nutritional Levels of **Oils and Fats**
10,000 = Level of Optimal Health e.g. a healthy newborn baby / hunter/gatherer tribes	10,000	Organic cold-pressed oils, such as olive, walnut, flax seed, grape seed, sesame, sunflower, coconut • Lard and butter from grass-raised cattle • Fat from wild and organically-raised animals
	9,500	Kerry Gold butter (Ireland) • Organic safflower oil
	9,000	
	8,500	Refined sesame oil • Refined grape seed oil
	8,000	Second-press olive oil • Refined sunflower oil • Lard from conventionally-raised cattle • Horizon organic butter
	7,500	Earth Balance spread
	7,000	
	6,500	Refined olive oil
AVERAGE LEVEL OF HEALTH IN USA Inflammation	6,000	Hollywood Safflower Oil • PAM Olive Oil Spray • Promise Spread • Smart Balance Butter Spread
Arthritis starts to manifest	5,500	Land O' Lakes Butter
Heart Disease starts to manifest	5,000	Smart Balance Spread (canola & soy oils) • Mazola Corn Oil • Land O'Lakes Light Butter Spread with canola oil
Cancer cells form: Breast, Prostate, Lung, Colon, Pancreas	4,500	Crisco Corn Oil • Peanut Oil
Diabetes • Osteoporosis	4,000	PAM Original • Wesson Vegetable Oil (soy bean) • Crisco Soybean Oil • Land O'Lakes Margarine • Fleichmann's Margarine • "I Can't Believe It's Not Butter" Spread
Lymphoma • Leukemia • Dementia	3,500	Peanut Oil
Congestive heart disease Brain cancer • Multiple sclerosis	3,000	Wesson Canola Oil • Crisco Pure Canola • PAM Butter Flavor (canola & soy) • Omega-9 canola oil
Breast cancer metastasizes	2,500	
Prostate cancer metastasizes • Common cold/ flu	2,000	Crisco All-vegetable Shortening • Burger King Frying Oil
Melanoma	1,500	Cottonseed Oil • Frying Oil: McDonald's, Wendy's, KFC and Dunkin' Donuts
Metastatic bone and lung cancer	1,000	
	500	
	50	
Decay and Death	0	

BETTER HEALTH ↑ / WORSENING HEALTH ↓

Measured in Bovis Units of Life Force Energy

How We Have Been Manipulated into Thinking We Need Statin Drugs to Stay Healthy

Much of our understanding of the supposed dangers of saturated fat in the diet has come from the media, who are mostly passing on information fed to them by the pharmaceutical companies. Though study after study has failed to find any correlation between dietary fat consumed and either cholesterol levels or heart disease, the theory became conventional wisdom, if not "wishful science," and drug companies rushed to develop statin drugs to lower blood levels of cholesterol. Fifty years later this unproven idea still influences the medical profession, not to mention the drug companies. But the *British Medical Journal* recently reported the results of a new study showing that for every heart attack prevented by a statin drug, two or more people suffered liver damage, kidney failure, cataracts, or extreme muscle weakness as a result of taking the drug. Statin drugs, in other words, harm far more people than they help.

Lipitor® (atorvastatin) is the best known of a group of cholesterol-lowering drugs called statins, which also includes Zocor® (simvastatin) and Pravachol® (prava-statin). Lipitor® is the best-selling prescription drug in the world. Annual sales for Lipitor®, made by Pfizer, are worth about $8 billion per year in the U.S. and $11 billion worldwide. Small wonder, then, that statins are promoted as the savior against heart disease. But unfortunately, the side effects from taking statins are serious, and the benefits minimal. Statin drugs *do* block cholesterol production in the body, but they also have the effect of blocking the body's natural production of coenzyme Q-10 (CoQ10), which is essential for heart health. Supplementation with CoQ10 is necessary to avoid the very heart disease that statins seek to avoid. In a small number of cases, the statin drug's depletion of CoQ10 also led to liver disease. But how many doctors will tell you that?

Dr. Beatrice Golomb, M.D., PhD, an associate professor of medicine at the University of California at San Diego, has shared shocking information about the truth about drug trials and how the scientific methods used are manipulated and distorted by the drug industry. Apparently, drug companies publish only a fraction of the studies they fund—the ones they find advantageous to the product they plan to promote. And often those studies are submitted multiple times, obscured by different authors and details in such a way that the reader won't realize it's the same study. She also explains that in order for scientific studies to take place, someone has to pay for them, and often the funds for a drug trial are provided by the same pharmaceutical company that makes it. She states that all of the major statin drug studies were funded exclusively by the drug industry. The second-highest funder of drug studies is the National Institute of Health (NIH), which, she says, accepts sums of money from the pharmaceutical industry.

The Importance of Essential Fatty Acids

As mentioned many times elsewhere in this book, essential fatty acids are fats that cannot be synthesized by the body and are therefore "essential" parts of our diet. Animal life first originated in the sea, where there was an abundance of omega-3 fatty acids—the same fatty acids that now form the essential components of our cell membranes. EFAs are crucial for building healthy cell membranes throughout the body, and for brain cells, healthy hair and skin, for maintaining bone health, regulating metabolism, and in the function of the reproductive system.

EFAs are found in all types of fat. The two main types of EFAs are alpha-linolenic acid, an omega-3 fatty acid, and linoleic acid, an omega-6 fatty acid. Omega-3 EFAs are found in organically-raised eggs, grass-fed beef, oily cold-water fish such as salmon, sardines, herring, and mackerel, flax seeds, chia seeds, walnuts, sea vegetables, and green leafy vegetables.

Food sources of omega-6 linoleic acid include sunflower, soy, corn, and sesame oils, while black currant, borage, and evening primrose oils are good sources of omega-6 gamma-linolenic acid (GLA), considered a "conditionally essential" fatty acid. GLA is responsible for normal functioning and growth of cells, nerves, muscles, and organs throughout the body. While most omega-6 EFAs are pro-inflammatory, GLA is thought to reduce inflammation.

Unfortunately, there are now increasingly limited sources of omega-3 EFAs in our modern diets, but, by contrast, sources of omega-6 EFAs have become more numerous. Omega-6 fatty acids are everywhere in our food supply and this is causing a major problem—vegetable oils, such as soybean oil, are used in

"The long-established dietary recommendations have created epidemics of obesity and diabetes, the consequences of which dwarf any historical plague in terms of mortality, human suffering and dire economic consequences. Despite the fact that 25% of the population takes expensive statin medications and despite the fact we have reduced the fat content of our diets, more Americans will die this year of heart disease than ever before."

— *Dr. Dwight Lundell, heart surgeon, former Chief Resident at Yale University Hospital, and author of* **The Cure For Heart Disease** *and the e-book,* **The Great Cholesterol Lie**

> "Trans fats are really like plastic, and when we eat them they incorporate in our cells and the cells cannot communicate or talk to one another. In turn, hormones are disturbed, weight gain follows but more troubling, the risk for heart disease, cancer, stroke, and infertility goes up."
> — *Dr. Michael Aziz, from his book* **The Perfect 10 Diet**

most of the snack foods, cookies, crackers and bakery goods in the American diet. Soybean oil is now so ubiquitous in fast foods and processed foods that 20 percent of the calories in the American diet are estimated to come from this single source.

Before processed foods were a major part of our diets, humans consumed omega-3 and omega-6 EFAs in roughly equal amounts. Omega-6 fatty acids tend to increase inflammation, blood clotting, and cell proliferation in the body, while those from omega-3 fatty acids decrease those functions.

A dietary imbalance between these fatty acids is believed to be the cause of many modern-day disorders which appear to stem from inflammation in the body, such as asthma, coronary heart disease, autoimmunity, neurodegenerative diseases, and many forms of cancer. Experts also believe that the imbalance between omega-3 and omega-6 fatty acids may contribute to obesity, depression, dyslexia, hyperactivity, and even a tendency toward violence.

To ensure you have the right balance of EFAs in your diet, chose a diet of whole, natural foods and reduce your intake of refined vegetable oils such as corn, sunflower, safflower, soy, peanut, and cottonseed oils. Commercially-produced mayonnaise and salad dressings are big culprits—they are nearly all made with soy bean oil. Eliminating fast foods and processed foods from your diet will also dramatically reduce your intake of omega-6s.

Fish oil supplements are good source of omega-3 fatty acids in principle, but finding high quality fish oil is difficult since it can easily become rancid by the time it gets to the store. Some fish oils can be contaminated with environmental toxins, especially if the oil is from larger fish, so krill oil is a safer choice.

One way to make sure you get a good supply of omega-3 fats is to eat a can of sardines or kipper snacks a few times a week. Drain the can well and mash the fish up with a mustard-vinaigrette or mayonnaise (preferably homemade), season with chopped olives or capers, maybe a touch of lemon juice, and spread it on crackers.

EFAs and the Link with Depression

The human brain is made up of 60 percent docosahexaenoic acid (DHA), a type of omega-3 fatty acid. Low levels of omega-3 fats in the diet are known to affect levels of serotonin and dopamine in the brain, as well as compromising the blood-brain barrier which normally protects the brain from unwanted matter gaining access to its fragile tissues. Omega-3 deficiency can also decrease blood flow to the brain, which ties in with earlier studies that show that people with depression have compromised blood flow to a number of brain regions.

Scientists at the National Institutes of Health have associated the increase in the rate of depression in the U.S. during the last century with the decline in consumption of DHA (docosahexaenoic acid) in our diet during the same period. The scientists, Joseph R. Hibbeln, M.D., and Norman Salem, Jr., Ph.D., concluded that the "relative deficiencies in essential fatty acids may also intensify vulnerability to depression." They also found lower rates of depression in societies that consume large amounts of fish, a major dietary source of DHA. North American and European populations showed cumulative rates of depression 10 times greater than a Taiwanese population that consumed a lot of fish. The Japanese, whose diet is rich in fish, have a significantly lower prevalence of depression compared to North America and Europe. And researchers in Belgium found that seriously depressed patients had lower omega-3 fatty acid levels than mildly depressed patients.

Researchers have also found that suicide risk was greatest among individuals with the lowest levels of DHA when analyzing a sample of suicide deaths among U.S. military personnel on active duty between 2002 and 2008. Studies have shown that as omega-3 EFA levels rise, symptoms of depression fall, and, in fact, omega-3 fats have actually been found to work just as well as antidepressants in preventing the signs of depression, but without any of the side effects.

All the evidence points to the fact that the increase in depression and corresponding explosion of anti-depressant drugs over the past few decades could well be a result of the decrease in consumption of saturated fat and the increase in consumption of vegetable oils over that period.

How Vegetable Oils & Trans Fats Came to Be Part of Our Modern Diet

Hydrogenated fats were first introduced into the American diet at the end of the 19th century when cheap substitutes for butter began to appear on the market. Called margarine, they were made from a mix of cheaper fats and colored yellow to look like butter. At first they were made of beef suet, milk, and water, and later included lard, whale oil, and vegetable oils such as soybean oil. Soon, a method for refining cottonseed oil was discovered, and Crisco was born. This marked the beginning of a radical change in the types of fat Americans consumed in their diets.

Later, when scientists insisted that vegetable oils reduced the amount of cholesterol in blood, the food industry was off and running, capitalizing on this new hypothesis and touting butter substitutes as a healthy food, and incidentally, raising the price.

Hydrogenated fats are made by heating vegetable oils such as soybean oil in the presence of a metal catalyst and forcing hydrogen into it under pressure. This "saturates" the oil, lending stability and shelf-life to a product that would otherwise spoil quickly. The end result is partially-hydrogenated vegetable oil, with a by-product of the process being trans fat in the oil. Margarine is also made in this manner to produce a solid that can be spread. The majority of the five billion pounds of trans fats Americans consume each year comes from partially-hydrogenated cooking oils used to fry foods.

Despite evidence to the contrary, the medical profession and pharmaceutical companies continue to advise the populace to avoid cholesterol and eat more "heart-healthy" fats like vegetable oils—but vegetable oils have never been proven to be beneficial, in fact, quite the opposite. There are countless scientific studies refuting this fact, including research that found that these fats actually increase the risk of developing certain kinds of cancer. Most significantly, French researchers found that dietary trans fatty acids make their way into the myelin of brain cells, where they changed the electrical conductivity of the cells.

The Dangers of Refined Vegetable Oils

Refined vegetable oils have only been part of our diets for the past 40 to 50 years. There are no records of indigenous peoples who ever ate such oils as cottonseed or rapeseed, and many nutritionists believe these seed oils should have no place in our diet.

Ray Peat, Ph.D., a physiologist who has studied hormones and dietary fats since 1968, says that polyunsaturated fatty acids in vegetable seed oils are the bane of human health and can cause cancer, diabetes, obesity, aging, thrombosis, arthritis, and immunodeficiencies. Their only appropriate use, he says, is as ingredients in paints and varnishes.

Studies have shown that the more unsaturated a vegetable oil is, the more specifically it suppresses tissue response to thyroid hormones. Omega 6 polyunsaturated fat impairs thyroid function as well as the ability of thyroid hormones to connect with their receptor sites and stimulate the mitochondria at the cellular level. It was discovered that these unsaturated fats also contain naturally-occurring toxins and enzyme suppressors that block protein digestive enzymes in the stomachs of mammals. Plants developed these naturally-occurring substances to protect their seeds from being eaten by predators and to prevent germination until conditions are optimal for sprouting. It's no coincidence that the millions of people who eat these thyroid-damaging toxins and enzyme suppressors are experiencing an epidemic of chronic diseases.

The Truth About Canola Oil

By the late 1970s, the oil industry had a problem since it had been discovered that polyunsaturated fats (such as corn oil and soybean oil) caused an increase in cancer, while monounsaturated fatty acids, such as olive oil, were proven to be more healthy. The obvious oil to promote was olive oil, but it was too expensive to use for mass-produced products such as margarine, crackers, mayonnaise, and salad dressings.

Meanwhile, two Canadian plant breeders had developed a new genetically-modified hybrid of the rapeseed plant, a naturally toxic plant of the mustard family. This is a plant so toxic that grazing animals will not eat it. Natural rapeseed oil contains high levels of a toxic substance called erucic acid and it is grown for commercial use in paints and coatings as a drying oil. The newly developed hybrid was thought to be healthier because it had lower levels of erucic acid. The word "canola" was invented to describe this new oil: Canadian oil, low acid = can-ol-a. But in fact, canola oil is anything but healthy—it is extracted and refined at temperatures as high as 300 degrees F, treated with toxic petroleum solvents such as hexane, and undergoes a chemical process of degumming, bleaching, and deodorization—and after that kind of refining process, there simply isn't much that's nutritious left in it.

Chemically, canola oil contains 5 percent saturated fat, 57 percent oleic acid, 23 percent omega-6, and 10 to 15 percent omega-3 essential fatty acids. Even though it has a smaller percentage of omega-3 over omega-6 EFAs, some manufacturers, in a stretch of the truth, advertise canola oil as being a good source of omega-3s, such as in the product Ensure.

Canola oil has been shown to cause some serious health issues. It was found in animal experiments to retard the growth of young animals and it is for this reason that canola oil is not allowed to be used in infant formula. In 1996, the Japanese announced a study that showed a canola oil diet had killed laboratory animals, and it has also been shown to deplete the body of vitamin E. It's also bad for cell membranes—researchers at the University of Florida in Gainesville determined that as much as 4.6 percent of the fatty acids in canola oil are "trans" isomers (aka plastic) due to the refining process. It is this plastic fat that is so devastating for our health—when our body uses these plastic trans fats to build cell walls, the cell membranes become impermeable, meaning nutrients cannot get into the cells and waste products cannot exit. This causes a breakdown in the functioning of the body's cells, leading to disease.

Phase Oil

Phase oil is a "liquid butter alternative," or fake butter. When you order an item in a restaurant that requires melted butter, you are more than likely to get this oil rather than the real thing. According to the Domino's Pizza website, phase oil, which they term "butter flavored oil," contains: liquid and hydrogenated soybean oil, salt, soy lecithin, natural and artificial flavor, beta carotene (color), TBHQ and citric acid, and dimethylpolysiloxane.

A food service website describes it thus: "Phase oil is the food industry's most versatile alternative to butter. It has a unique heat-activated flavor system that provides great buttery taste in all applications." But what a shame to dunk your plump steamer clams or fresh boiled lobster into what is basically hydrogenated soybean oil! Next time, make sure you ask for real melted butter.

Omega-9 Oils are Now On The Market

An omega-9 oil derived from canola and sunflower oils has been developed by Dow AgroSciences. Although omega-9 oils are not essential fatty acids since they can be manufactured in the body from vegetable oils, this oil is being described as healthier than the partially-hydrogenated oils that the fast-food industry currently uses for frying foods. Omega-9 is the most abundant fatty acid in nature, and is found in animal fat and vegetable oils, including rapeseed, wallflower seed, and mustard seed. Bear in mind that canola oil, made from rapeseed, is already a manufactured (genetically-modified) oil.

The website www.omega-9oils.com, maintained by Dow AgroSciences, states that "trans-fat consumption alone is responsible for an estimated 30,000 premature deaths in the United States each year." Well, why don't they suggest going back to using lard, which is far healthier than this new omega-9 oil, which calibrates at the level of congestive heart disease, just the disease they are trying to avoid.

They continue: "Healthier Oils. Healthier Eating. Omega-9 Canola and Sunflower Oils represent the 'next generation' in healthier oils because they have zero trans fat, the lowest saturated fats and high heart-healthy monounsaturated fats (omega-9) without affecting great taste or functionality. More and more restaurants, food service operations and food manufacturers, concerned about the health of their food items, are making the switch to Omega-9 Oils." This gives us yet one more reason to avoid junk food, fast food, and processed food.

Choosing Healthy Fats

The best fats to eat are the ones that were consumed by our ancestors. Many nutritionists are now advising that we eat only extra-virgin olive oil and butter, and use coconut oil for frying or cooking at high heat, since it does not oxidize at a high temperature. Lard is making a comeback—it has been used traditionally for frying for centuries and can safely be heated to a high temperature so that it sears the food on the outside and therefore does not absorb much of the fat.

Coconut oil, once mistakenly believed to be unhealthy because of its high saturated fat content, is now acknowledged to possess many health giving properties. It is touted as a nutritious health food and has been described as "the healthiest oil on earth." Coconut oil has been prominent in the diets of millions of people for thousands of years, and those who still follow their traditional diet, such as Pacific Islanders, enjoy long, healthy lives. However, as a tropical oil, it is not a natural part of the diet of a person from temperate climes, so each person should see how they tolerate it.

Oils & Fats

The Bottom Line

THE GOOD: Fats from pasture-raised animals (cream, butter, lard) • extra-virgin olive oil • nut oils such as walnut and hazelnut • organically-grown fresh plant seed oils such as borage, sesame, flax, safflower, evening primrose and black currant • good quality fish oils

THE BAD: Peanut oil

THE DOWNRIGHT DANGEROUS: Refined vegetable oils, including corn, canola, soybean, and cottonseed • all oils made from GM seeds • solid vegetable fats such as margarine, Crisco, and other alternative-to-butter spreads

CHAPTER 22

Salad Dressings & Mayonnaise

IT IS QUITE SHOCKING TO LOOK AT THE CHART ON THE RIGHT and see how unhealthy bottled salad dressings are—even the sainted Paul Newman's Own dressings are made with soybean oil. I don't know if it has to do with cost or shelf life, or chutzpah on the part of the manufacturers who assume we don't know the difference, but not one of these dressings is made with 100 percent olive oil. Some advertise that they are "made with olive oil," but when you read the label, they are in fact a blend of soy, canola and olive, and the healthy olive oil is degraded by mixing it with refined vegetable oils. The truth is, it's so easy to make our own dressing, and so much cheaper too, that these prepared dressings should have no place in our shopping carts.

A crisp fresh salad deserves no less than a dressing made from virgin olive oil. And with Trader Joe's selling a one liter bottle (33.8 oz.) of extra-virgin olive oil for $5.99, there is no excuse not to make it at home. To make a salad dressing your family will love, follow this recipe: Choose a clean glass jar with a tight-fitting lid and fill it about 1/5 full with balsamic or apple cider vinegar. Add seasonings to taste such as sea salt, ground pepper, a teaspoon of Dijon mustard, a crushed garlic clove, and maybe a touch of honey or maple syrup, and shake well. Pour in olive oil to almost fill the jar and shake vigorously to blend all the ingredients. You may prefer to use fresh lemon juice instead of vinegar, and you may also want to change the proportion of oil to vinegar to suit your own personal taste. A one pint bottle (16 oz.) of balsamic vinegar, such as Monardi, sells for around $2.50 to $3, and the same amount of apple cider vinegar costs $1.19. This works out at about $2.88 for a 16 oz. bottle of balsamic vinaigrette, and $2.24 for the salad dressing made with apple cider vinegar—cheaper than Kraft Balsamic Vinaigrette, for instance, which costs $3.89 for a 16 oz. bottle at most retail outlets, and Wishbone, which costs $2.99 a bottle, both of which are made with soybean oil.

Another offender is commercially-produced mayonnaise—it is a low-grade product made from soybean oil, and after seeing where it calibrates on the chart, I banished it from my kitchen. Making mayonnaise at home is not difficult, but maybe we don't need to eat it at all—the U.S. is the only country I know of where it's the custom to make sandwiches with mayo and not butter, and by doing so, we are merely spreading soybean oil on our bread. Instead of using commercial mayo, try butter—it's healthier and tastier, and can be spread very thin when at room temperature. The best part is that the bread doesn't get soggy because the butter acts as a barrier between the bread and the sandwich ingredients.

Also really unhealthy are reduced fat or fat-free dressings, because when manufacturers cut down on the oil, they compensate by adding sugar. At the bottom of the list are the fruity dressings, nothing more than sugary concoctions with which to drench healthy salads. Remember that healthy fats like olive oil are good for you—they will not make you fat, but sugar will, so don't be fooled into buying "low fat" processed foods thinking they are healthier.

The Bottom Line

THE GOOD: Salad dressings and mayonnaise made from extra-virgin olive oil or nut oils (walnut, hazelnut) and natural sweeteners in small amounts (honey, maple syrup)

THE BAD: Most bottled salad dressings

THE DOWNRIGHT DANGEROUS: Salad dressings and mayonnaise made with soy-bean oil, which is most likely to be GM • low-fat and honey-mustard dressings made with sugar and HFCS • Sandwich Spread

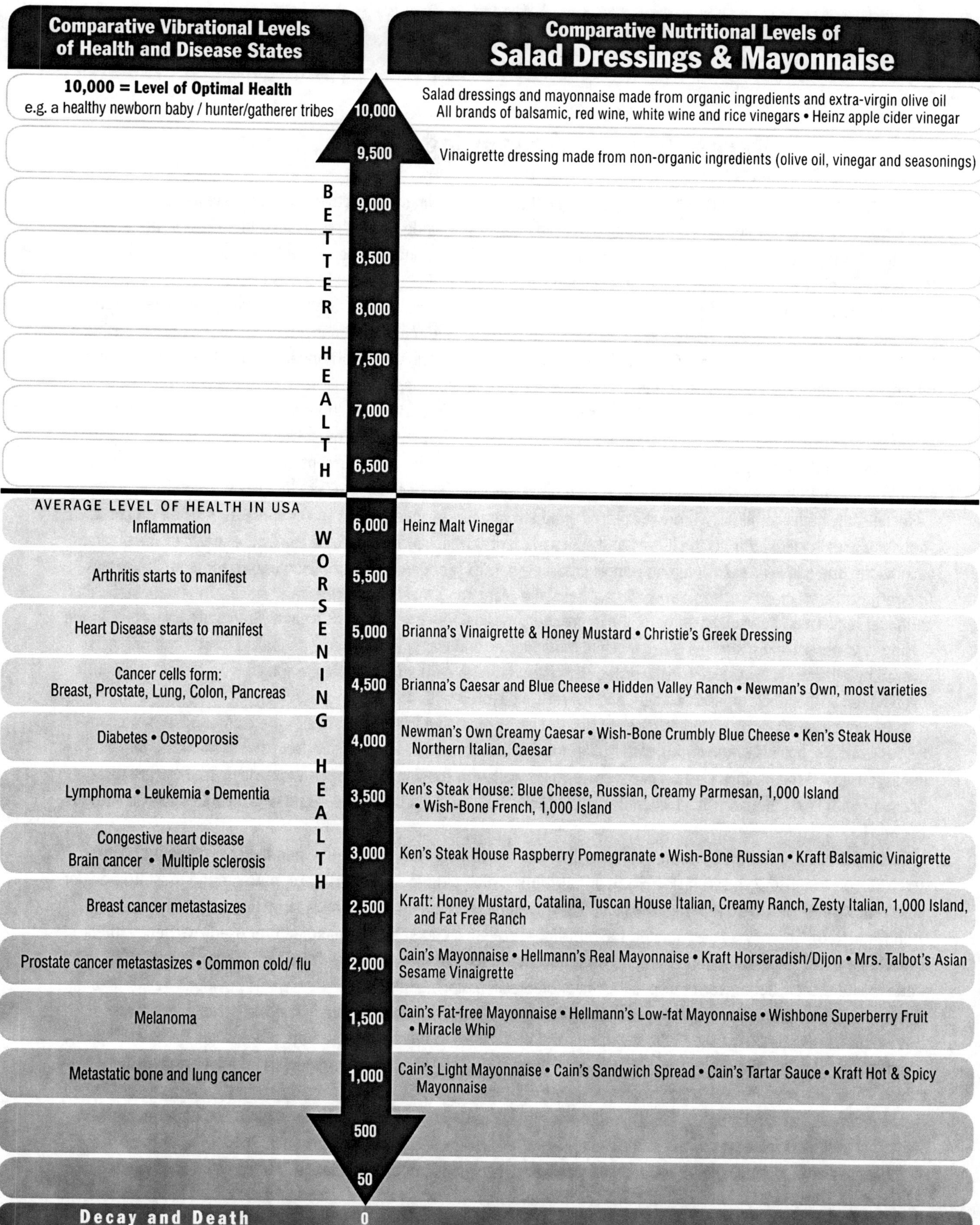

Comparative Vibrational Levels of Health and Disease States
Comparative Nutritional Levels of Salad Dressings & Mayonnaise
10,000 = Level of Optimal Health
e.g. a healthy newborn baby / hunter/gatherer tribes
10,000
Salad dressings and mayonnaise made from organic ingredients and extra-virgin olive oil
All brands of balsamic, red wine, white wine and rice vinegars • Heinz apple cider vinegar
9,500
Vinaigrette dressing made from non-organic ingredients (olive oil, vinegar and seasonings)
9,000
8,500
8,000
7,500
7,000
6,500
BETTER HEALTH
AVERAGE LEVEL OF HEALTH IN USA
Inflammation
6,000
Heinz Malt Vinegar
Arthritis starts to manifest
5,500
Heart Disease starts to manifest
5,000
Brianna's Vinaigrette & Honey Mustard • Christie's Greek Dressing
Cancer cells form:
Breast, Prostate, Lung, Colon, Pancreas
4,500
Brianna's Caesar and Blue Cheese • Hidden Valley Ranch • Newman's Own, most varieties
Diabetes • Osteoporosis
4,000
Newman's Own Creamy Caesar • Wish-Bone Crumbly Blue Cheese • Ken's Steak House Northern Italian, Caesar
Lymphoma • Leukemia • Dementia
3,500
Ken's Steak House: Blue Cheese, Russian, Creamy Parmesan, 1,000 Island • Wish-Bone French, 1,000 Island
Congestive heart disease
Brain cancer • Multiple sclerosis
3,000
Ken's Steak House Raspberry Pomegranate • Wish-Bone Russian • Kraft Balsamic Vinaigrette
Breast cancer metastasizes
2,500
Kraft: Honey Mustard, Catalina, Tuscan House Italian, Creamy Ranch, Zesty Italian, 1,000 Island, and Fat Free Ranch
Prostate cancer metastasizes • Common cold/ flu
2,000
Cain's Mayonnaise • Hellmann's Real Mayonnaise • Kraft Horseradish/Dijon • Mrs. Talbot's Asian Sesame Vinaigrette
Melanoma
1,500
Cain's Fat-free Mayonnaise • Hellmann's Low-fat Mayonnaise • Wishbone Superberry Fruit • Miracle Whip
Metastatic bone and lung cancer
1,000
Cain's Light Mayonnaise • Cain's Sandwich Spread • Cain's Tartar Sauce • Kraft Hot & Spicy Mayonnaise
500
50
WORSENING HEALTH
Decay and Death
0
Measured in Bovis Units of Life Force Energy

CHAPTER 23

Herbs, Spices, Seasonings & Flavorings

HERBS AND SPICES ADDED TO OUR FOODS generally enhance their culinary attractiveness and make palatable some foods that otherwise would taste bland. They are used all over the world because of their distinctively aromatic and sometimes pungent flavoring qualities, which come from volatile oils, and also because of their healing qualities. In fact, the age-old use of herbs and spices in our food is where the culinary and healing arts intersect.

Plants evolved with the ability to synthesize chemical compounds to help defend themselves against attack from a wide variety of predators such as herbivorous mammals, insects, and fungi, and many of these compounds have been found to be beneficial to humans. These include natural antivirals, antibiotics, antifungals, and anti-inflammatories which are found in such as plants as garlic, oregano, mustard and turmeric.

It is thought that the use of herbs and spices in food developed in part as a response to the threat of food-borne pathogens. Recipes are the most highly spiced in tropical climates where food is most likely to "go off," and invariably the spices with the most potent antimicrobial action are used with foods most susceptible to spoilage, such as meat. In all cultures, vegetables tend to be less spiced than meat, presumably because they are less likely to spoil.

Technically, herbs come from aromatic plants grown in temperate zones, while spices come from tropical plants. Herbs are usually derived from the leaves and stalks of plants, while spices can come from other parts of the plants, such as the bud (cloves), seeds (cumin, poppy, sesame), berries (peppercorn), bark (cinnamon), roots and rhizomes (ginger), or the stamens (saffron.) Sometimes, the same plant can provide both herbs and spices, for example, fresh coriander leaves can be used as an herb, while ground coriander seeds are used as a spice. Spices are important in the cuisine of warmer climes, such as Mexican chili, Indian curry, and Cajun food, and in the baked goods and desserts favored by Western cultures, such as Danish pastry flavored with cardamom, apple pie spiced with cloves, raisin muffins flavored with cinnamon and nutmeg, and ice cream flavored with vanilla.

Different cuisines rely on different types of herbs, mostly plants which grow native or are cultivated in that country: for example, basil is synonymous with Italian food, while coriander/cilantro is widely used in Mexican, Indian and South-east Asian dishes. Certain herbs seem to go well with specific foods, such as parsley with new potatoes, rosemary with lamb, thyme with chicken, sage with pork, bay leaf with beef stew—and what would pizza be without oregano?

These naturally-occurring flavorings enhance the nutritional content of food, but when they are combined with sugar or high fructose corn syrup (HFCS), their nutritional value plummets. For instance, pure ground mustard powder mixed with water calibrates at a healthy 10,000, but when a food manufacturer mixes it with a sweetener to make "honey mustard," it ends up very low on the nutritional scale. Of course, if the manufacturer used *real* honey, then it would be a healthful condiment. French's Honey Mustard, for instance, contains "distilled vinegar, water, HFCS, #1 grade mustard seed, sugar, corn syrup, salt, carrot oleoresin (color), honey, spices, and garlic powder." Yes, it actually contains HFCS, sugar *and* corn syrup—and of course, just a touch of honey to satisfy truth-in-advertising laws.

It would be nice to think that all the flavorings and seasonings in our food came from wholesome herbs and spices, but in fact most of the flavorings used in processed foods consist of chemically-engineered additives and artificial colorings. There are more than 3,000 different additives that can legally be added to food products, and some are known to cause cancer. Testing for safety has been done for individual additives, but not for combinations of additives, and the risk of ill effects increases with multiple numbers of additives used in any one product. They do have to be listed on the ingredients, but being able to read them and decipher them can be a challenge. You can look them up in *Food Additives: A Shopper's Guide To What's Safe And What's Not.* Or just avoid processed and packaged foods altogether.

Comparative Vibrational Levels of Health and Disease States		Comparative Nutritional Levels of **Herbs, Spices and Seasonings**
10,000 = Level of Optimal Health e.g. a healthy newborn baby / hunter/gatherer tribes	10,000	Naturally grown and/or organic herbs and spices • Colman's mustard powder • Unprocessed sea salt, e.g. Himalayan salt, La Baleine sea salt, Morton's Natural sea salt
	9,500	Colman's Horseradish Sauce
	9,000	
	8,500	
	8,000	
	7,500	
	7,000	
	6,500	Diamond Crystal Salt • McCormick Garlic Powder • McCormick Sliced Garlic
AVERAGE LEVEL OF HEALTH IN USA		
Inflammation	6,000	Kosciusko's Mustard • Grey Poupon Deli Mustard • Morton's Salt • Howard's Garlic Juice
Arthritis starts to manifest	5,500	Maille Old-Style Dijon Mustard • Grey Poupon Dijon Mustard • Morton's Light Salt • French's "No Salt"
Heart Disease starts to manifest	5,000	Gulden's Yellow Mustard
Cancer cells form: Breast, Prostate, Lung, Colon, Pancreas	4,500	French's Mustard: Spicy Brown and Dijon • Morton's Kosher Salt
Diabetes • Osteoporosis	4,000	French's Honey Mustard • Emeril's NY Deli Style Mustard
Lymphoma • Leukemia • Dementia	3,500	Gulden's Spicy Brown Mustard • Hellman's Creamy Dijon Mustard
Congestive heart disease Brain cancer • Multiple sclerosis	3,000	
Breast cancer metastasizes	2,500	
Prostate cancer metastasizes • Common cold/ flu	2,000	Hellman's Honey Mustard • Chef Prudhomme's Magic Seasonings • Bell's Seasonings • Mrs. Dash
Melanoma	1,500	Koop's Horseradish • Koop's Arizona Heat
Metastatic bone and lung cancer	1,000	Olde Cape Cod Honey Mustard • Koop's Honey Mustard • Boar's Head Honey Mustard
	500	McCormick Bac'n Pieces bacon flavored chips
	50	Gulden's Honey Mustard Dipping Sauce • McCormick Imitation Vanilla and Almond Extracts • Liquid Smoke
Decay and Death	0	

BETTER HEALTH ↑ / WORSENING HEALTH ↓

Measured in Bovis Units of Life Force Energy

The Spice Trade of Earlier Times

The importance of obtaining spices for use in preparing food created a huge demand for these products in the earlier days of Western civilization. They were highly prized, especially for flavoring foods in the days before refrigeration when it was difficult to keep meat fresh.

The spice trade brought exotic spices and foods from the East to the West by following the path of the Silk Route from Asia to the Middle East and on to Greece and Italy. This lucrative trade initiated the Age of Exploration, when intrepid sailors set off around the world to seek their fortunes in gold and spices. Magellan's personal documents indicated his desire to find "the golden islands of Tarshish and Ophir," and in 1492 Christopher Columbus set sail to discover sources of valuable spices.

The fight to control the flow of cloves, nutmeg, black pepper, gold, silver, and other commodities from the East to the West led to the discovery of the route around the southern tip of Africa, and the exploration of the Western hemisphere and the Pacific Ocean. Black pepper was one of the most profitable trade items shipped to Europe. In 1585, ships from the West Indies arrived in Europe with the first cargo of Jamaican ginger, a root originating in India and South China, and the first Asian spice to be grown successfully in the New World.

However, the arrival of refrigeration in the 19th century resulted in a decline in the demand for fresh spices and signaled the end of this global trade.

Herbs and Spices as Medicine

The use of plants as medicines predates written human history, and they have certainly been used since prehistoric times. By the Middle-Ages in Europe, it was well-known that herbs and spices had medicinal qualities. The word drug comes from the Dutch word "droog," which means "dried plant." Some examples of plants used as medicines today are inulin from the roots of dahlias, quinine from the cinchona tree, morphine and codeine from the opium poppy, and digoxin/digitalis from the foxglove. Aspirin is derived from salicin, the active ingredient in willow bark, which is converted in the body into salicylic acid. Once prescribed by Hippocrates, aspirin was originally a brand name patented by Bayer AG, and is still a protected trademark in some countries.

The most effective antimicrobial herbs and spices include thyme, garlic, onion, cinnamon, cloves and sage. Thyme has a characteristic smell and flavor due to the chemical thymol. It has antiseptic properties and low toxicity so is used as an antiseptic in dental mouth washes, and was used to dress wounds in days gone by. Sage contains cirisiliol, a potent inhibitor of an enzyme (arachidonate, 5-lipoxygenase) involved in metabolizing fats, and there is some suggestion that it might protect against prostate cancer.

The allicin in garlic has been scientifically proven to be a powerful natural antibiotic, antiviral and anti-fungal agent, and has also been shown to kill highly resistant MRSA infections in human clinical studies. In addition to its potent infection-fighting abilities, garlic also helps lower blood pressure, promotes balanced intestinal health, and is a powerful immune system booster. Allicin also acts as an antimicrobial agent, as does the allyl isothiocyanate present in mustard.

Herbs and spices have numerous chemical constituents—some are irritants, some are toxic, and others have medicinal properties—but most have a relatively low toxicity level, and eating food seasoned with herbs and spices generally does not cause any problems. However, the nutmeg and the clove might be an exception.

The nutmeg comes from the *Myristica fragrans*, an evergreen tree indigenous to the Banda Islands in the Moluccas (or Spice Islands) of Indonesia. The nutmeg has a number of pharmacologically active chemicals, including pinene, camphene, dipentene and trimyristin, which are used as perfumes and flavouring agents, but it also contains myristicin, a naturally occurring insecticide that can have neurotoxic and hallucinogenic effects. The intoxicating effects of myristicin can lead to a physical state somewhere between waking and dreaming; euphoria is reported and nausea is often experienced. Nutmeg also contains the hallucinogen, elemicin—however, it would take a lot of elemicin to get any effect.

Cloves are the dried flower buds of a small tropical tree, *Syzygium aromaticum*, and contain a substance called eugenol, which not only gives cloves their characteristic taste and smell, but is also an anesthetic. Clove oil was used by dentists as an anesthetic until quite recently, and in fact some people still use it—when you chew on a clove, you will feel your mouth get numb. But despite its pharmacological effect, eugenol has low toxicity, plus it is not actually eaten, just used for flavoring. Eugenol is also used commercially in the manufacture of vanillin, the chemical that gives vanilla its characteristic flavor and smell.

Mustard—the Most Popular Spice in the World

Used the world over, mustard it is one of the most popular and widely used of all the spices. Prepared mustard is a popular accompaniment for meats and cheeses, including hamburgers, bratwurst, and hot dogs, as well as in the preparation of sandwiches. The use of mustard as a hot dog condiment was first seen at the 1904 St. Louis World's Fair, when the bright yellow French's mustard was introduced by the R. T. French Company.

Mustard may have originally been used because of its antibacterial properties—it will not grow mold, mildew or harmful bacteria, and is a good preservative, and for this reason, it does not require refrigeration.

Mustard is a condiment made from the seeds of a mustard plant (white or yellow mustard, brown or Indian mustard, or black mustard). The seeds—whole, ground or cracked—can be mixed with water, salt, lemon juice, wine, mayonnaise or other liquids, and sometimes other flavorings and spices, to create a paste or sauce ranging in color from bright yellow to dark brown. English mustard is among the strongest, usually a simple mix of mustard flour and water, while French mustard, or *moutarde de Dijon*, has added vinegar, and is milder. German mustard or senf is milder still. Homemade mustards are often far hotter and more intensely flavored than commercial preparations. A strong mustard can cause the eyes to water, sting the palate, and inflame the nasal passages and throat. Mustard can also cause allergic reactions: since 2005, products in the European Union must be labelled as potential allergens if they contain mustard.

Romans were probably the first to experiment with the preparation of mustard as a condiment. A recipe for mustard appears in a Roman cookbook from the late 4th or early 5th century which consists of a mixture of ground mustard, pepper, caraway, lovage, grilled coriander seeds, dill, celery, thyme, oregano, onion, honey, vinegar, fish stock and oil, and was intended as a glaze for spit-roasted boar.

Mustard is an emulsifier which can stabilize a mixture of two or more unblendable liquids such as oil and water. Added to Hollandaise sauce and mayonnaise, mustard can reduce the possibility of curdling. Mustard is also used as an ingredient in salad dressings, marinades and barbecue sauce.

One of the factors that determines the strength of a prepared mustard is the temperature of the water, vinegar, or other liquid mixed with the ground seeds: hotter liquids reduce the strength-producing compounds of the mustard, so using hot water will result in a milder mustard while cold water will produce a hotter mustard. In the same way, if added to a dish during cooking much of the effect of the mustard is lost.

It Turns Out that Salt is Good for Us!

Salt is one of the most effective and widely used of all food seasonings and natural preservatives, and is the only food item we consume that is not animal or vegetable—it is a mineral. Our Paleolithic ancestors ate salt, but not the refined salt we buy in our supermarkets today. This refined salt, or table salt, is 99.9 percent sodium-chloride, a chemical as pure as heroin or white sugar, and is mined from underground deposits of rock salt. On the other hand, natural sea salt is a healthful product that supplies trace amounts of about 80 mineral elements that the body needs.

Sea salt is harvested from ancient sea beds or obtained by evaporation of sea water. The traces of magnesium, calcium, potassium, manganese, phosphorous and iodine present in sea salt provide our bodies with minerals essential for good health. For example, magnesium is necessary for proper immune, brain and nerve cell function, as well as being a component in metabolism; calcium and phosphorous are essential to bone formation; iodine is important to the cell metabolism required for normal growth and development; and salt is vital for the generation of hydro-electric energy in cells in the body.

If we dissolve unprocessed sea salt in water in the proper ratio, we get sea water, which has the same salinity as human blood and most other body fluids, such as tears and sweat. When we eat it, natural sea salt acts like reconstituted seawater in our body, aiding in energy metabolism in our cells. During World War II, Navy doctors would use sea water for blood transfusions when blood supplies ran out, and many lives were saved.

Humans are not the only beings to have consumed natural salt since time began—mammals around the world crave salt, seeking out salt licks wherever they can. I remember that the cows on our family farm were given a hunk of pink sea salt to lick in their barn during the winter.

For the past 25 years, we have been advised by the medical profession to avoid salt because it was thought to cause high blood pressure and heart disease, but an article published recently in the *Journal of the American Medical Association* cites a new European study that shows that people who ate a lot of salt were *not* more likely to get high blood pressure, and were in fact *less likely* to die of heart disease than those with a low salt intake. And participants with the lowest salt intake actually had the highest rate of death from heart disease during the follow up. Says study author Dr. Jan Staessen of the University of Leuven in Belgium: "The findings certainly do not support the current recommendation to lower salt intake in the general population."

In the refining of rock salt, beneficial minerals are removed and sold for other purposes, then chemicals such as aluminosilicate of sodium or yellow prussiate of soda are added to bleach the salt, prevent water absorption, and to make it easier to pour. The problem is that the chemicals added to salt to prevent water absorption can also prevent it from being properly absorbed in

---

"There must be something strangely sacred in salt.
It is in our tears and in the sea."
— *Kahlil Gibran*

"Some people claim that since salt is not a live food, one cannot obtain the minerals from salt. This is simply not true. The minerals may not be as bio-available as they are in foods . . . however, the body has quite an ability to chelate or bind inorganic minerals, especially those found in some sea salts."

— *Lawrence Wilson, M.D., author of* **Nutritional Balancing and Hair Mineral Analysis**

the body so that it will be unable to combine with human body fluids. This can cause problems with edema (water retention) and other health disturbances. Many nutritional experts think it is this kind of salt that causes problems in the body, not natural sea salt, which provides the body with important minerals.

Be sure to buy *natural* sea salt, not sea salt that has gone through a refining process but is still labeled sea salt. Unprocessed sea salt will generally have a darker color—a dirty off-white, or brown, or even pink, though some French sea salt is naturally very white. Good brands are Celtic Sea Salt, Baleine Sea Salt, Le Tresor Grey Sea Salt, Hawaiian Jade Sea Salt, Pacific Salt, and Himalayan Salt, which is pink. Genuine sea salt generally tastes less "salty" and has a more robust, umami flavor than refined salt.

Flavor Enhancers

One of the side effects of factory-farmed, processed and low-fat foods is that the resulting food products are so bland they often taste like cardboard. Many people have no idea what a free-range chicken or a freshly-picked tomato tastes like. But the food industry has found a way to overcome the problem that they created in the first place. No, not by providing more nutritious and better tasting food, but by "enhancing" the flavors of processed foods.

About 90 percent of the money that Americans spend on food is now spent on processed food, and an entire industry has arisen to make this food palatable. In his book *Fast Food Nation*, Eric Schlosser writes that without this "flavor industry," today's fast food would not exist. "Look at the labels on your food . . . you'll find 'natural flavor' or 'artificial flavor' in just about every list of ingredients. The similarities between these two broad categories are far more significant than the differences. Both are man-made additives that give most processed food most of its taste," he writes. He goes on to explain that people usually buy a food item the first time because of its packaging or appearance, but the taste of the product usually determines whether they buy it again. So a lot of money and time is spent on making sure that the added flavors are instantly appealing. As would be expected, the flavor industry is highly secretive: "The fast-food chains, understandably, would like the public to believe that the flavors of the food they sell somehow originate in their restaurant kitchens, not in distant factories run by other firms. The rise and fall of corporate empires—of soft-drink companies, snack-food companies, and fast-food chains—is often determined by how their products taste," writes Schlosser.

Until the 1950s, man-made flavorings were used mostly in sodas, baked goods and candy. But as the sales of processed food began to soar, the invention of machines such as gas chromatographs and mass spectrometers that were capable of identifying more subtle flavors dramatically increased the number of flavors that could be synthesized. These companies were soon manufacturing compounds that provided the "taste" to a huge array of highly-processed foods, including orange and grapefruit juice.

The sad truth is, the more our food is factory-farmed and manufactured from refined ingredients, the less inherent flavor it has and the more artificial flavor enhancers are needed to give it any kind of taste at all. These additives and colorings can cause problems in sensitive individuals, including allergic reactions and hyperactivity/ADD in children, and may contribute to visual and learning disorders or cause nerve damage.

Monosodium Glutamate (MSG)

MSG is marketed as a flavor enhancer under the brand name of Accent. MSG is now used by most fast food chains and is found in many foodstuffs, particularly processed foods.

A human being has five basic taste sensations: sweet, salty, sour, bitter, and savory, also called umami, which is the taste produced by glutamates commonly found in fermented or aged foods. The food additive MSG is a umami substance. Usually only compounds that enhance umami are considered and referred to as taste flavorants. Some examples of a savory taste are parmesan and roquefort cheese, soy sauce, and fish sauce.

MSG is the salt version of glutamic acid, one of a chain of 20 amino acids that make up a protein molecule. It's made by bacterial or microbial fermentation where the bacteria used are often, if not always, genetically engineered. "In this method, bacteria are grown aerobically in a liquid nutrient medium. The bacteria have the ability to excrete the glutamic acid they synthesize outside of their cell membrane into the liquid nutrient medium in which they are grown. The glutamic acid is then separated from the fermentation broth by filtration, concentration, acidification, and crystallization, and, through the addition of sodium, converted to its monosodium salt," states the website www.TruthInLabelling.org.

Glutamic acid is a pro-inflammatory amino acid to which many people seem to have an adverse reaction, often called Chinese restaurant syndrome. Scientific studies have been carried out but with no definitive results one way or the other, and the FDA has concluded that MSG is safe for most people when "eaten at customary levels." The Truth in Labelling website states: "By FDA definition, processed free glutamic acid is 'naturally occurring,' because the basic ingredients are found in nature. 'Naturally occurring' does not mean that a food additive is being used in its natural state . . . it only means that the food additive began with something found in nature. By FDA definition, the ingredient 'monosodium glutamate' is natural. So is hydrochloric acid. So is arsenic. 'Natural' doesn't mean 'safe.' "

Even if toxicologists believe that MSG is a harmless ingredient for most people, it is not a natural food and should be avoided. Many people are sensitive to the effects of MSG, and children are four times more sensitive than adults. Neonatal exposure to MSG can cause a permanent reduction in the secretion of growth hormone, leading to stunted growth and irreversible obesity. Other reactions include headaches, nausea, weakness, a burning sensation in the back of the neck and forearms, wheezing, changes in heart rate, and difficulty breathing. To eliminate MSG from your diet, avoid foods with the following ingredients in their label: Monosodium glutamate, free glutamate, hydrolyzed proteins (any type), autolyzed yeast, yeast extract, caseinate, and "natural or artificial flavors."

Herbs, Spices, Seasonings & Flavorings

The Bottom Line

THE GOOD: All naturally-grown herbs and spices • natural unrefined sea salt

THE BAD: Refined table salt • some processed mustards, especially "honey mustard"

THE DANGEROUS: Chemical food flavorings and additives • MSG • artificial flavorings such as vanilla extract, almond extract, and smoke flavoring

CHAPTER 24

Snack Foods and Nuts

WE ALL LOVE SOMETHING CRUNCHY TO SNACK ON—whether it's potato chips, Cheetos, nuts, celery sticks or M&Ms, they all satisfy that craving for something salty, savory or sweet, and all the better if they are instantly available. But with snack foods, as with all food categories, there are the good ones, the not-so-good ones, and the really bad ones. As far as our health goes, what's important is the quality of the ingredients of the snacks we eat, rather than *what* we eat, as well as *how much of them* we eat. And apparently we are eating a lot more of them than we used to. A government survey shows that during the last decade, the average American adult ate nearly one-third more than they did in the late 1970s, and they ate more frequently.

Barry Popkin, Ph.D., a professor of nutrition at the University of North Carolina at Chapel Hill, has said: "The frequency of eating is probably, for the average overweight adult, becoming a huge issue. Why are we snacking . . . and munching all the time? The food is there, it's available all the time . . . it's not very healthy, but it's tasty. It's sweet, it's salty, it's fatty—it's all the things we love."

Ready-to-eat snack foods are ubiquitous, and now tempt us at supermarket check-outs, gas stations, vending machines, and convenience stores, and are hard to resist. Designed to be less perishable and more portable than prepared foods, they contain substantial amounts of preservatives, sweeteners, and appealing ingredients such as chocolate, peanuts, and specially-designed flavors. Packaged snack foods are often classified as junk food because they typically have little or no nutritional value, and nutritional experts are now recommending that people make a conscious effort to eat more healthy snacks such as fruit, sliced vegetables, nuts, and whole grain products while avoiding high-calorie, low-nutrient junk food.

Maybe one of the reasons we are snacking more is that advertising from food manufacturers has given us the idea that it's normal to do so. And we seem to have got the message loud and clear: frequent—and often mindless—snacking now seems to be the norm. But when we visit other countries, we'll notice that people are not constantly snacking—on the streets in Europe, for instance, we don't habitually see people eating out of packets of chips and cookies or nursing goblets of coffee or cans of Coke. Snacking in this way is a habit, and habits can be broken. The key to breaking this particular habit is really quite mundane—eat satisfying meals that fill us up. If we eat a nutritious meal in the morning, we can usually navigate the time span from breakfast to lunch without the need for a snack. However, the long stretch between lunch and dinner is more of a challenge, which is why it's a good idea to schedule a substantial snack, or mini-meal, around 4 p.m., as the British do at "teatime."

When we feel hunger pangs, we tend to reach for the nearest and most convenient thing, even if it's a donut—anything to fill us up. So plan ahead—always have a healthy snack on hand, such as a baggie of mixed nuts in the car or a container of hummus and veggie sticks in the fridge, so you don't get caught short and are tempted by junk food. And beware of meals composed of snack foods! Think of Superbowl parties, where the table is liberally spread with chips and dips, Buffalo wings and cookies, and people stand around nibbling mindlessly as they chat. It's fun, but not a good thing to do on a regular basis. It's one thing to snack on some Cheetos while you enjoy a beer, but quite another to dine on them!

"Chips and fries are soaked in soybean oil; processed foods are manufactured with [these inflammatory oils] for longer shelf life. The inflammatory process that begins with junk food turns into a vicious cycle over time that creates heart disease, high blood pressure, diabetes and, finally, Alzheimer's disease, as the inflammatory process continues unabated."

— Dr. Dwight Lundell, heart surgeon, former Chief Resident at Yale University Hospital, and author of **The Cure For Heart Disease**

Comparative Vibrational Levels of Health and Disease States		Comparative Nutritional Levels of Snack Foods & Nuts
10,000 = Level of Optimal Health e.g. a healthy newborn baby / hunter/gatherer tribes	10,000	Organic vegetables, nuts, fruit, cheese, crackers and chips • Dips and salsa made from organic ingredients • Homemade potato chips made from organic potatoes fried in organic lard or oil
	9,500	
	9,000	Homemade potato chips made from supermarket potatoes fried in organic lard
	8,500	
	8,000	Homemade potato chips made from supermarket potatoes fried in regular lard
	7,500	Ben & Jerry's vanilla ice cream
	7,000	Ben & Jerry's chocolate ice cream
	6,500	
AVERAGE LEVEL OF HEALTH IN USA Inflammation	6,000	
Arthritis starts to manifest	5,500	Green Mountain Gringo Salsa • Haagen Dazs Vanilla Ice Cream
Heart Disease starts to manifest	5,000	Tostitos Salsa • Planter's Walnuts • Terra Sweet Potato Chips
Cancer cells form: Breast, Prostate, Lung, Colon, Pancreas	4,500	Planter's Dry-Roasted Peanuts and Roasted Almonds
Diabetes • Osteoporosis	4,000	Matador Beef Jerky • Green Mountain Gringo corn chips • Yoplait yogurt • Ben & Jerry's Cherry Garcia
Lymphoma • Leukemia • Dementia	3,500	Jiffy-Pop butter-flavored popcorn • Pirate's Booty Puffs, Veggie • Garden of Eatin' blue corn chips Cape Cod potato chips • Utz reduced-fat potato chips • Ben & Jerry's Cheesecake Brownie ice cream
Congestive heart disease Brain cancer • Multiple sclerosis	3,000	Ley's & Utz potato chips • Tostitos Creamy Spinach Dip, Salsa con Queso • Slim Jim beef jerky
Breast cancer metastasizes	2,500	Pirate's Booty Puffs, Cheddar Flavor • Planter's cashews • Kettle Krinkle Cut Potato Chips
Prostate cancer metastasizes • Common cold/ flu	2,000	Cheese pizza • Rold Gold Pretzels • Bachman Pretzels • Snyder's Pretzels • Utz Salsa con Queso
Melanoma	1,500	Planter's cocktail peanuts, sunflower seeds • Quaker Rice Cakes • Buffalo chicken wings • Wheat Thins
Metastatic bone and lung cancer	1,000	Frito-Lay French Onion Dip • Utz Potato Chips • Pringles Originals • Ritz Crackers
	500	Cheetos • Doritos tortilla chips, most flavors • Utz Creamy Onion Dip • Soft-serve ice cream
	50	Snyder's pretzels: Honey-Mustard and other flavors • Stacey's pita chips • Flavored Pringles • Granola bars • Candy & chocolate bars • Planter's honey-roasted peanuts • Quaker rice cakes, apple-cinnamon
Decay and Death	0	

BETTER HEALTH / WORSENING HEALTH

Measured in Bovis Units of Life Force Energy

Why Are We So Addicted to Snacking?

The popularity of snacks has increased dramatically over the past 40 years, and one reason may be due to the misguided dictates from the U.S. Government that we should reduce our intake of animal protein and increase our intake of carbohydrates. But a meal high in carbohydrates, which are easily and quickly assimilated by the body, can leave us feeling hungry an hour or so afterwards—aka the "Thai restaurant syndrome." The more protein and fat in a meal, the longer it will give us a feeling of fullness and satisfaction afterwards, and the less likely we are to crave a snack.

Another reason we snack is out of habit—one of the worst things we can do is to get into the habit of mindlessly snacking throughout the day, especially when working at the computer or doing a repetitive task. And sometimes just spending too much time in the kitchen may tempt us to start snacking, and we all know from experience that once it starts, it's hard to stop. The results of a study published in the *Journal of the American Dietetic Association* shows that women who have a mid-morning snack lose less weight than their counterparts who ate a healthy breakfast and don't snack in the morning. In the study, snacks were defined as any food or beverage consumed between meals. "We think this finding may not relate necessarily to the time of day one snacks, but rather to the short interval between breakfast and lunch," says study researcher Anne McTiernan, MD, PhD. "Mid-morning snacking therefore might be a reflection of recreational or mindless eating habits rather than eating to satisfy true hunger."

So aim to eat three full meals a day, and if you absolutely need a snack, plan healthy snacks ahead of time.

The Nighttime Nibbler

Midnight snacking is often a response to feeling stressed, bored or lonely, or because dinner wasn't filling enough. Nutritional experts agree that late-night snacking can signal the start of a vicious cycle of weight gain. Some heavy snackers eat most of their calories at night for any of the above reasons—except for actually being hungry. For others, having a snack is part of their routine, such as when they get home late after work.

"For those who have finished their daily duties and are relaxing at home, snacking is giving in to a normal urge," says Dr. Donald Hensrud, Associate Professor of Preventive Medicine and Nutrition at the Mayo Clinic in Rochester, Minnesota. "And, when there is little reason to put the brakes on, it is easy to eat quite a lot."

Snacking at night also interferes with the night-time "fasting" period, which usually lasts from 10 to 12 hours. Recent research has found that the body stores sugar as glycogen in the liver but only stores enough to last for 6-8 hours. After this time, the glycogen store has been used up, and this forces the body to metabolize fat stored elsewhere, leading to weight loss.

To prevent bingeing at night, experts recommend increasing the size of the evening meal. But don't eat it too late—one problem with eating later in the evening or after dark is that if you go to sleep full, you'll wake up fuller in the morning, and so will be tempted to skip breakfast—triggering a serious snack-attack around 11 am.

What Exactly is in Processed Snack Foods?

Processed snack foods are made from the cheapest, most highly refined, most "altered" of all the food items we consume. Predominantly made of wheat, corn, soy and sugar, these are the crops that are the most adulterated and all are now genetically modified (GM). The latest reports show that 94 percent of all soybeans, 93 percent of canola oil, 93 percent of cottonseed oil, and 86 percent of corn are GM. Approximately 25 percent of all milk and yoghurt contains genetically engineered recombinant bovine growth hormone (rBGH).

By law, GM foods sold in the U.S. do not have to be labelled. GM foods have been banned in many countries around the world, but in the U.S., unless food is labelled "organic," we don't even know that we are eating GM ingredients in our food. GM crops are also drenched in pesticides and herbicides, so the result is food that might seem innocuous but is in fact incredibly dangerous, especially for growing children. GMOs and plants treated with pesticides have been shown again and again to affect the health, fertility and brain function in animals and humans.

And then there are the "additives" which give snack foods their distinctive color and flavor, and which can include any from a long list allowed by the FDA and many that are not, either in such small quantities that they do not need to be included in the list of ingredients, or are added illegally. The result is highly engineered foods made from dangerous ingredients and chemical additives that add up to anti-nutrition.

The list of ingredients on the label of Cheetos, a popular snack food, reads: "Enriched corn meal, vegetable oil (corn, soybean, or sunflower oil), cheese seasoning, partially hydrogenated soybean oil, canola oil, sour cream, maltodextrin, artificial flavor, monosodium glutamate, lactic acid, salt, artificial colors (including Yellow 6), and citric acid."

The label that gives us the Nutrition Facts of Cheetos says that each portion contains 10 g. of fat, 2 g. of saturated fat, 0 g. of cholesterol, 290 mg. of sodium, 15 g. of carbohydrates and 2 g. of protein. But it doesn't tell us whether it's actually good for us or not. And in fact, it isn't—it's highly dangerous, with at least four of the ingredients being genetically modified and at least four being manufactured chemicals, and but you wouldn't know that from the food label. So we have to ask ourselves, isn't there something very wrong with these nutritional labels when we can't decipher whether a food is actually good for us or not?

"Make no mistake: junk food is convenient, economically alluring, and engineered to appeal to your primal drive for calories, fat, sugar, and salt."
—*Dr. Joseph Mercola, editor of mercola.com Health Newsletter*

Food Colorings in Snack Foods

From the Doritos website: "Color is an important property of food that can add to the enjoyment of eating. Frito-Lay uses plant-based or synthetic dyes to enhance the color of some of our snacks." Yes, color is an important property of food so we can tell if it's fresh! When food loses its color, it's not fresh anymore. Think of a dead lettuce leaf. So really, they are putting color back into dead food, rather like painting a corpse ready for its wake.

Food manufacturers in the U.S. can use nine dyes in all, though Red 40, Yellow 5 and Yellow 6 make up 90 percent of the market. They are everywhere in our food, including packaged snacks, candy, boxed cereals, pickles, cough syrup, processed meats, waffles, and crackers. More than two dozen studies point to problems with the dyes, according to Dr. David Wallinga of the Institute for Agriculture and Trade Policy, who says, "They're really ubiquitous in this food supply that we've created."

Many children diagnosed with Attention Deficit Hyperactivity Disorder, or ADHD, have improved when foods containing food dyes have been eliminated from their diets. Though a statement from the FDA says it does not believe that artificial food dyes cause hyperactivity in children in the general population, they have admitted that food dyes may exacerbate problems in susceptible children diagnosed with ADHD because they may have a unique intolerance to them. The FDA has voted against putting warning labels on foods and believes that more research is needed. Still, some grocery chains, like Whole Foods Market, won't sell foods containing synthetic dyes. Warning labels are required in much of Europe, and American companies like Kraft, General Mills, and Kellogg's have had to remove artificial dyes from the products they sell overseas. Some foods familiar in the U.S. look different in Europe, such as the candy snack M&M's, where the colors aren't as bright—and are probably a lot safer to eat.

The Snack Food Industry

"Snacking is an important part of a healthy diet, whether you want to lose weight, sustain energy or simply live a better lifestyle."
—*from the Frito-Lay website*

With the spread of suitable retail outlets, packaged snack foods are now a significant business, and there is actually a Snack Food Association, whose purpose is to promote the snack food industry. According to the 2011 State of the Snack Food Industry Report, performed by analytical group Symphony IRI, the sectors that saw the largest increases in sales volume were snack bars, granola bars, and yogurt. "We see that snacks are playing more diverse roles . . . and are way more than chips and pretzels. Consumer are trying to eat healthier with 71% surveyed claiming to be on the healthier journey," says the report. "Healthier segments are outpacing indulgent snacks 4 to 1 . . . with 28% of consumers purchasing snacks to satisfy immediate hunger. Consumers, 40%, are now viewing snacks as an important part of a healthy eating plan all day presenting new product development opportunities for food entrepreneurs. Why? Consumers viewing snacks as not just a 'snack' but as a mini meal on the go that delivers high value."

It seems that consumers are asking for healthier snack foods, which is certainly a move in the right direction, but when the snack food industry uses healthier ingredients, we don't necessarily get a better product. By the time the food processors are done with healthy items such as nuts, fruit, yogurt, and whole grains, we get products like fruit roll-ups, pasteurized sweetened yogurt, sugar-coated nuts, and granola bars, all highly processed food items that are no healthier than the maligned chips and pretzels. Such high-carbohydrate snacks give a quick jolt of energy followed by a crash that can leave us feeling hungry, cranky, sleepy, and unable to concentrate. The idea of a "mini-meal on the go" is one we can all embrace, but it has to be healthy otherwise it defeats the purpose, which is to get us through to the next main meal, not to spike our blood sugar and give us a hypoglycemic crash.

Kids and Snacks

Growing children need regular meals and healthy snacks for optimal performance and development. They need a good breakfast to keep them going until lunch time, a nutritious lunch in the middle of the day, and a healthy snack at the end of the school day to get them through until dinner. After-school snacks are especially important when students have an early lunch period, and when their evening meal may be delayed or of poor quality. A study in 2010 showed that children in the U.S. snacked on average six times per day, approximately twice as often as they did in the 1970s, which might be a result of children not getting adequate nutrition at home, or in school for the infamous school lunch (for more on this see the chapter on Children's Food). The after-school snack is really a mini-meal, and should be considered one, with protein as its main component, rather than the time-honored packet of cookies and a glass of milk.

Nuts—The Most Nutritious Snack of All

Nuts are nature's most convenient power snack. They are highly nutritious, full of protein and beneficial fats, and give us the feeling of being full, unlike carbohydrates, which can make us feel hungry again soon after eating them. There are many studies showing that nuts are good for us, including a recent report that shows that consuming one ounce of nuts every day reduces the risk of developing diabetes. However, nuts roasted in inferior oils, such as cottonseed oil, are not good—it's best to eat nuts raw or dry-roasted.

The most common nuts we can purchase include almonds, Brazil nuts, cashews, coconuts, hazelnuts or filberts, macadamias, pecans, pistachios, and walnuts. Walnuts are especially nutritious, being a good source of omega-3 essential fatty acids which are in short supply in the average American diet. In scientific experiments, eating walnuts has been shown to reverse brain aging in rats, and reduce prostate and breast cancer in mice. They can taste a little bitter when eaten alone, but when scattered in a Waldolf salad or chopped up and added to pancakes and fruit breads, they add a delicious flavor as well as valuable nutrients. As a snack, they are good eaten with banana or apple slices and raisins.

Those who are watching their weight should know that certain nuts, such as pistachios and cashews, have higher amounts of carbohydrates than other nuts.

And we must not forget the peanut—not actually a nut, but a legume. Dry-roasted are best—avoid peanuts roasted in cottonseed oil, such as Planter's, they are virtually poisonous. Peanuts have the reputation of being one of the most pesticide-laden foods on the market, and most peanuts are contaminated with aflatoxin, a carcinogenic mold, so buy only organic peanuts. Both peanut and almond butter make a great snack on a slice of toast, crackers, or a rice cake, but make sure the peanut butter is made without added sugar—brands such as Skippy have added sugar and calibrate low on the chart.

The Hall of Shame

The Quaker Oats Company, for managing to make a simple rice cake, supposedly a "health food," that calibrates at the low level of 1500.

Snack Foods

The Bottom Line

THE GOOD: Organic vegetables, nuts, fruit, cheese, crackers, popcorn • dips, hummus and salsa made from organic ingredients • potato chips and corn chips fried in lard or coconut oil

THE BAD: Commercially-roasted nuts • artificially-flavored popcorn

THE DOWNRIGHT DANGEROUS: Packaged snack foods such as corn chips, potato chips, and pretzels, e.g. Cheetos, Doritos, Pringles • packaged snacking cakes and cookies • granola bars and breakfast bars • all snack foods containing refined sugar and/or HFCS, such as "honey" roasted nuts, chocolate-covered raisins, peanut M&Ms, and sweetened yogurt • candy and chocolate

CHAPTER 25

Breakfast Foods

WE ALL KNOW THE OLD ADAGE, "Breakfast like a king, lunch like a prince and dine like a pauper," and in fact most nutritionists do consider breakfast to be the most important meal of the day. Breakfast literally means "breaking the fast" of the night before, and as the first meal after the "night's fast," it provides the body with fuel for the first half of the day. Studies show that eating a nutritious breakfast can have beneficial effects on energy metabolism, regulating appetite, and insulin resistance, and that people who skip breakfast are likely to have problems with concentration, metabolism, and weight-gain.

The best foods to start the day are quality proteins and healthy fats supplemented with complex carbohydrates that can include whole-grains and potatoes. However, *refined* carbohydrates, such as boxed breakfast cereals, muffins, bagels, donuts, pancakes, pastries, processed fruit juice and most packaged breads are not good choices for breakfast, and will spike both blood sugar and insulin levels in the body. They are even worse when eaten with syrup, jelly or jam.

When I first came to this country, I was amazed to see Americans eat what to me seemed like dessert for breakfast—I had never seen anyone eat bacon soaked in maple syrup or pancakes for breakfast, let alone a donut. Where I came from, breakfast was a hearty three-course meal of oatmeal, bacon and eggs, or an omelette, or kippers (smoked herring), followed by whole wheat toast. I have stayed at country inns in the U.S. where I have been served items for breakfast I could not imagine eating—sweet casseroles such as bread and butter pudding, or waffles covered in whipped cream. Although these might seem like pure indulgence, in fact our idea of what constitutes a healthy breakfast has been planted in our brains through relentless advertising by corporations who make highly-profitable breakfast foods. Those ads with images of a stack of pancakes swimming in syrup or toaster pastries covered in icing subliminally give us license to accept them as appropriate breakfast foods. Remember those ads that showed a bowl of sugary cereal floating in milk accompanied by a glass of juice, with the caption, "Part of a healthy breakfast?" It makes you wonder what they consider to be the healthy part.

The saddest thing of all is that some mothers actually think that feeding their children Froot Loops or Pop Tarts for breakfast is good for them. How hard is it to scramble an egg and toast a slice of whole wheat bread? Even sadder is that one in five children does not eat breakfast at all.

According to the market research company NPD Group, the average American spends about 13 minutes a day preparing and eating breakfast. It's good to remember that we are not just what we eat, we are what we *digest* of what we eat—so it's important to schedule the time to not only to prepare breakfast, but to sit down and enjoy it in a calm atmosphere, conducive to good digestion, as nothing interferes with digestion more than stress. This is also a good time to have a quiet moment of gratitude, maybe light a candle and center yourself before you set off to work or school. It takes just a few moments but can set your mood for the rest of the day—and the same goes for the entire family, too.

"Eating breakfast is important for everyone, but is especially so for children and adolescents. According to the American Dietetic Association, children who eat breakfast perform better in the classroom and on the playground, with better concentration, problem-solving skills, and eye-hand coordination."

—*from the WebMD website*

What Makes a Healthy Breakfast?

Breakfast is a meal like any other, an opportunity to fuel the body with quality food, not a license to eat donuts or pancakes first thing in the morning. The typical American breakfast that consists of cold cereal with toast or a pastry, accompanied by orange juice and a cup of coffee or tea, is a jolt to the system—a perfect storm of highly-refined carbohydrates and caffeine which over-revs the body in the morning and leads to a hypoglycemic crash around 11 a.m., that dangerous time when many of us crave a muffin and a cup of coffee to keep us going.

Britain is famous for the "Full Monty," the hearty breakfast named for Field Marshall Montgomery who ordered it every morning even while fighting in North Africa during WWII. Consisting of bacon, eggs, sausage, grilled tomato, sauteed mushrooms, baked beans and toast, a meal like that will keep you going all day. American versions, usually called a country breakfast in restaurants, consist of any combination of eggs, sausage, bacon, and hash browns, served with toast, jam or jelly, and fruit juice, and sometimes offering pancakes and waffles. In Victorian times, breakfast would often be a mixed grill (sausage, bacon, lamb chop, lamb's kidneys), or smoked fish, a serious meal that kept the system stoked up until at least lunch time.

And in fact, researchers at the University of Alabama have found that a breakfast fit for a king is a great way to start the day. They report that a meal with a higher fat content first thing in the morning appears to program the body's metabolism for the rest of the day. They found that mice fed a high fat meal after waking remained healthy, but those given a breakfast rich in carbohydrates did not fare as well. They put on weight and had trouble processing sugar, raising their risk of diabetes. Blood tests also showed an elevated risk of heart disease and strokes.

One of the researchers, Dr. Martin Young, says, "This study suggests that if you ate a carbohydrate-rich breakfast it would promote carbohydrate utilisation throughout the rest of the day, whereas if you have a fat-rich breakfast, you (can) transfer your energy utilisation between carbohydrate and fat." The researchers advocate a hearty breakfast of proteins and fats for optimum health, followed by a smaller lunch and a light evening meal. They are not alone in their findings: a South American study found that women who ate half of their daily calories first thing in the morning lost more weight in the long-term than those who ate a small breakfast.

There's no "rule" that says we have to eat conventional breakfast foods for breakfast. Maybe it's time to start a healthy breakfast tradition of your own. There's nothing wrong with having a thin-cut steak, smoked fish, or even leftovers from the night before—but try to avoid left-over pizza! And don't skip breakfast altogether—another study revealed that obesity and insulin resistance syndrome rates were 35 percent to 50 percent lower among people who ate breakfast every day, compared to those who frequently skipped it.

Ready-to-Eat Breakfast Cereals Are Not the Best Way to Start the Day

The custom of eating cereals for breakfast goes back hundreds of years in places like Russia and Northern Europe, where porridge, made from oats, was a traditional food. In days gone by, people would often eat some version of bread soaked in milk and made into a kind of gruel. One uniquely American addition to breakfast is corn, especially popular in the South where hominy, first eaten by Native Americans, was eaten along with corn meal mush, corn pone and grits.

Flaked cereals have been popular in America since their creation in the early 1900s, but they have only been consumed widely since WW II, when more nutritious food was reserved for fighting soldiers. The first modern cereal foods were created by Seventh-day Adventists who formed the Western Health Reform Institute in the 1860s in Michigan. The Institute was later renamed the Battle Creek Sanitarium after its location in Battle Creek and the Adventists manufactured, promoted, and sold wholesome cereals. Will Keith Kellogg, the founder of the W. K. Kellogg Foundation, was a Seventh-day Adventist who started the Battle Creek Toasted Corn Flake Company in 1906 as a way to promote the benefits of a vegetarian diet. But in the last 40 years, flaked and dried cereals have been transformed into anything BUT a health food as they have become ever more heavily processed and sugared. Frosted flakes, corn flakes coated in sugar, were first introduced in 1951 by the Kellogg company, and a recent report from the Environmental Working Group reveals that many popular children's cereal brands now contain more sugar than snack cakes and cookies.

Most major players in the food industry are in the business to make a profit, and so they create and promote products that are highly palatable to most people, especially kids—and to appeal to their palates, the food is loaded with sugar and artificial flavors. According to a report from the USDA, "In the 1980s and the first half of the 1990s, the ready-to-eat cereal industry was one of the most profitable of all food manufacturing industries, with profits averaging 17 percent of sales." But many of the iconic brands of cereal are less popular with the public these days—sales of breakfast cereals are declining due to changing breakfast tastes and concerns about high sugar consumption. Symphony/IRI, a retail tracking company, reports that six of Kellogg's cereal brands—Corn Flakes, Cheerios, Raisin Bran, Rice Krispies, Special K and Corn Pops—have all seen declining

Comparative Vibrational Levels of Health and Disease States	Level	Comparative Nutritional Levels of **Conventional Breakfast Foods**
10,000 = Level of Optimal Health e.g. a healthy newborn baby / hunter/gatherer tribes	10,000	Organic eggs, bacon, sausages, home fries, yogurt, cereals, oatmeal, bread etc. • Organic tea • Maple syrup • Raw honey • Jams & jelly sweetened with fruit juice • Fresh-squeezed organic fruit juice
	9,500	Pete & Jerry's organic eggs • The Organic Hen eggs • Kerry Gold Irish butter • Organic coffee
BETTER HEALTH	9,000	Home Fries (regular potatoes sauteed in lard, olive oil or coconut oil)
	8,500	Tropicana grapefruit juice • Kate's Pure Butter
	8,000	Tropicana orange juice • Horizon organic butter • Regular tea made with tap water, no cream or sugar
	7,500	Hood orange juice • Average supermarket eggs • Earth Balance spread
	7,000	Shady Brook Farms Turkey Breakfast Sausage
	6,500	Lactaid milk • Regular coffee made with average tap water, no cream or sugar
AVERAGE LEVEL OF HEALTH IN USA Inflammation	6,000	Grits • Pepperidge Farm Whole Wheat Bread • Vermont Bread Whole-wheat • Arnold's Health Nut, 12 Grain
WORSENING HEALTH Arthritis starts to manifest	5,500	Oscar Meyer Breakfast Sausages • Hood Milk • Land O'Lakes Butter
Heart Disease starts to manifest	5,000	Average supermarket milk, pasteurized & homogenized • Hodgson Mills Pancake Mix • Jimmy Dean Breakfast Links • Oscar Meyer bacon • Plumrose bacon
Cancer cells form: Breast, Prostate, Lung, Colon, Pancreas	4,500	Ocean Spray orange juice • Eggs Benedict (average ingredients) • Minute Maid orange juice
Diabetes • Osteoporosis	4,000	Land O'Lakes Margarine • "I Can't Believe It's Not Butter" Spread • Home fries (in corn or peanut oil)
Lymphoma • Leukemia • Dementia	3,500	Dunkin Donuts coffee with cream (no sugar) • Home fries (in canola or soybean oil)
Congestive heart disease Brain cancer • Multiple sclerosis	3,000	Egg Beaters 100% Egg Whites • McDonald's Egg McMuffin • Starbuck's coffee with cream & sugar
Breast cancer metastasizes	2,500	McDonald's Cappuccino
Prostate cancer metastasizes • Common cold/ flu	2,000	Bagels, croissants, donuts, white bread toast, English muffins • Libby's corned beef hash (canned)
Melanoma	1,500	
Metastatic bone and lung cancer	1,000	Eggo Frozen Waffles, cinnamon & brown sugar • Bisquick pancake mix • Aunt Jemima pancake mix
	500	Muffins (non-organic): raisin, corn, blueberry • Pancakes/waffles with Aunt Jemima syrup
	50	Glazed donuts • Danish pastries • Pop Tarts • Toaster pastries • Carnation Breakfast Essentials, chocolate and vanilla flavor • Jelly, jam & marmalade made with sugar
Decay and Death	0	

Measured in Bovis Units of Life Force Energy

sales. Sales of Post Honey Bunches of Oats, one of its flagship brands, fell by nearly 12 percent in the last year. The CEO of Dean Foods, the largest U.S. processor and distributor of milk, recently blamed "soft" milk sales partly on "a weak cereal category, which drives roughly 30 percent of milk use."

Food producers have been reducing the amount of sugar in their breakfast cereals because of government threats to restrict the use of cartoon characters to sell these products over concerns about childhood obesity. But the manufacturers have developed other ways of selling sweetened cereals, such as breakfast bars, sales of which are soaring. Unfortunately, breakfast bars are no better than eating a candy bar for breakfast.

But in fact cereals were never intended to be the whole breakfast, they were the starter, to be followed by a more serious course, such as bacon and eggs, much as pasta was originally the first course, not the entire meal.

Why Are Boxed Cereals So Expensive?

That's a good question, because ready-to-eat breakfast cereals are not good value for money—they are dangerous to your health, with few redeeming qualities. Packaged breakfast cereals are simply highly processed grains laced with sweeteners and synthetic vitamins—they are manufactured food products made from the cheapest ingredients that should be revealed for what they really are: seriously bad nutrition.

The money you pay for a box of cornflakes does not translate into providing good nutrition for you and your family—you are paying mostly for packaging and advertising, and providing General Mills or Kellogg's with a big, fat profit. The breakfast cereal industry has gross profit margins of around 40 to 45 percent. Corn is a cheap commodity and sells for around $2.50 per bushel, which is 56 pounds. That works out to be 4.5 cents per pound. A 12 oz. box of Kellogg's cornflakes sells for around $3.79, which means we are paying about $5 per pound for corn! That's a mark-up of 1000 percent, quite a profit margin for milling the corn, adding sugar and vitamins, and packaging it in a cardboard box.

But it really makes you wonder why people buy these products when they are such bad value for money. Perhaps it's an addiction, and maybe that is the point of all those additives and "special flavorings," to get the consumer hooked on their own favorite brand so they'll buy them at any price.

Yes, I know—sometimes there's nothing better than a bowl of crunchy cereal with milk, but make it an occasional treat, not a regular part of your daily breakfast.

Whole Grains Can Be Part of a Nutritious Breakfast

By looking at the chart opposite, it's clear to see that the more grains are processed, they more they lose their nutritional value. However, simple whole grains such as oatmeal (porridge) can provide a nutritious breakfast, but buy organic products, they cost only a small amount more. Other nutritious cereals can include grits, granola, and cream of wheat, at least for those who don't have an allergy to wheat. And of course, toast is an integral part of breakfast, but make sure it's organic whole wheat.

Milled oats used to be sold in bulk, but it was the Quaker Oats company which changed the way we now buy cereals. Registered as a cereal trademark in 1877, Quaker Oats soon started to sell oats pre-packaged in cardboard boxes. "Quick Oats" were introduced in 1922, "Instant" oatmeal in 1966, and in the 1970s, flavored oatmeal in individual packets was introduced. But this is a very expensive way to buy oats—the flavored varieties, such as apple and cinnamon, sell for around $3.49 for a box of 10 packets, with a total weight of 15.1 ounces, which works out to be $3.70 per pound. Quaker Quick Oats are $4.59 for a tub weighing 2 pounds and 10 ounces, which is only $1.76 per pound, so the consumer is paying an extra two dollars per pound for flavorings. Even organic oats are cheaper than the flavored kind: an 18 ounce container of organic oats (e.g. Stop & Shop's Nature's Promise) sells for around $2.59, which works out to $2.91 per pound, 80 cents per pound cheaper than the packets.

You can also get good value by buying oats in bulk from your local health food store. However, I do prefer quick oats myself, rather than munching my way through the old-fashioned kind, and kids would probably prefer them, too. The best way to prepare oatmeal is to mix it with a good amount of water, add salt to taste (yes, that's important, to enhance the flavor, and then you'll need to add less sweetener), cook it until it's good and soupy (keep adding water as necessary), then pour into serving bowls. Melt in a little butter, swirl some milk or cream on top, and top with a drizzle of maple syrup—just delicious!

GM Grains in Breakfast Cereals

Another problem with processed breakfast cereals, apart from the high sugar content and lack of nutritional value, is that many of them are made from genetically-modified (GM) ingredients. Currently, about 86 percent of the corn grown in the U.S. is genetically modified, along with about 95 percent of sugar beets, and more than 90 percent of soy. What this means is that just about every processed food on sale at our local supermarket that is not labeled "100 Percent USDA Organic" is likely to contain at least one GM component. And breakfast cereals are loaded

Comparative Vibrational Levels of Health and Disease States	Bovis Units	Comparative Nutritional Levels of **Breakfast Cereals**
10,000 = Level of Optimal Health e.g. a healthy newborn baby / hunter/gatherer tribes	10,000	Organic oats and other grains • Organic oatmeal
	9,500	Quaker Old-Fashioned oatmeal & instant oatmeal
	9,000	Stop & Shop Quick Oats • Erewhon Organic Crispy Brown Rice
	8,500	Quaker Instant Grits • Wheatena • Cascadian Farms Organic Granola
	8,000	Cream of Wheat, instant • Cascadian Farms Organic Cinnamon-Raisin cereal
	7,500	Cascadian Farms Organic Oats & Honey cereal
	7,000	
	6,500	
AVERAGE LEVEL OF HEALTH IN USA Inflammation	6,000	"Newman's Own" Vanilla Almond Whole Grain Cereal
Arthritis starts to manifest	5,500	Kellogg's Smart Start Toasted Oat • Cascadian Farms Organic Dark Chocolate Almond Cereal
Heart Disease starts to manifest	5,000	Kellogg's Granola with Raisins • Barbara's Shredded Oats
Cancer cells form: Breast, Prostate, Lung, Colon, Pancreas	4,500	Kellogg's Corn Flakes, Special K, All Bran, Fiber Plus • Stop & Shop Cinnamon Roll instant oatmeal
Diabetes • Osteoporosis	4,000	Kellogg's Rice Krispies, Raisin Bran • Quaker Life • Post Wheetabix, Grapenuts, Shredded Wheat
Lymphoma • Leukemia • Dementia	3,500	Post Honey Bunches of Oats • Post Cocoa Pebbles • GM Kix
Congestive heart disease Brain cancer • Multiple sclerosis	3,000	Erin Baker's Organic Peanut Butter Breakfast Cookies
Breast cancer metastasizes	2,500	Cap'n Crunch Peanut Butter • GM Rice Chex, Corn Chex • Barbara's Honey Rice Puffins
Prostate cancer metastasizes • Common cold/ flu	2,000	Cap'n Crunch • Kellogg's Apple Jacks • GM Trix • GM Wheaties • Post Marshmallow Pebbles, Cupcake Pebbles
Melanoma	1,500	Kellogg's Frosted Flakes • GM Lucky Charms, Froot Loops, Reese's Puffs, Trix Frutalicious Swirls
Metastatic bone and lung cancer	1,000	Kellogg's Frosted Mini-Wheats • Cascadian Farm Peanut Butter Breakfast Bar
	500	Kashi Go-Lean, all types
	50	Kellogg's Krave Chocolate Cereal • Most breakfast bars: Kashi, Nutri-Grain, Nature Valley, Cliff's
Decay and Death	0	

BETTER HEALTH ↑ · WORSENING HEALTH ↓

Measured in Bovis Units of Life Force Energy

with sugar, corn and soy products. This is a sobering thought as GM corn and soy have been shown to reduce fertility in animals, and glyphosate, the active ingredient in Monsanto's weed killer Roundup, which is heavily used on GM crops, has also been shown to alter fertility. Glyphosate can build up in the body so its toxic effects are accumulative, a serious concern for the next generation, as children growing up today are eating processed foods containing GM ingredients on a daily basis, whether their parents are aware of it or not.

But it's not only the regular fare we have to worry about—according to a report entitled "Cereal Crimes" from the Cornucopia Institute, an organic food watchdog based in Wisconsin, many GM ingredients have also been found in so-called all-natural foods. The Cornucopia Institute sent samples of breakfast cereals to an accredited GMO testing laboratory which found that several cereal manufacturers that market their foods as "natural," even some that claim to avoid GM ingredients and are enrolled in the Non-GMO Project, were selling foods that contained high levels of GM ingredients. Tests of Kashi brand cereals (owned by Kellogg's) revealed that 100 percent of the soy used was GM soy. Mother's brand cereals (owned by PepsiCo) was also shown to contain high levels of GMOs. Over 50 percent of the corn in Whole Foods Market's 365 brand Corn Flakes was GM corn, and samples of Barbara's Bakery Puffins cereal were found to contain more than 50 percent GM corn. Other "natural products" that contained 100 percent GM grains included: Kashi GoLean®, Nutritious Living®, General Mills Kix®, Bumpers®, and Hi-Lo®. Avoid them all. Incidentally, the report found that Nature's Path organic products live up to what they promise: their products are all certified organic and they appear to be made with entirely non-GM ingredients.

So it turns out that even when we try to avoid consuming GM foods, we are being deceived. This is one of the main reasons why labeling foods containing GM ingredients is so important.

False Advertising Class Action Lawsuit Against Kellogg & Kashi

According to a federal class action lawsuit, Kashi Co. and Kellogg Company mislabeled their products as free of artificial ingredients, even though they knew that some of their GoLean and TLC products are "composed almost entirely of synthetic and unnaturally processed ingredients." According to the lawsuit, "Defendants inserted a spectacular array of unnaturally processed and synthetic ingredients to its so-called 'all-natural' products. For example, Kashi's so-called 'All Natural' GoLean Shakes are composed almost entirely of synthetic and unnaturally processed ingredients."

Some of the ingredients in Kashi's "All Natural" products are alleged to include synthetic substances listed as prescription drugs, irradiated substances, pesticides that are a by-product of uranium mining, and federally declared hazardous substances. Kashi also adds several ingredients to its products that the FDA has declined to declare as a "safe" food additive, as well as several highly processed exitotoxins that are hidden sources of MSG.

The Kashi class action lawsuit was brought on behalf of all U.S. consumers who purchased falsely labeled Kashi products in the U.S. Kellogg has already settled at least two false advertising class action lawsuits concerning the nutritional claims of its Rice Krispies Cereal and its Frosted Mini Wheats. Kashi was purchased by the Kellogg Company in 2000 and is independently operated in La Jolla, California.

The Difference Between "Natural" and "Organic"

By now we know that it's important not to confuse the label "natural" with "organic." Many brands of cereal that are labeled "all-natural" are misleading customers into thinking they're buying from a small, environmentally-conscious company, when in fact they're owned by some of the largest processed food manufacturers in the world. The Cornucopia Institute warns: "Since breakfast cereals are popular with children, it is especially important for parents to be aware of the differences between 'natural' products, with conventional ingredients, and certified organic ones. Children are especially vulnerable to the harmful effects of synthetic pesticides and other inputs that are commonly used in 'natural' products but prohibited in organics."

The USDA certified organic label is the best guarantee that a food has been produced without toxic pesticides and GM ingredients. Products labeled "100% Organic" must contain only organically produced ingredients; products labeled "Certified Organic" must contain at least 95 percent organic ingredients; and a product labeled "Made with Organic Ingredients" can contain anywhere between 70 to 95 percent organic ingredients. This is really important for grains and boxed cereals, where many contain sugar, high fructose corn syrup, soybean oil, and corn, all of which are now largely grown from genetically-modified seeds in the U.S.

Fortified Foods

We must bear in mind that any food items that need to be "fortified" with minerals and vitamins have been stripped of them to begin with. All edible foods start off with their own nutrients. Manufacturers can only get away with saying such things in their marketing campaigns as "Good Nutrition From The Start" and "Balanced nutritional drink provides 375 calories per serving, 13 grams protein, and 26 vitamins and minerals to help meet daily nutritional needs" (Carnation Breakfast Essentials) because of the reductionist idea that food can be stripped of its nutrients and then fortified with what has been removed—vitamins, minerals, enzymes—and Hey Presto!—it's just as nutritious as when it was whole. *It is not,* and the basic idea that it can be is based on bad science. When food is processed, it loses its vitality, its life force energy, and ceases to be nutritious; in fact, according to Dr. Robert Lustig, author of *Sugar: The Bitter Truth,* it becomes a poison.

The Hall of Shame

There are so many to choose from! How about **Kellogg's**, for not only producing Frosted Flakes, but now **Krave Chocolate cereal**! From the Kellogg's web site: "Satisfy your inner chocovore with Kellogg's Krave™ Chocolate cereal. Inside each crunchy bite hides a smooth chocolate center. So what are you waiting for? Get crunching!" Main ingredients: Chocolate flavored filling (sugar, soybean oil, skim milk, cocoa, chocolate, soy lecithin, palm oil, vanilla extract,) sugar, whole grain oat flour, whole wheat flour, rice flour, oat fiber, corn bran. Obviously, Kellogg's wants us to feed candy to our kids for breakfast.

And also Kellogg's **Nutri-Grain Breakfast Bars**—they contain soybean oil, high fructose corn syrup, corn fiber, sugar, whey, wheat bran, soy lecithin, wheat gluten, and oats. If ever there was a mixture guaranteed to cause blood sugar problems and food allergies, this is it. But wait, that's just the outside! There's a filling—it contains: high fructose corn syrup, corn syrup, sugar, modified corn starch, colorings and flavoring additives. These breakfast bars calibrate at 50 units of total nutritional value, close to the level of weed killer. In fact, this "food" has just about the lowest calibration of any of the products that have been tested for this book, and is probably the *worst food* you can eat.

Also **Carnation**, for making "breakfast drinks" that are more expensive than plain milk, but calibrate at the same low nutritional level as pure sugar. Of course, no surprise that this offering is from Nestle, a company I have personally boycotted since the 1970s.

Breakfast Foods

The Bottom Line

THE GOOD: Organic eggs, meats, fish, cereals, fruit, nuts, vegetables and dairy products can all contribute to a healthy breakfast • bread, bagels, English muffins and croissants made from organic flour

THE BAD: Highly processed milk • coffee and tea with added sugar

THE DOWNRIGHT DANGEROUS: Sweetened ready-to-eat dry cereals • bread, bagels, croissants, pancakes and waffles made from conventional refined white flour • pastries, donuts and muffins made with refined white flour and sugar • artificially-flavored syrups, such as Aunt Jemima's "maple" syrup • chocolate milk

CHAPTER 26

Fast Food

IT WILL COME AS NO SURPRISE TO MOST PEOPLE to hear that fast food is bad for you, especially since the dangers have been well publicized in the popular media. In the documentary film "Supersize me," Morgan Spurlock heroically endeavored to survive for a month by feeding exclusively at McDonald's. Though his doctor advised him to abandon the diet after three weeks due to his rapidly deteriorating health, Spurlock persisted for 30 days but found that the diet had a drastic negative effect on his physical and psychological well-being. Not only was his general health affected and he gained 24 pounds, but he also started to suffer from depression, mood swings, lack of attention, and sexual dysfunction.

If fast food has this effect on a grown man, just think about the effect it must have on our children—on their ability to focus and learn, and to grow up into healthy, productive members of society. And this is where our fondness for fast food is taking us—towards a huge crisis for America where a combination of staggering health care costs and lost productivity could seriously damage the economy in the future.

The consumption of fast food is a primary driving factor of obesity and poor health and, sadly, it is mostly the uneducated and lower income groups who misguidedly think that fast food is nourishment. *Time* magazine reports that 75 percent of all health care costs are spent on *preventable* diseases. It's hard not to see a direct connection between these figures, as we now know that preventable diseases, also called life-style diseases, are largely the result of eating the wrong kinds of food, most particularly processed food and fast food.

There are now close to 50,000 fast-food outlets across the U.S., with McDonald's being the largest restaurant chain. They are everywhere. Fast food is cheap, and it's addictive, created with carefully engineered flavorings to appeal to our taste buds. But we know that cheap food is not cheap when you add in the costs of health care. The more of it we eat, the more we endanger our health, and when people eat fast food on a regular basis, they, and we as a society, are in big trouble. Americans spend nearly $100 billion on fast food every year, which leads one to believe that some people must be getting their entire food supply from these outlets. A regular diet of fast food leads to a host of serious diseases which are sending health care costs sky high, and this in turn is helping to raise health insurance rates to the point where they are crippling both private industry and state governments.

But what exactly causes fast food to be so bad for us? It's certainly a great business model: take cheap ingredients, fry in refined vegetable oil, add plenty of sugar, high fructose corn syrup and "flavor enhancers," and serve in an efficient manner for instant gratification. This creates a healthy bottom line for the food industry, but it's the inferior ingredients, the key to these huge profits, that are so bad for us.

Columnist Mark Bittman has written in the *New York Times*: "… the engineering behind hyperprocessed food makes it virtually addictive. A 2009 study by the Scripps Research Institute indicates that overconsumption of fast food 'triggers addiction-like neuroaddictive responses' in the brain, making it harder to trigger the release of dopamine. In other words the more fast food we eat, the more we need to give us pleasure; thus the report suggests that the same mechanisms underlie drug addiction and obesity."

If we need proof of how dangerous our Western diet is to our health, it is this: the average new immigrant to America has a calibration of 10,000 when they first arrive, the level of optimal health. After just one year in this country eating the standard American diet, which includes a large dose of fast food, that level drops to 8,000. After two years the level drops to 7,000, after six years it sinks to 6,500, and the next year it reaches 6,000, in effect, going from perfect health to inflammatory and degenerative illness in just seven years.

Comparative Vibrational Levels of Health and Disease States	Bovis Units	Comparative Nutritional Levels of McDonald's Food Products
10,000 = Level of Optimal Health e.g. a healthy newborn baby / hunter/gatherer tribes	10,000	
	9,500	
	9,000	
	8,500	
	8,000	
	7,500	Plain Angus Burger, no bun, no fixings
	7,000	Premium Roast coffee, black
	6,500	Southwest salad with grilled chicken
AVERAGE LEVEL OF HEALTH IN USA Inflammation	6,000	
Arthritis starts to manifest	5,500	Angus Burger with fixings, no bun
Heart Disease starts to manifest	5,000	Premium Roast coffee with milk or cream, no sugar
Cancer cells form: Breast, Prostate, Lung, Colon, Pancreas	4,500	Milk • Filet O'Fish • Burger with fixings, no bun
Diabetes • Osteoporosis	4,000	Double Cheeseburger • Minute Maid® Orange Juice and Apple Juice
Lymphoma • Leukemia • Dementia	3,500	Cheeseburger • Sausage McMuffin • Bacon, Egg & Cheese Bagel • Sausage Burrito
Congestive heart disease Brain cancer • Multiple sclerosis	3,000	Hamburger • Egg McMuffin • Sausage Biscuit • Big N' Tasty • Hot Cakes (no syrup) • McRib • Sausage McGriddle • Snack Size Fruit & Walnuts (candied walnuts & vanilla yogurt)
Breast cancer metastasizes	2,500	Big Mac • Bacon, Egg & Cheese Biscuit • Chicken Club Sandwich • Cappuccino • McDonald's fries
Prostate cancer metastasizes • Common cold/ flu	2,000	Chicken McNuggets • Chicken Strips • Mac Snack Wrap • Big Breakfast with Hot Cakes (no syrup) • McChicken • Hash Browns • Plain hamburger bun • Coca-Cola
Melanoma	1,500	McDonald's frying oil • Sprite
Metastatic bone and lung cancer	1,000	Dr. Pepper • Diet Coke • Apple Slices with Dipping Sauce
	500	Honey Mustard Snack Wrap • Vanilla milk shake • McFlurry • Fruit/yogurt parfait • Hot Cakes with syrup
	50	Cinnamon Melts • Apple Pie • Oatmeal Raisin Cookies • Ice Cream Sundaes • Chocolate Milk
Decay and Death	0	

BETTER HEALTH ↑ / WORSENING HEALTH ↓

Measured in Bovis Units of Life Force Energy

Inferior Ingredients are the Key to Profits

"If you value your health, you would be wise to avoid fast food restaurants at all costs. Not only does the fast food diet promote hypertension, heart attacks, obesity and diabetes; such foods are also laden with added chemicals, and virtually all animal based food comes from factory farms."

—*Joseph Mercola, M.D.*

Fast food is so cheap because the main ingredients used are the result of factory farming and/or government farm subsidies, mainly wheat, corn, and soy. The animal protein at fast-food restaurants is of a deplorably low standard, with eggs, beef, pork, and chicken all coming from concentrated animal feeding operations (CAFOs) via the meat packing industry which is manned by cheap immigrant labor.

Fortunately, there seems to be a growing awareness about this issue. A recent ABC "20/20" TV news program investigated the unhealthy conditions of egg-laying facilities at Sparboe Farms in Minnesota, one of the country's largest egg producers. The egg producer was cited for at least 13 violations of rules in place to prevent salmonella outbreaks. After the program aired, McDonald's and Target both announced they would cease purchasing eggs from Sparboe. Organic eggs have been proven to be safer than CAFO-raised eggs; in one study, more than 23 percent of farms with caged hens tested positive for salmonella, while just over four percent of organic flocks tested positive.

Eggs that come from chickens raised in inhumane and unsanitary conditions have no place in our diets; the same goes for animals and birds raised in factory farms—they are a disgrace. Beef cattle raised naturally on pasture have high levels of healthy omega-3 fatty acids, while beef raised on feed-lots, force-fed corn and antibiotics so that they put on weight, have high levels of inflammatory omega-6 fatty acids from the corn. This practice of feeding cattle corn turns what should be a healthy food into junk food.

When we look at the charts on the opposite pages, we see that the nutritional value of a food item goes up when there is higher proportion of animal protein, even if it's not high quality protein, and goes down when refined products such as sugar and white flour are added, for instance, if the item is encased in a bun or wrap, or doused in a sweet sauce.

The McDonald's Bun

The beef in the bun has for a long time taken the rap as being the unhealthiest part of a hamburger. But in fact, it is the bun that takes top honors for being the worse part of a Happy Meal or a Big Mac (you can read more in the Bread chapter about how very dangerous refined flour is for our health.) The McDonald's bun calibrates at a jaw-dropping 2,000 units of Life Force Energy, the same level as colon cancer. So, when the bun is removed from the Big Mac, you actually have a much healthier product.

According to McDonald's web site, their hamburger bun is made from: "Enriched flour (bleached wheat flour, malted barley flour, niacin, reduced iron, thiamin mononitrate, riboflavin, folic acid, enzymes), water, high fructose corn syrup, sugar, yeast, soybean oil and/or partially hydrogenated soybean oil, contains 2% or less of the following: salt, calcium sulfate, calcium carbonate, wheat gluten, ammonium sulfate, ammonium chloride, dough conditioners (sodium stearoyl lactylate, datem, ascorbic acid, azodicarbonamide, mono- and diglycerides, ethoxylated monoglycerides, monocalcium phosphate, enzymes, guar gum, calcium peroxide, soy flour), calcium propionate and sodium propionate (preservatives), soy lecithin."

In one neat little package McDonald's manages to serve up all the "bad guys": refined wheat flour, HFCS, sugar, and partially-hydrogenated soybean oil. It is the cumulative effect of eating this kind of food every day, sometimes three times a day, that is making people so sick.

Bland Foods Need "Flavor Enhancers"

"The canning, freezing, and dehydrating techniques used in processing destroy most of food's flavor—and so a vast industry has arisen in the United States to make processed food palatable. Without this flavor industry, today's fast food would not exist."

— *Eric Schlosser, author of* **Fast Food Nation**

In his book *Fast Food Nation*, investigative journalist Eric Schlosser dedicates a chapter to the science of the flavorings and color additives that are used in processed foods to make them look and taste appealing. The FDA does not require companies to disclose color or flavor additives on the list of ingredients so long as the chemicals used are considered to be generally recognized as safe (GRAS). At Burger King, Wendy's, and McDonald's, coloring agents are added to many of the soft drinks, salad dressings, cookies, condiments, chicken dishes and sandwich buns, but these are not listed on the list of ingredients.

Schlosser reveals the ingredients in a typical artificial strawberry flavor, such as the kind found in a Burger King strawberry shake: "Amyl acetate, amyl butyrate, amyl valerate, anethol, anisyl formate, benzyl acetate, benzyl isobutyrate, butyric acid, cinnamyl isobutyrate, cinnamyl valerate, cognac essential oil, diacetyl, dipropyl ketone, ethyl acetate, ethyl amyl ketone, ethyl butyrate, ethyl cinnamate, ethyl heptanoate, ethyl heptylate, ethyl lactate, ethyl methylphenylglycidate, ethyl nitrate, ethyl

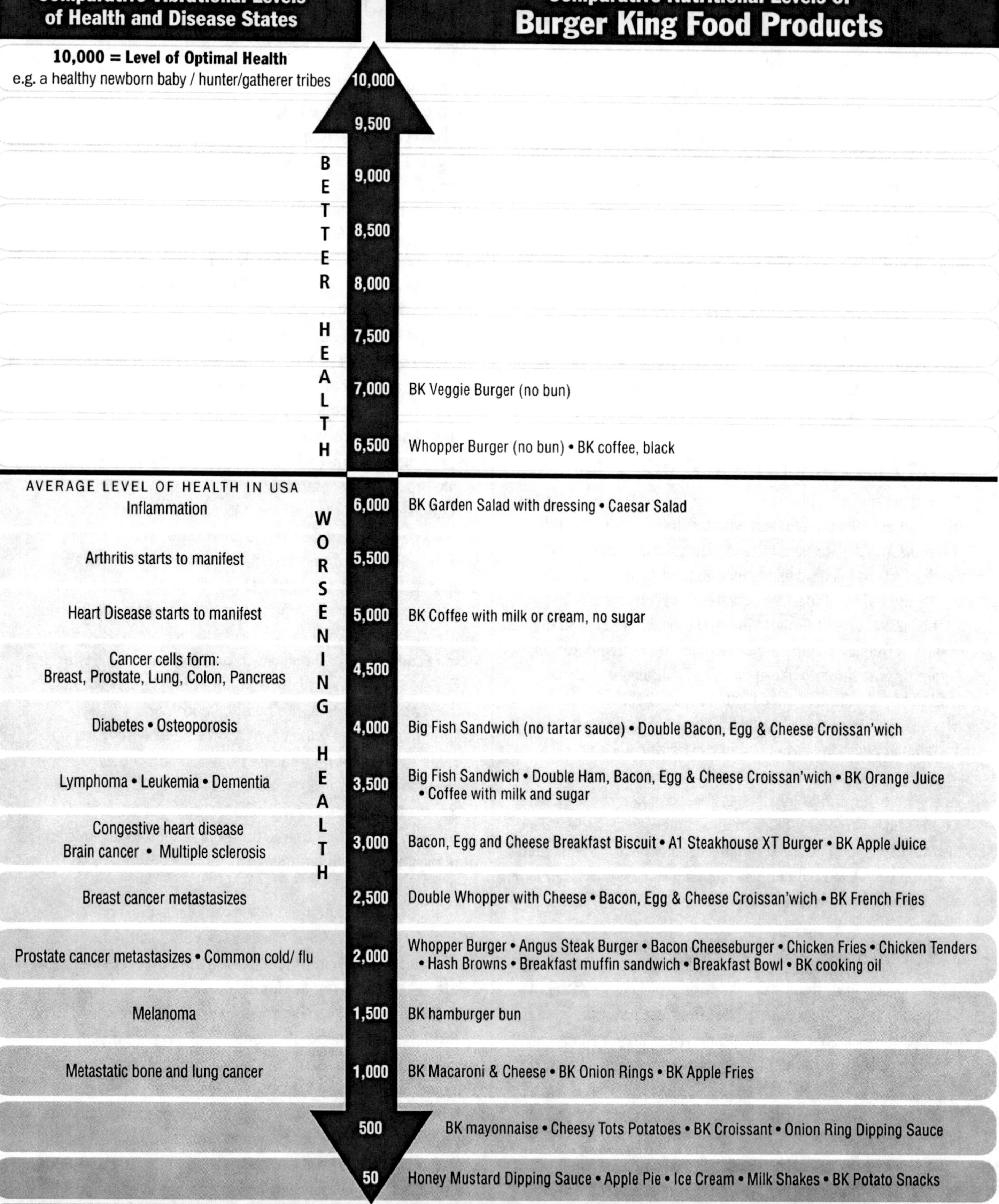

Comparative Vibrational Levels of Health and Disease States	Measured in Bovis Units of Life Force Energy	Comparative Nutritional Levels of Burger King Food Products
10,000 = Level of Optimal Health e.g. a healthy newborn baby / hunter/gatherer tribes	10,000	
	9,500	
BETTER HEALTH	9,000	
	8,500	
	8,000	
	7,500	
	7,000	BK Veggie Burger (no bun)
	6,500	Whopper Burger (no bun) • BK coffee, black
AVERAGE LEVEL OF HEALTH IN USA		
Inflammation	6,000	BK Garden Salad with dressing • Caesar Salad
WORSENING HEALTH		
Arthritis starts to manifest	5,500	
Heart Disease starts to manifest	5,000	BK Coffee with milk or cream, no sugar
Cancer cells form: Breast, Prostate, Lung, Colon, Pancreas	4,500	
Diabetes • Osteoporosis	4,000	Big Fish Sandwich (no tartar sauce) • Double Bacon, Egg & Cheese Croissan'wich
Lymphoma • Leukemia • Dementia	3,500	Big Fish Sandwich • Double Ham, Bacon, Egg & Cheese Croissan'wich • BK Orange Juice • Coffee with milk and sugar
Congestive heart disease Brain cancer • Multiple sclerosis	3,000	Bacon, Egg and Cheese Breakfast Biscuit • A1 Steakhouse XT Burger • BK Apple Juice
Breast cancer metastasizes	2,500	Double Whopper with Cheese • Bacon, Egg & Cheese Croissan'wich • BK French Fries
Prostate cancer metastasizes • Common cold/ flu	2,000	Whopper Burger • Angus Steak Burger • Bacon Cheeseburger • Chicken Fries • Chicken Tenders • Hash Browns • Breakfast muffin sandwich • Breakfast Bowl • BK cooking oil
Melanoma	1,500	BK hamburger bun
Metastatic bone and lung cancer	1,000	BK Macaroni & Cheese • BK Onion Rings • BK Apple Fries
	500	BK mayonnaise • Cheesy Tots Potatoes • BK Croissant • Onion Ring Dipping Sauce
	50	Honey Mustard Dipping Sauce • Apple Pie • Ice Cream • Milk Shakes • BK Potato Snacks
Decay and Death	0	

Measured in Bovis Units of Life Force Energy

propionate, ethyl valerate, heliotropin, hydroxyphenyl-2-butanone (10 percent solution in alcohol), a-ionone, isobutyl anthranilate, isobutyl butyrate, lemon essential oil, maltol, 4-methylacetophenone, methyl anthranilate, methyl benzoate, methyl cinnamate, methyl heptine carbonate, methyl naphthyl ketone, methyl salicylate, mint essential oil, neroli essential oil, nerolin, neryl isobutyrate, orris butter, phenethyl alcohol, rose, rum ether, g-undecalactone, vanillin, and solvent." And these ingredients are not listed on their website, or anywhere for that matter.

Other popular fast foods derive their flavor from unexpected ingredients. McDonald's Chicken McNuggets contain beef extracts, as does Wendy's Grilled Chicken Sandwich. Companies such as Red Arrow make a commercial product called Liquid Smoke so that other companies can sell food that seems to have been cooked over a fire. This smoke flavor is added to barbecue sauces, snack foods, processed meats, and fast-foods, including Burger King's BK Broiler Chicken Breast Patty.

Most Fast Food is Fried Food

You'd think the main problem with fast food is that much of it is fried, but actually the problem with fast food is *the oil in which it is fried.* The latest scientific research, published in the *British Medical Journal*, is now telling us that fried food is not bad for us, it's the frying oil used that creates the problems.

The French fries at Burger King, the chicken at KFC and the donuts at Dunkin' Donuts are all fried in refined vegetable oil. Before the witch-hunt against all things containing cholesterol, food used to be fried in animal fat—usually beef tallow or lard, which is actually a much healthier option. Vegetable oils are unstable at high temperatures and can be carcinogenic. McDonald's fries cooked in vegetable oil, for instance, calibrate at a very unhealthy 2,500, while fries cooked in lard calibrate at 9,000. And when *organic* lard from pasture-raised cattle is used, they calibrate at 10,000, the optimal level of health. Foods fried in olive oil are also healthier than foods fried in refined vegetable oils such as corn, canola and soy.

Fast Food for Family Meals

It is a tragedy that, thanks to advertising and media manipulation, many people now think of fast food is a nourishing family meal. And we can hardly blame them when they are bombarded with ads showing that a family meal is a shared giant pizza or a bucket of KFC fried chicken, and a birthday treat is a visit to McDonald's—or even worse, when it's served in school for their child's lunch.

On the KFC web site, they excitedly tell us that a family of five can have dinner for just $15: "Unbeatable Feast for an Unbeatable Price — KFC's Unbeatable Feast is an affordable family dinner solution for five for only $3 per person. It includes everything needed for a family meal: 10 pieces of Original Recipe chicken, two family-size orders of mashed potatoes with gravy, one large order of coleslaw and five biscuits for $14.99. KFC is committed to offering a wide variety of finger lickin' good choices with zero grams trans fat per serving at unbeatable prices." This meal calibrates at 2,000, the level of colon cancer.

But the truth is, feeding five people at $3 each amounts to $15, an amount for which you can in fact cook a healthy, even organic, meal for your family. A four-pound Bell & Evan's free-range chicken costs around $13, and organic chicken from Trader Joe's costs about $5 per pound. Served with organic carrots (99 cents per pound) and organic potatoes ($5.99 for a 5 pound bag), you can feed a family of five for about the same price, giving them optimum nutrition and leaving a carcass or bones for a tasty soup. And a Perdue chicken costs even less. It's not that fried chicken in itself is bad, it's the ingredients that are the problem—KFC uses factory-farmed chicken and highly-processed vegetable oils.

Astonishingly, there are over 14,000 KFC outlets in more than 80 countries and territories around the world, serving some 12 million customers each day, which adds up to a lot of people eating really unhealthy food. What this tells us is that it's all about education. A huge number of people are just not aware of what constitutes healthy food. We are not teaching Home Economics in schools any more, and what a disaster that has been. The average high school graduate knows virtually nothing about nutrition, nor how to choose and purchase healthy food, nor how to cook it. And obviously they are not learning at home. A new survey from England shows that fewer than half of young adults aged 16 to 23 know that butter comes from a dairy cow, and a third do not know that eggs come from hens. More than a third did not know bacon comes from pigs and four in ten failed to link milk with an image of a cow.

The most important life skill we can give a person is the ability to feed themselves and their family with healthy food. There is a pervasive notion in America these days that we should hire "experts" to do everything for us—weed our garden, paint our walls, wash our car, cook our food. People feel they need to go to restaurants where "professionals" will prepare their food for them. But good food is so easy to prepare and cook at home. You don't need to bury food under a blanket of melted cheese or fancy sauces to make food taste appealing; you just need to buy good quality ingredients to start with. Naturally-raised food *tastes good.* People have become so used to the bland taste of mass-produced food that they have forgotten what the real thing tastes like.

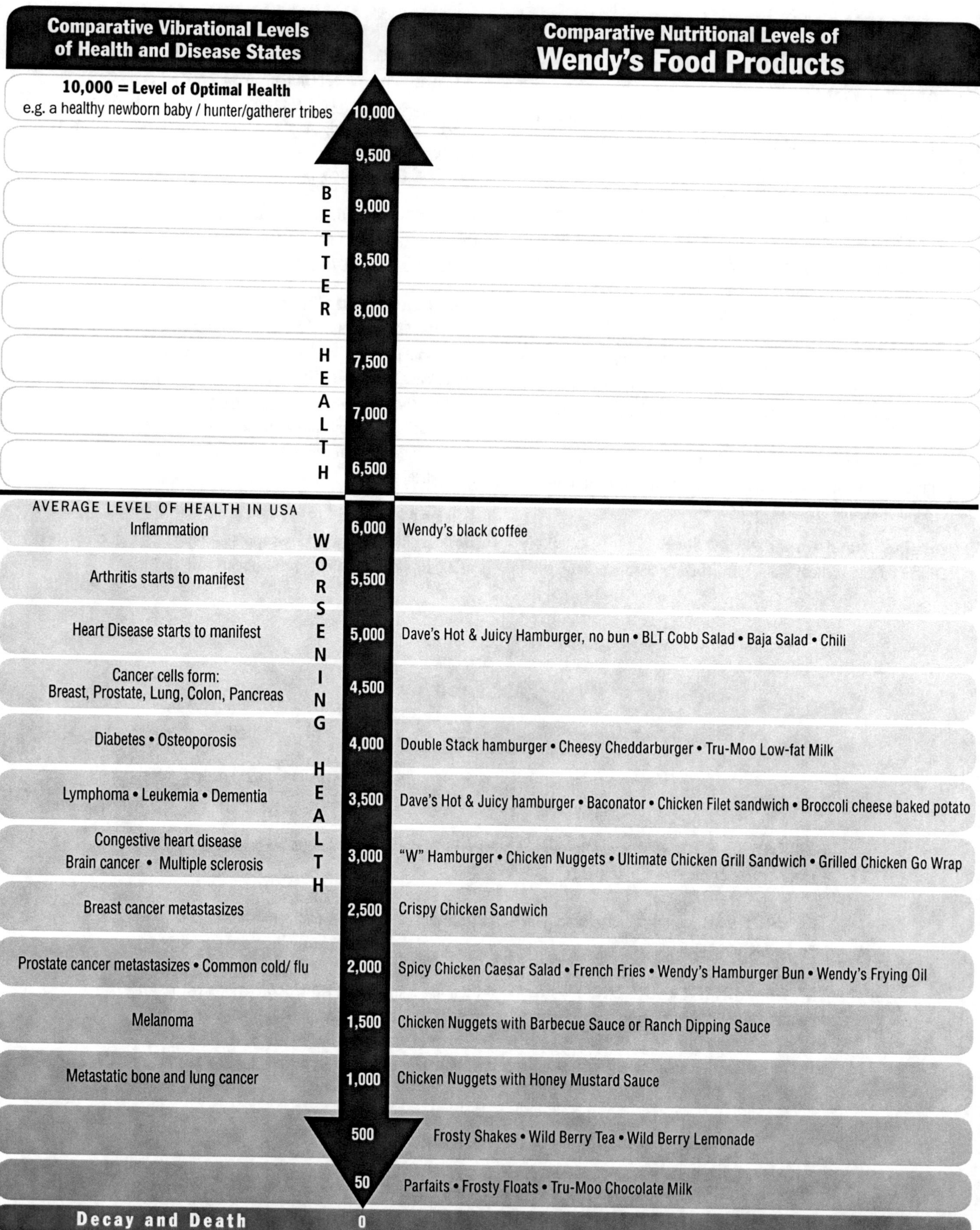

Comparative Vibrational Levels of Health and Disease States
Comparative Nutritional Levels of Wendy's Food Products
10,000 = Level of Optimal Health
e.g. a healthy newborn baby / hunter/gatherer tribes
10,000
9,500
9,000
8,500
8,000
7,500
7,000
6,500
BETTER HEALTH
AVERAGE LEVEL OF HEALTH IN USA
Inflammation
6,000
Wendy's black coffee
Arthritis starts to manifest
5,500
Heart Disease starts to manifest
5,000
Dave's Hot & Juicy Hamburger, no bun • BLT Cobb Salad • Baja Salad • Chili
Cancer cells form:
Breast, Prostate, Lung, Colon, Pancreas
4,500
Diabetes • Osteoporosis
4,000
Double Stack hamburger • Cheesy Cheddarburger • Tru-Moo Low-fat Milk
Lymphoma • Leukemia • Dementia
3,500
Dave's Hot & Juicy hamburger • Baconator • Chicken Filet sandwich • Broccoli cheese baked potato
Congestive heart disease
Brain cancer • Multiple sclerosis
3,000
"W" Hamburger • Chicken Nuggets • Ultimate Chicken Grill Sandwich • Grilled Chicken Go Wrap
Breast cancer metastasizes
2,500
Crispy Chicken Sandwich
Prostate cancer metastasizes • Common cold/ flu
2,000
Spicy Chicken Caesar Salad • French Fries • Wendy's Hamburger Bun • Wendy's Frying Oil
Melanoma
1,500
Chicken Nuggets with Barbecue Sauce or Ranch Dipping Sauce
Metastatic bone and lung cancer
1,000
Chicken Nuggets with Honey Mustard Sauce
500
Frosty Shakes • Wild Berry Tea • Wild Berry Lemonade
50
Parfaits • Frosty Floats • Tru-Moo Chocolate Milk
Decay and Death
0
WORSENING HEALTH
Measured in Bovis Units
of Life Force Energy

The Hall of Shame

Domino's Pizza

The headline on Domino's website page for Nutritional Information reads: "We're about to divulge our oldest secret to success and the key to a delicious meal: Really good ingredients."

Sadly, there are few to none "really good ingredients" in a Domino's Pizza. Although on their Nutritional Info page the items are broken down into the amounts of fat, carbohydrates, sodium, sugar and protein, and the added chemicals, preservatives, flavor enhancers, and colorings each one contains, they don't add up to good nutrition. It is still junk food. If Domino's made their pizza dough from organic flour and added the same cheese, tomato sauce and toppings, the pizza would calibrate at a healthy 8,000, nowhere near junk food level. And if all the toppings were organic, a Domino's pizza would calibrate at the optimal level of health.

Here are the ingredients for a Domino's pizza crust compared with the recipe for a pizza crust from the Sunrise Flour Mill, an organic flour mill in North Branch, Minnesota:

Domino's Hand-Tossed Pizza Dough

Enriched Flour (Wheat Flour, Iron, Thiamine Mononitrate, Niacin, Riboflavin, Folic Acid), Water, Vegetable Oil (Soybean), Sugar, Salt, Yeast, Vital Wheat Gluten, Less than 1% Dough Conditioners [Sodium Stearoyl Lactylate, Whey, Enzyme (with Wheat Starch), Ascorbic Acid, L-cysteine, and Silicon Dioxide added as processing aid]

This calibrates at 2,000, the level of colon cancer.

Sunrise Flour Mill Pizza Dough Recipe

Organic wheat pizza flour, water, fresh yeast, sea salt

This calibrates at 10,000, the highest level of nutritional value

Kentucky Fried Chicken

From the FKC web site: "We strive to proactively improve the nutritional profile of our high quality food while providing great taste. We always will offer a variety of menu options at each of our branches that can be part of a balanced diet."

KFC sells just about the worst food you can eat. Their "original recipe" fried chicken calibrates at 3,000, the level of congestive heart disease.

Burger King

How can BK manage to serve apple juice for kids that calibrates at 3,000, the equivalent level as heart disease?

Fast Food

The Bottom Line

THE GOOD: Nothing

THE NOT-SO-BAD: BK Veggie Burger (no bun) • McDonald's plain Angus burger (no bun) • black coffee at most establishments

THE BAD: Most food products containing animal protein from CAFOs (concentrated animal feeding operations)

THE DOWNRIGHT DANGEROUS: Any foods fried in vegetable oil • any foods made with conventional refined white flour and/or sugar, such as bread, buns, pizza, pasta, biscuits, pastries, cookies, pancakes, desserts, coffee, shakes, sodas, ketchup, gravy, barbecue sauce, and honey-mustard sauce • all salad dressings containing soy bean oil • phase oil (artificial "melted butter")

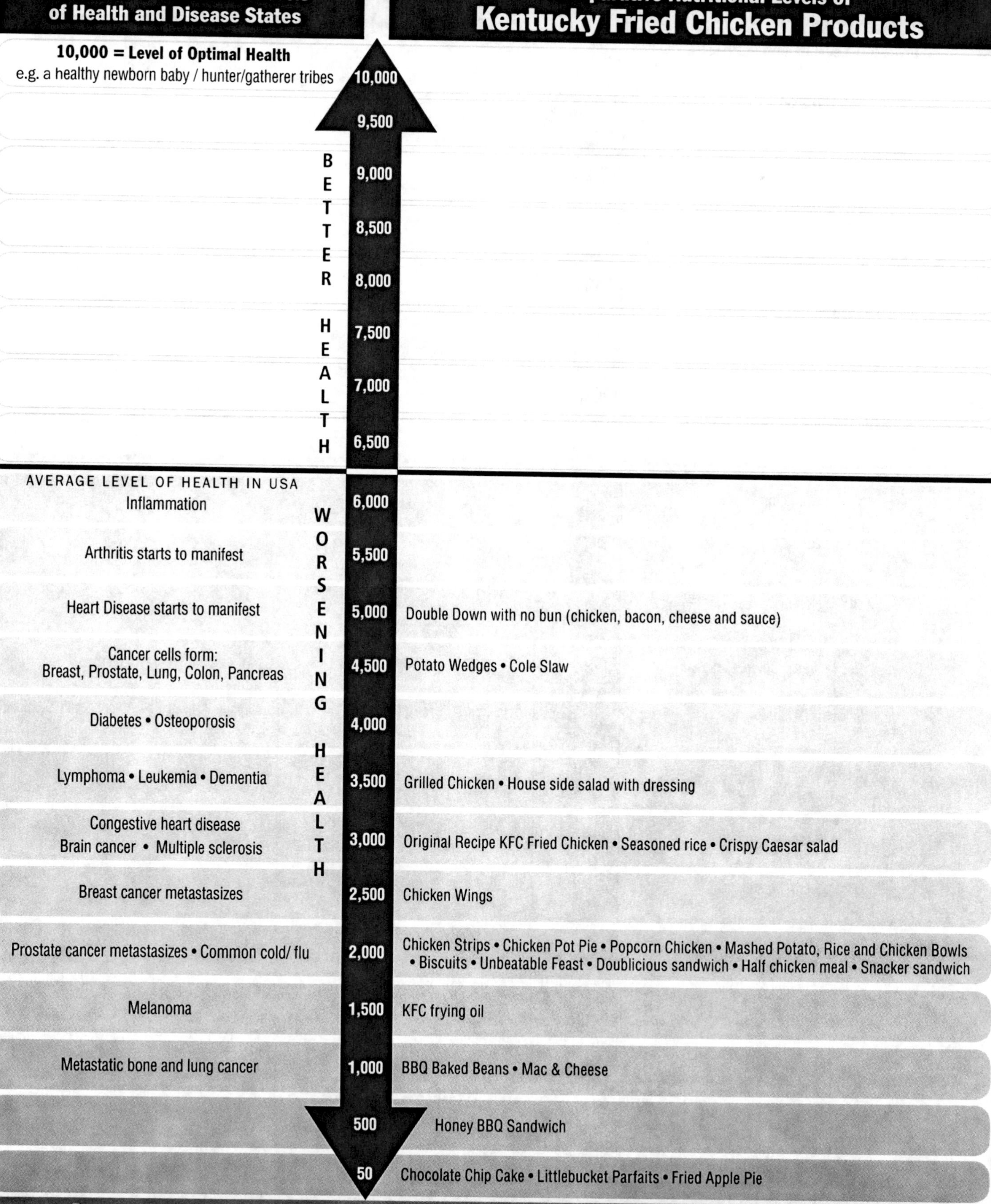

Comparative Vibrational Levels of Health and Disease States
Comparative Nutritional Levels of Kentucky Fried Chicken Products
10,000 = Level of Optimal Health
e.g. a healthy newborn baby / hunter/gatherer tribes
10,000
9,500
9,000
8,500
8,000
7,500
7,000
6,500
BETTER HEALTH
AVERAGE LEVEL OF HEALTH IN USA
WORSENING HEALTH
Inflammation
6,000
Arthritis starts to manifest
5,500
Heart Disease starts to manifest
5,000
Double Down with no bun (chicken, bacon, cheese and sauce)
Cancer cells form: Breast, Prostate, Lung, Colon, Pancreas
4,500
Potato Wedges • Cole Slaw
Diabetes • Osteoporosis
4,000
Lymphoma • Leukemia • Dementia
3,500
Grilled Chicken • House side salad with dressing
Congestive heart disease
Brain cancer • Multiple sclerosis
3,000
Original Recipe KFC Fried Chicken • Seasoned rice • Crispy Caesar salad
Breast cancer metastasizes
2,500
Chicken Wings
Prostate cancer metastasizes • Common cold/ flu
2,000
Chicken Strips • Chicken Pot Pie • Popcorn Chicken • Mashed Potato, Rice and Chicken Bowls • Biscuits • Unbeatable Feast • Doublicious sandwich • Half chicken meal • Snacker sandwich
Melanoma
1,500
KFC frying oil
Metastatic bone and lung cancer
1,000
BBQ Baked Beans • Mac & Cheese
500
Honey BBQ Sandwich
50
Chocolate Chip Cake • Littlebucket Parfaits • Fried Apple Pie
Decay and Death
0
Measured in Bovis Units of Life Force Energy

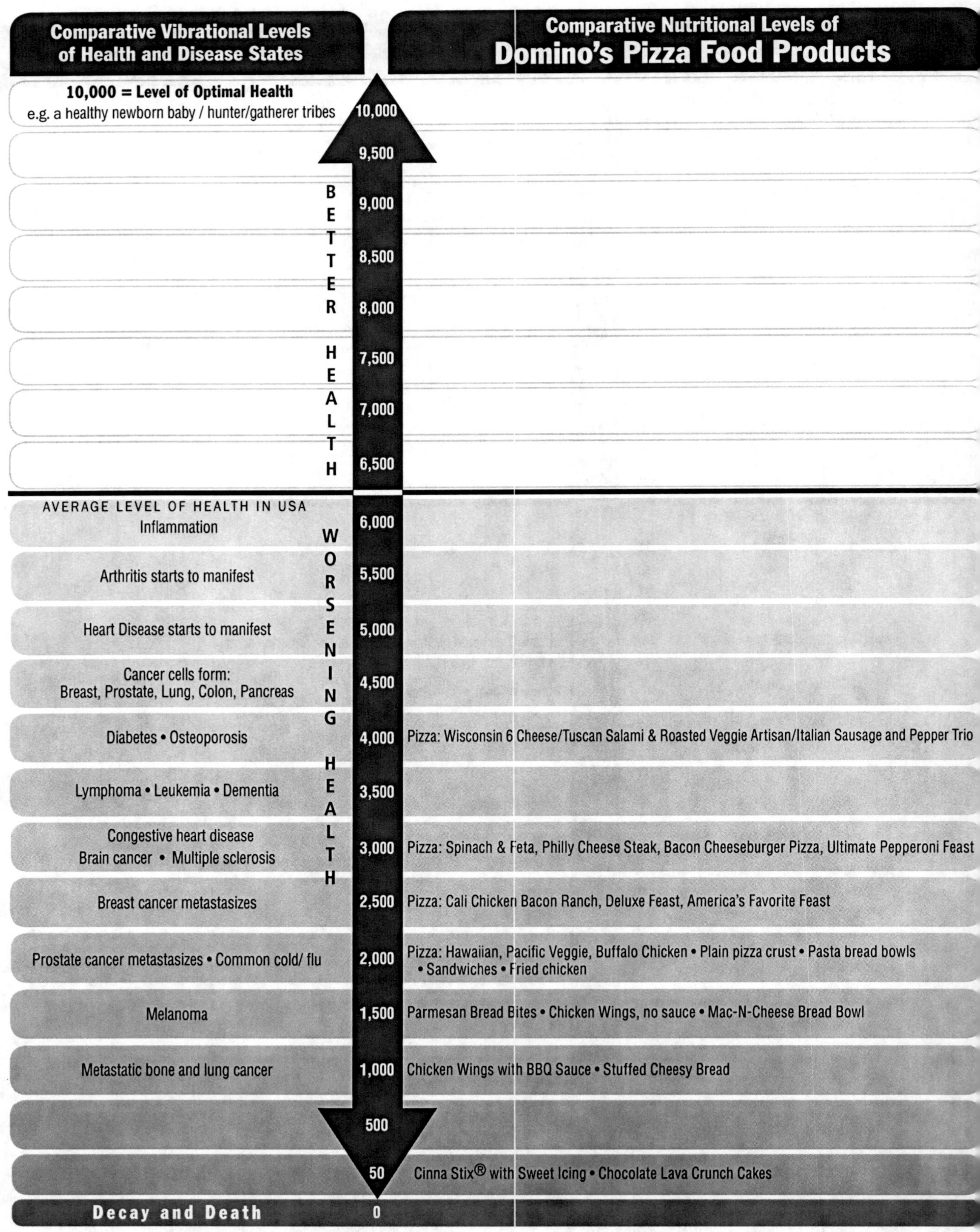
Comparative Vibrational Levels of Health and Disease States
Comparative Nutritional Levels of Domino's Pizza Food Products
10,000 = Level of Optimal Health
e.g. a healthy newborn baby / hunter/gatherer tribes
10,000
9,500
9,000
8,500
8,000
7,500
7,000
6,500
BETTER HEALTH
AVERAGE LEVEL OF HEALTH IN USA
Inflammation
6,000
Arthritis starts to manifest
5,500
Heart Disease starts to manifest
5,000
Cancer cells form: Breast, Prostate, Lung, Colon, Pancreas
4,500
Diabetes • Osteoporosis
4,000
Pizza: Wisconsin 6 Cheese/Tuscan Salami & Roasted Veggie Artisan/Italian Sausage and Pepper Trio
Lymphoma • Leukemia • Dementia
3,500
Congestive heart disease
Brain cancer • Multiple sclerosis
3,000
Pizza: Spinach & Feta, Philly Cheese Steak, Bacon Cheeseburger Pizza, Ultimate Pepperoni Feast
Breast cancer metastasizes
2,500
Pizza: Cali Chicken Bacon Ranch, Deluxe Feast, America's Favorite Feast
Prostate cancer metastasizes • Common cold/ flu
2,000
Pizza: Hawaiian, Pacific Veggie, Buffalo Chicken • Plain pizza crust • Pasta bread bowls • Sandwiches • Fried chicken
Melanoma
1,500
Parmesan Bread Bites • Chicken Wings, no sauce • Mac-N-Cheese Bread Bowl
Metastatic bone and lung cancer
1,000
Chicken Wings with BBQ Sauce • Stuffed Cheesy Bread
500
50
Cinna Stix® with Sweet Icing • Chocolate Lava Crunch Cakes
WORSENING HEALTH
Decay and Death
0
Measured in Bovis Units of Life Force Energy

CHAPTER 27

Diets & Weight-Loss Products

FOR THE PAST 40 YEARS OR SO, doctors and nutritional experts have been giving us advice about what to eat and what not to eat, even though much of it was a direct contradiction of what humans had been eating since the beginning of time. We were told to avoid eggs, butter and animal fats as they were "bad for our hearts," and to instead eat more vegetable oils and carbohydrates. But has it done us any good? After spending two years researching the information for this book, reading countless books on diet and nutritional science, and reviewing admonitions from doctors, nutritional experts and TV diet gurus, I would say that the answer is NO. In fact, that advice has probably caused far more illness and death than if we hadn't been told to alter our diet in the first place, as obesity and life-style diseases such as cancer, diabetes and heart disease have become epidemic during that same time frame.

The truth is, we don't need a doctor to tell us what we need to eat to be healthy, or to be a biochemist to figure out which foods contain phytonutrients or antioxidants or other health-giving components. Human beings got along just fine figuring it out by themselves—in fact they flourished and thrived. We knew that we needed nourishing food to grow healthy bodies; life was tough, and only healthy people could survive the labors of growing and finding food and maintaining shelter in the days before modern conveniences. Our bodies intuitively knew what they needed to be healthy; if they didn't, we wouldn't have survived this long.

Yes, we do know what's good for us—*as long as we don't get seduced by processed foods*. And that's the problem, because processed foods now constitute about 90 percent of the average person's diet in America, mainly because they are cheap, readily available—and addictive. But it's also the solution—because by eliminating processed and refined foods from our diet, especially sugar and wheat, we can avoid and/or cure many of the diseases we have come to expect with advancing age, such as heart disease, arthritis, diabetes, cancer and osteoporosis. It's a simple idea, but not one that gets much press, because it would be difficult to make money from it. It's far more profitable to tell people that by going to meetings, eating pre-packaged meals and taking vitamin pills and supplements, they can still eat the sugary foods they crave AND lose weight. If that's true, then I've got a bridge in New York to sell you . . .

In the U.S., over 70 percent of men and women are overweight, and one in 10 are obese. By the year 2020, eight out of 10 are expected to be overweight. Even more alarmingly, one third of children are now overweight, and over half of them are obese. This is a national catastrophe. Not unexpectedly, weight-loss aids are big business. But do they work? Well, certain aspects might, such as support groups, but if we look at some the packaged weight-loss products that are being touted today, we see that most of them are no more than junk food in different packaging. Knowing that people are paying good money to eat this substandard fare thinking it's healthy is just heartbreaking—it's one thing to go to weight-loss meetings for group support, but quite another to get suckered into buying their food products. They are a waste of money and dangerous for your health.

The chart on the next page shows the level of nutritional health that a person would attain if they followed several different popular diets, and demonstrates yet again that nothing compares to eating a healthy diet of whole foods. It is also evidence of the importance of eating quality animal protein, something that has been out of vogue for some years now, and which many experts now realize was a great mistake. Many primitive tribes count their wealth in the number of camels, cattle or goats they own. These animals have a value for a reason—they are the source of high quality protein, an essential part of the human diet, and representative of life itself.

Do Diets Work?

Dieting is a multi-million dollar industry, with powerful marketing and advertising campaigns promoting cookbooks, diet-plans, and weight-loss groups. Conventional wisdom accepts that to lose weight we must eat less and exercise more. But is that true? And just how effective are these diets?

In an article titled, "Diets Don't Work," Dr. Joseph Mercola writes, "Studies are clear that 90 to 95 percent of dieters gain back the weight they lose, and THEN some. You may lose 10 pounds on a diet, but you'll gain back 15 or 20—dieting is a physiologically flawed concept and sets you up for failure. Dieting is a temporary fix . . . do you want to be temporarily healthy? Of course not! You want to be permanently healthy. So, you have to make some permanent lifestyle changes."

When we lose weight by dieting, our body will be triggered into adding on extra body fat as a way of protecting us from the effects of a lack of food, which creates a sort of biological flash-back to previous eras when famine was a real possibility. The body sees this as a threat, so it adds on weight as insurance against possible lack of food in the future.

The Importance of Leptin in Maintaining Healthy Weight

One of the reasons diets often don't work is that a person who has been accustomed to eat a large proportion of carbohydrates in their diet can become resistant to leptin. Leptin is a hormone that works in tandem with insulin to regulate the body's energy intake and output. Leptin is produced by fat cells, and this hormone signals the brain to tell it whether it needs to eat food to make more fat, or whether to expend energy on cell maintenance and repair. Leptin resistance is associated with obesity, and it is the impairment of the ability of fat cells to be able to transfer correct information to the brain that is the true cause of most chronic degenerative diseases.

Leptin controls energy storage by controlling hunger, which is a powerful drive that signals the body to eat food to store more energy. And it's these feelings of hunger that cause people to eat more than they really need.

"The only way to eat less in the long-term is to not be hungry," says Dr. Joseph Mercola, "and the only way to do this is to control the hormones that regulate hunger, the primary one being leptin."

Resistance to leptin happens in the same way as resistance to insulin—by constant dietary exposure to high levels of the hormone from a diet high in refined carbohydrates, primarily sugar, HFCS, grains, and processed foods. As the body is exposed to too much leptin over time, it will become resistant, just as the body's cells can become resistant to insulin.

The only way to reestablish proper leptin and insulin function is by a prudent diet. As Dr. Mercola asserts, "Diet can have a more profound effect on your health than any other known modality of medical treatment."

It's ironic that we are the wealthiest nation in the world, yet many of us chose to eat a diet that poor nations embraced because they could not afford animal protein, such as pasta, pizza, and polenta (from Italy,) rice (from Asia), and corn (from Central America)—these foods may be cheaper than buying animal protein, but it results in a high-carbohydrate diet. Much healthier is a whole-food diet that includes good fats and a minimum of refined carbohydrates. This will ensure that leptin can once again influence the brain in the correct manner to maintain a healthy balance of energy input and output—that is, a healthy body weight.

The Best Way to Maintain a Healthy Weight

The best way to change our diet so we can maintain a healthy weight is to cut down on grains, or not eat them at all. They are ubiquitous in modern Western diets, but are known to be a major cause of inflammation and create an acidic condition in the body. Contrary to what we have been told, a reasonable level of animal protein in the diet has NOT been shown to cause obesity—quite the opposite, as the high-protein Atkins diet has proven. Many primitive tribes and communities can and do thrive on a diet consisting almost entirely of animal protein.

The main culprits in weight gain are grains, sugar and high fructose corn syrup, and most people will find they cannot lose weight without kicking the refined grains/sugar/soda habit. These food products are highly addictive, and some people will need to eliminate them from their diets altogether, otherwise food cravings will sabotage their attempts to control their diet. Eliminating carbohydrates from your diet can be tough in the beginning, but after that you will feel and look so good, you won't want to go back to your old dietary habits. And once you have kicked the habit, the cravings will fade.

Yes, not eating wheat can be inconvenient at times, but there are now plenty of healthy wheat substitutes in the stores, even in restaurants. If you are trying to lose weight, it's also best to avoid alcohol and fruit juices, as they are concentrated forms of carbohydrates.

This really is the only solution to losing weight, and if you find it hard to kick the refined carb habit, then it's a good idea to hire a nutritional consultant to coach you through it, the extra cost will be well worth it. It's essential to have someone you can contact who can help you get through the tough times when you are tempted to eat a packet of chocolate-chip cookies or a pint of ice cream, or whatever your trigger might be.

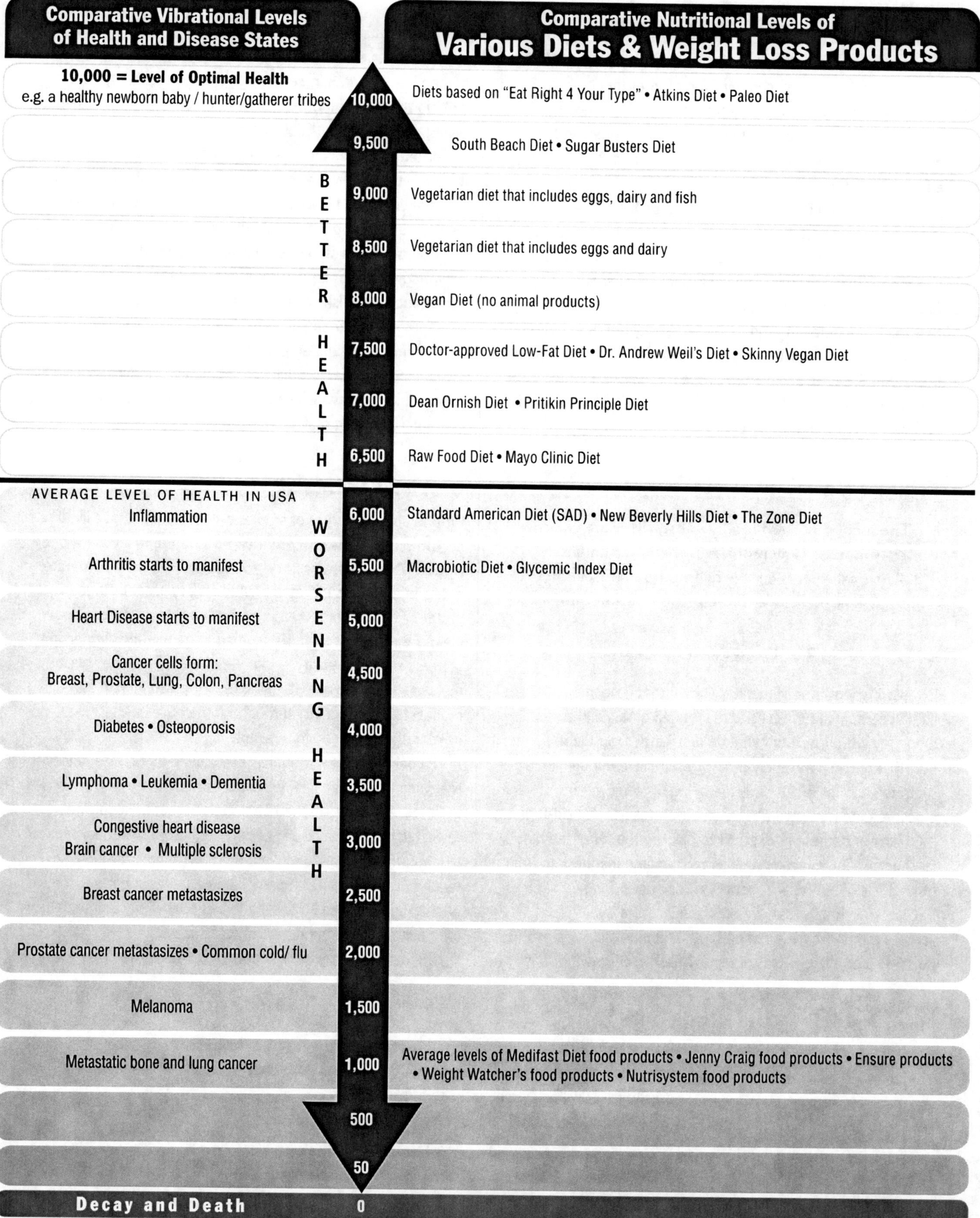
Comparative Vibrational Levels of Health and Disease States
Comparative Nutritional Levels of Various Diets & Weight Loss Products
10,000 = Level of Optimal Health
e.g. a healthy newborn baby / hunter/gatherer tribes
10,000
Diets based on "Eat Right 4 Your Type" • Atkins Diet • Paleo Diet
9,500
South Beach Diet • Sugar Busters Diet
BETTER HEALTH
9,000
Vegetarian diet that includes eggs, dairy and fish
8,500
Vegetarian diet that includes eggs and dairy
8,000
Vegan Diet (no animal products)
7,500
Doctor-approved Low-Fat Diet • Dr. Andrew Weil's Diet • Skinny Vegan Diet
7,000
Dean Ornish Diet • Pritikin Principle Diet
6,500
Raw Food Diet • Mayo Clinic Diet
AVERAGE LEVEL OF HEALTH IN USA
Inflammation
6,000
Standard American Diet (SAD) • New Beverly Hills Diet • The Zone Diet
WORSENING HEALTH
Arthritis starts to manifest
5,500
Macrobiotic Diet • Glycemic Index Diet
Heart Disease starts to manifest
5,000
Cancer cells form:
Breast, Prostate, Lung, Colon, Pancreas
4,500
Diabetes • Osteoporosis
4,000
Lymphoma • Leukemia • Dementia
3,500
Congestive heart disease
Brain cancer • Multiple sclerosis
3,000
Breast cancer metastasizes
2,500
Prostate cancer metastasizes • Common cold/ flu
2,000
Melanoma
1,500
Metastatic bone and lung cancer
1,000
Average levels of Medifast Diet food products • Jenny Craig food products • Ensure products • Weight Watcher's food products • Nutrisystem food products
500
50
Decay and Death
0
Measured in Bovis Units of Life Force Energy

A body that is well-nourished is less susceptible to food cravings, so increase your nutritional level by eating only the highest quality organic food you can get. Don't forget that high-fat foods make you feel full and help counteract food cravings, so make sure you eat a good amount of healthy protein and fats—and that includes nuts, avocados, olive oil, meat, fish, chicken, eggs, and butter.

The information in the book *Eat Right for Your Type* by Peter D'Adamo is very useful—sticking to a diet that is right for your blood type has been shown to help maintain a healthy weight and reduce food cravings. And in his book *The Fat Switch*, Dr. Richard J. Johnson discusses important new research showing that fructose-containing sugars cause obesity not by calories but by turning on a "fat switch" so we gain weight. Dr. Johnson believes that this is an ancient protective mechanism that we share with virtually all animals, and that this "switch" can be turned off, allowing us to return to a normal weight.

Vitamin-Deficient Diets

"The more processed food you eat, the more vitamins you need. The problem is that the standard American diet is energy dense (too many calories) but nutrient poor (not enough vitamins and minerals)."

—*Dr. Mark Hyman, author of* **The Blood Sugar Solution**

Extensive scientific research has shown that if people eat a diet high in carbohydrates, specifically refined grains and sugars, then they will suffer from vitamin deficiencies. So the problem isn't that we aren't getting enough vitamins in our diets, it's that the vitamins in our body are being depleted when we digest refined carbohydrates. Carbohydrates are an acid-forming food, so our bodies, in an effort to balance the pH of the blood, leaches alkaline minerals such as calcium and magnesium from other parts of our body, most often the bones and teeth.

Of course, it's best to get our vitamins from quality food sources rather than vitamin pills, but vitamins and supplements do serve a purpose when someone is sick, run-down, or has a severe vitamin deficiency. Most vitamin deficiencies are the direct result of a deficient diet—scurvy, rickets, pellegra and beri beri are all vitamin deficiency diseases caused by eating a diet high in refined foods—and the "cure" is to restore them to health on a diet of nutritious whole foods.

Certain restricted diets can cause vitamin deficiencies, for instance, those on vegetarian and vegan diets often have low levels of vitamin B12, which comes from animal protein. Low levels of B12 have been linked with an increased risk of Alzheimer's disease, and a study from Finland published in the journal *Neurology* found that people who consumed foods rich in B12 may reduce their risk of Alzheimer's in their later years. Those who follow vegetarian and vegan diets are usually advised to take vitamin B12 supplements. Raw-food and vegan diets can result in a state that is much like self-induced famine, causing vitamin deficiencies which can lead to such conditions as memory loss, infertility, and skeletal problems.

Diet and Longevity

Writing about a survey of studies on people who have lived to be 100 years of age or more, Deepak Chopra, M.D., in his book *Ageless Body, Timeless Mind,* found that they were moderate eaters whose diets included a wide variety of foods high in protein. Eating in moderation and maintaining a steady body weight throughout their life seemed to be the most important factors in their longevity, and none of them followed special diets or took a slew of vitamin pills. They also all had fairly modest levels of activity throughout their lives—there were no ex-marathon runners, for example.

The only thing so far that has been found to increase longevity is a calorie-restricted diet. Research carried out by Dr. Clive McKay of Cornell University in the 1930s showed that by supplying a restricted but nutritious diet of only 60 percent of normal calories to laboratory animals, a method he called "undernutrition," extended the maximum life span of animals. It was found that mice on this regimen lived 20 percent longer than average mice, which, for a human, would represent about 15 years.

Alternatively, they were kept on a restricted diet only every

"Food cravings are usually a very strong signal that something is out of balance nutrition-wise. That's why they accompany most weight-loss diets that restrict certain food groups. Low-fat dieters will crave things like pizza or ice cream. Low-carb dieters will crave the candy and sweets."

—*Dr. David Williams, medical researcher, biochemist, chiropractor, one of the world's leading authorities on natural healing and editor of* **Alternatives** *newsletter* other day, which was found to be a highly effective way to increase life span. Another noted gerontologist, Dr. Leonard Hayflick, pointed out that maybe "the restricted mice are merely being allowed to reach the limit of their life span. It's overfeeding that kills the control group."

Intermittent fasting is now being adopted by some people, either fasting for one day a week, or restricting food every other day, in an attempt to stay fit and healthy and hopefully live a longer life. But for most people, it's enough to fast between dinner and breakfast, which is about 12 hours—just remember to avoid mid-night snacks if you wake in the night.

One report states that there are currently about 90,000 individuals in the U.S. who are 100 years or older but none of them are vegetarians. However, in the UK a couple named Karam and Kartari Chand, who met 87 years ago on the day of their marriage in Punjab, India, and moved to Britain in 1965, are both centenarians—Karam is 107 and his wife is 100 years old. Says Kartari, "We are vegetarian so I bought lots of fresh vegetables and made sure he was eating healthy food. Health is very important and I wanted to look after him so we could grow old together." It's true that this example reflects a strong cultural heritage, but it is also an indication that we need to determine which kinds of food suit us best, as we are all different.

Where the "Experts" Were Wrong

One of the reasons the general level of health in the U.S. is so low right now is the misinformation we were given by nutritional scientist, and doctors over the past 30 to 40 years. But the pendulum is beginning to swing back in the direction of sanity, and many of the food items we were told to avoid are being given the all-clear. Just remember that your doctor most probably did not study nutrition in medical school, and may not be the best source of advice on how to eat.

Here is some of the **bad nutritional advice** we were given:

1. Eggs are bad for you—limit them to two per week
2. Animal protein/saturated fat is bad for you
3. Margarine is healthier than butter
4. One diet is right for everyone
5. A healthy diet should be based on whole grains, as per the FDA food pyramid
6. Salt should be banished from your diet
7. Stay out of the sun

These have all been proven to be FALSE and the consequences dire, in some cases fatal.

The Truth is:

1. Eggs are good for us

Eggs are a valuable and easily digestible source of nutrition. Eat as many as you want, unless you are allergic to eggs. It's best to choose eggs from free-range chickens fed an organic diet; in most communities, there are neighbors and local farms who raise chickens who provide fresh eggs.

2. Animal protein is good for us

But it has to be *healthy* animal protein, not from confined feedlot animals fed grains instead of grass. Some doctors are reported to be curing cancer by putting their patients on high protein diets which starve cancer cells of sugar, their favorite food. Some primitive tribes live on a diet made up almost entirely of animal fats.

3. Butter is healthier than margarine

It saddens me when I think about this one. My own father was robbed of the last years of his life by doctors who insisted he substitute margarine for butter, avoid eggs, and stay out of the sun, a regime they'd had him on for 20 years. The truth is, butter made from grass-fed cows is one of the healthiest foods we can eat, while margarine contains deadly trans-fats, which the medical profession is now realizing. Even New York City has banned it in restaurant food.

4. One diet is not right for everyone

We all have different diatetic needs. Research has shown that, generally, those with type O and type B blood do best on a diet with a higher proportion of animal protein, smaller amounts of vegetables, fruit and nuts, and virtually no grains, while those with type A blood generally need more vegetables, fruit, beans and nuts, and can get by with less animal protein, or even none in some cases. Vegetarians should remember that vegetables are definitely a good choice, but a diet too high in grains is not healthy. Many people have been shamed into eating a vegetarian diet, which is okay for some people, but not good for everyone. We all need to find out what's best *for us.*

5. Our diets should not be based on whole grains

One of the things that we can eliminate from our diets with no ill effects is grains. There are no animals on earth whose natural food is grains. In nature, only birds eat grains, which are basically grass seeds—they have special organs called gizzards that can grind them up. Grains cause inflammation and are heavily implicated in causing blood sugar problems such as diabetes and metabolic syndrome. Most people are much better off never eating wheat, and eating corn and rice only occasionally. But the farmers are growing them, the government is subsidizing them, and we are urged to eat them.

6. Our bodies need salt

Scientists now realize that salt isn't the evil villain it has been made out to be. Every system in our body needs salt to function optimally. Natural sea salt is best—refined table salt is highly processed and lacks beneficial minerals, resulting in almost pure sodium chloride which can alter fluid balance in the body and overburden elimination systems. On the other hand, natural sea salt contains up to 84 trace elements which promote a healthy balance in the body.

7. Sunlight is GOOD for us

Sunlight is an important nutrient. When it shines on our skin, it nourishes us with a form of vitamin D that cannot be obtained from any other source—not from fortified milk, nor vitamin pills. And it's best not to use sun-screen—not only is it carcinogenic (remember: *don't put anything on your skin you wouldn't eat*), but it blocks the skin from absorbing vitamin D. Having a low level of vitamin D has been shown to increase the risk for cancer, so, far from preventing cancer, staying out of the sun can actually cause it. Stay in the sun as long as you can without burning, and then move to the shade or wear a hat and light-weight protective clothing for the rest of the day. The longer you stay in the sun, the more you will build up a natural tan that protects from burning.

The Hall of Shame

It's hard to choose, but the worst offender may be the product **Ensure**—marketed to people who seek to gain weight in a healthy way. Sadly, it's nothing but an expensive blend of sugar, soy, and chemicals, low in nutrition and high in inflammatory substances and empty calories. I noticed that Ensure is advertised as containing "omega-3s to support heart health" and I wondered what ingredient in the list on the container contributed those omega-3 fatty acids. I contacted the producer, Abbott Laboratories, and they told me it was from canola oil. The truth is, canola oil is processed at 300 degrees F, so it's very doubtful that any beneficial omega-3s would survive. Canola oil also has twice as many omega-6 oils as omega-3s, which in itself would cancel out any benefit at all.

The Bottom Line

A good guideline is to eat what our ancestors ate. Beyond that, as much as possible, eat a diet of naturally-raised whole foods, grown locally, and eaten in season. Avoid processed foods, especially refined carbohydrates and all foods containing sugar and wheat. Favor organically-grown foods and animals that are pasture-raised or fed an organic diet for the simple reason that it is the only way we can know that they are free of genetically-modified organisms, pesticides and herbicides. If we do this, we will be healthy and can maintain a normal weight.

It's good to prepare food with gratitude and eat food with gratitude, and to bless the food, water and wine that we eat and drink.

"I mind my own business, and I don't eat junk food."

—Besse Cooper of Monroe, Georgia, who celebrated her 116th birthday in 2012 and is believed to be the world's oldest documented living person

CHAPTER 28

Children's Food

THE NUTRITIONAL LEVEL OF CHILDREN IN THE U.S. is at a crisis point. It is estimated that nearly 50 percent of children's diets now comes from refined sugar, refined flour, and unhealthy vegetable fats and oils. This is a recipe for disaster and disease, and a primary reason why today's kids are dramatically less healthy than the previous generation. Diseases that usually show up in middle age, such as diabetes and heart conditions, are now being seen in children. The U.S. Center for Disease Control and Prevention estimates that by 2050, one in three people in the U.S. will have diabetes. And many behavioral and learning problems in children can be traced to food sensitivities and allergies caused by highly processed foods made from low-quality ingredients, often genetically modified, grown with the aid of pesticides, fungicides, and growth hormones, and laced with additives, colorings and artificial flavorings.

It is essential that children learn healthy eating habits—and their parents too. We need to educate ourselves and our community about proper nutrition and the dangers of eating processed foods in order to change the food culture of an entire generation of America's children. Children need a high quality diet because more of the food they eat is converted to build organs and tissues, whereas adults convert more of their food into energy. It's imperative that we feed our children naturally-raised food, locally grown if possible—it's the single best investment we can make in their future. It doesn't have to be expensive; in fact, packaged processed foods, also called convenience foods—though there's nothing convenient about its effect, which can lead to such things as insulin injections and chemotherapy treatments—can be more expensive than organic. If we choose wisely, we can feed a family mostly organic fare for not much more than conventionally-grown food.

Children that are well fed are generally healthier, miss less school due to sickness, are able to think more clearly, and get better grades. The dropout rate from high school has now reached alarming levels, we are told on the news, and the cost to our economy in lost tax revenue and welfare payments will be in the billions. Wouldn't it be cheaper and more humane to fully fund the School Lunch Program so these kids' brains are properly nourished so they can actually learn in school? A diet high in refined carbohydrates such as candy, soda, snack foods and white flour products has been shown to cause diminished reasoning power and behavioral and emotional problems—and so kids are disruptive in school, denying both themselves and others in the class the chance of an education and a future, and driving gifted teachers from the profession.

Judging by the chart on the next page, it's obvious that much of the food produced and marketed for children is just plain garbage. In the 1930s, Dr. Weston A. Price reported in his book, *Nutrition and Physical Degeneration*, that many primitive cultures around the world reserve their community's most nutritious foods for the young and the betrothed so they can produce the healthiest youngsters possible to keep the tribe strong. And now here we are feeding our kids junk like McDonald's Happy Meals and KFC chicken and Costco hot-dogs and expecting them to grow and learn. But children cannot build sound bodies and functional brains on a diet of junk food. Providing healthy food for our children is the foundation of a responsible society, and if we don't do something fast to solve the problems of malnutrition and declining health in America's children, we are threatening the very future of the country.

> "With the increase in the number of working parents and the ubiquity of fast-food establishments, children are eating more meals away from home than ever before. One study found that children in urban areas obtain more than half their calories outside the home. Fast foods, although convenient, increase children's risk of becoming obese and of developing various chronic diseases in adulthood."
>
> —*Children's Nutrition and Learning National Health/Education Consortium*

Children and Milk

Children consume a disproportionately large amount of milk compared to other members of the community. We are relentlessly told in the media and in advertising that milk is good for our children—supposedly it makes them grow up to be hale and hearty, with strong bones and perfect teeth. Well, research into milk consumption in children has shown quite the opposite. To start with, the vast majority of milk consumed by children in the U.S. is highly processed—pasteurized at a high temperature that virtually destroys any useful nourishment, including the enzymes that enable milk to be digested, and then homogenized so tiny fat particles can enter parts of the body they are not meant to. If children had access to raw pasture-fed cow's milk, as they did before mechanized dairies and the demise of small family farms, they probably wouldn't have so many difficulties digesting milk. But we don't live in that world anymore.

The various recommendations for dairy intake in children established by a variety of organizations suggest two cups of milk for one- to three-year-old children, two to three cups for four- to eight-year-olds, and three to four cups for those nine to eighteen years of age, depending on the recommending agency. There's no suggestion as to what *type* of milk is best, it's all lumped into one product—MILK.

But there are many different qualities of milk, and that's what makes the difference. The kind of milk you buy in the supermarket, let's call it generic milk, is super-heated and highly homogenized, and it has been shown that this type of milk causes allergies and digestive problems in a large proportion of the people who consume it. If you want to give your child milk, track down organic raw whole milk from pasture-fed cows. If you can't get raw milk, then purchase organic milk from your local dairy that is not homogenized (which is NOT required by law), and is pasteurized only up to the minimum temperature allowed by law. This preserves more of the nutrients and enzymes that naturally occur in the milk.

In the United States, dairy products mostly come from cows held in CAFOs which are treated with antibiotics and often with the Monsanto-developed genetically engineered bovine growth hormone (rbGH). This milk contains increased amounts of hormones and antibiotics and an altered nutritional content. According to a paper published in the *Journal of the Royal Society of Medicine*, infants drinking milk containing rbGH could be exposed to a dose of insulin-like growth factor 1 (IGF-1) that is 12.5 times the recommended minimum. Samuel Epstein, chairman of the Cancer Prevention Coalition and an expert on the health effects of rbGH, says that risks of high exposure to IGF-1 are "of particular concern . . . to infants and children in view of their high susceptibility to cancer-causing products and chemicals." He also suggests that regular exposure might promote "premature growth stimulation in infants [and] gynecomastia [development of abnormally large breasts on males] in young children." This bovine growth hormone is also linked to the development of breast, prostate and colon cancers in humans.

The industry reckons that about 30 percent of milk sales in the U.S. is driven by breakfast cereals, so serving children high-protein breakfasts is one way of cutting down on milk consumption. For more on the dangers of pasteurized and homogenized milk, see the chapter on Dairy Products.

Refined Grains Are Not a Healthy Food For Kids

Many nutritional experts now agree that processed grains, especially corn and wheat, are not a healthy food for children, and especially not for breakfast. Processed breakfast cereals have been a tradition in America since Kellogg's first introduced their Corn Flakes in 1906. But how healthy are they really? The truth is, not at all. The only really healthy breakfast cereal is oatmeal, which, when organic, calibrates at the full level of life force energy. A great many people have developed an allergy, sensitivity or digestive reaction to wheat products, now grown from highly hybridized seeds, and most of the corn used in processed foods in the U.S. has been genetically-modified.

A child's diet is critically important for proper brain development and cognitive functioning, and two recent studies highlight just how important this is, one showing that rice is better for brain function than wheat, and the other showing that the higher the carbohydrate consumption, the lower the child's IQ. In the first study, Japanese researchers analyzed the relationship between breakfast staples and intelligence in children. They divided 290 healthy children into three groups according to their breakfast staple—rice, bread, or both. They found that children in the rice group had significantly more gray matter in their brains and showed a higher perceptual organization index, which is a component of intelligence, than those fed wheat. This supports the theory that children's breakfast choices affect their cognitive function. The second study was done in Tehran, Iran, and examined the relationship between long-term refined carbohydrate intake and non-verbal intelligence among school children aged from six to seven. Researchers found that the consumption of refined carbohydrate and non-verbal IQ were inversely related—in other words, the more refined carbohydrates the children ate, the lower their non-verbal IQs.

Excellent "brain food" consists of protein and healthy fats, such as quality butter, eggs, animal protein, and fish—foods which provide a steady supply of nutrition to the brain cells.

Comparative Vibrational Levels of Health and Disease States	Bovis	Comparative Nutritional Levels of **Food Marketed to Children & Toddlers**
10,000 = Level of Optimal Health e.g. a healthy newborn baby / hunter/gatherer tribes	10,000	Organic meat, poultry, fish, vegetables, unprocessed cow & goat milk, oats, brown rice and fruit
	9,500	Quaker Old-Fashioned Oatmeal & Instant Oatmeal
BETTER HEALTH	9,000	Gerber Smart Nourish Organic Oatmeal
	8,500	Average supermarket fruit and vegetables, non-organic • Bird's Eye frozen peas • Wheatena
	8,000	Cream of Wheat, instant • Gerber Graduates purified water with minerals
	7,500	
	7,000	
	6,500	
AVERAGE LEVEL OF HEALTH IN USA Inflammation	6,000	
WORSENING HEALTH — Arthritis starts to manifest	5,500	
Heart Disease starts to manifest	5,000	Sprout Organic Apples & Blueberries, and Roast Turkey & Vegetables
Cancer cells form: Breast, Prostate, Lung, Colon, Pancreas	4,500	Dreyer's Rocky Road Ice Cream
Diabetes • Osteoporosis	4,000	Average School Lunch • Kellogg's Rice Krispies • Sprout Organic Bananas & Brown Rice
Lymphoma • Leukemia • Dementia	3,500	Average School Breakfast • Post Coco Pebbles • GM Kix
Congestive heart disease Brain cancer • Multiple sclerosis	3,000	Cheerios • Campbell's Condensed Tomato Soup • Sprout Organic Pasta with Lentils Bolognese • Sprout Vegetables: Butternut Squash, Baked Sweet Potato, Carrots • Sprout Fruit
Breast cancer metastasizes	2,500	Cap'n Crunch Peanut Butter cereal • Barbara's Honey Rice Puffins • Baskin Robbins ice cream: Chocolate, Butter Pecan, Rum Raisin, Egg Nog flavors
Prostate cancer metastasizes • Common cold/ flu	2,000	Similac Go & Grow Soy • Kellogg's Apple Jacks • Gerber Graduates Grabbers Squeezable Fruit • Beech Nut Steamies: Vegetable/Beef, Rice/Chicken, Corn/Rice • Sprout Organic Veggie Lasagna
Melanoma	1,500	Gerber Graduates Breakfast Buddies • Enfagrow Toddler, Older Toddler • Sprout Organic Peach Pumpkin Pie, Creamed Vegetables, Minestrone • PediaSure & Cottontails Pediatric nutritional drink
Metastatic bone and lung cancer	1,000	Kellogg's Frosted Flakes • Campbell's Spaghetti Os • Gerber Graduates Spaghetti Rings in Meat Sauce • Mini Teddy Grahams • Barnum's Animals Crackers
	500	Campbell's Healthy Kids Canned Soups: Mega Noodle, Double Noodle, Chicken/Stars • Gerber Graduates Fruit Splash, Mac & Cheese, Ravioli, Cookies, Cereal Bars • Soft-serve ice cream
	50	Candy • chocolate • Gerber Graduates Yogurt Melts, Lil' Crunchies Corn Snacks & Puffs • Beech Nut Goodies Toddler Snacks • Kellogg's Crave Chocolate Cereal
Decay and Death	0	

Measured in Bovis Units of Life Force Energy

Research has shown that a good breakfast helps a child do better in school. A high protein breakfast for kids, such as a vegetable omelette or bacon and eggs, will mean that they can go for longer periods of time without getting hungry and can concentrate better. A study published in the *Archives of Pediatrics & Adolescent Medicine* showed that children who ate breakfast regularly had higher reading and math scores, lower levels of depression, anxiety, and hyperactivity, better school attendance, improved attention spans, and fewer behavior problems than those who didn't.

A high-protein breakfast has also been shown to be beneficial for children with ADHD. In a study published in the *Journal of Psychiatric Research,* scientists at George Washington University tested three breakfast types (high-carbohydrate, high-protein, and no breakfast at all) on 39 children with ADHD and 44 kids without the condition. For the hyperactive children, performance on several tests, including a test for attention, was significantly worse with the high-carbohydrate breakfast, as compared with the scores of the children who ate the high-protein breakfast.

Marketing Junk Food to Children

There's this idea in the U.S. that children should eat different food from the "grown-ups." But kids can and should eat the same food as adults. Food is food. Okay, they will need to have it mashed up when they are little, but soon they'll be onto the real thing, chomping through chicken and tackling more advanced fare as their teeth grow in. That's how strong teeth and jaws develop, by chewing. Children do not need a diet of mac & cheese, hot dogs, and pizza, they need nutritious REAL FOOD.

Processed foods are made from the cheapest ingredients and the food companies stand to make huge profits by selling them in quantity, which is why these foods are so heavily advertised. Food and beverage companies spend $2 billion a year promoting unhealthy foods to kids. Because of the dramatic increase in childhood obesity, Congress in 2009 instructed the FDA, the CDC, the Federal Trade Commission, and the Department of Agriculture to form an Interagency Working Group to examine child-targeted advertising and recommend standards for marketing food to children under 18. When the Working Group published its draft voluntary guidelines in April, it suggested that food companies should adopt two principles, but they are not legally enforceable by any regulatory agency.

They suggested that food advertised to children should:

- make "a meaningful contribution to a healthful diet" by containing a significant amount of dairy products, fish, meat or poultry, eggs, fruit, vegetables, whole grains, nuts and seeds, and beans
- have only "minimal quantities of nutrients that could have a negative impact on health and weight"

But the processed food industry is only interested in the bottom line, so the industry is lobbying the government and calling on the Working Group to throw out its voluntary proposal and use the industry's own guidelines for "responsible advertising."

Though we have no control over what the food industry decides to do, it's important that we support all measures to curtail advertising to kids, and also that we vote with our pocketbook by purchasing healthy food. Eating a little junk food occasionally when away from home is to be expected, but the healthy eating habits kids learn from their families will last a lifetime, which will be a long one, we hope. After all, if no one bought Kellogg's breakfast cereal, Kellogg's would go out of business. And in fact, sales of breakfast cereals were down significantly last year, a reflection of changing times in America. Sales of such cereals as Fruit Loops, Raisin Bran and Special K fell in the single digits, and sales of Kellogg's Corn Pops dropped by 19 percent. Let's hope this is just the beginning of the awareness of the junk food status of sugared breakfast cereals and a movement away from processed foods.

Children's Menus in Restaurants

One of the worse offenders when it comes to marketing junk food to kids is "family" restaurants, with their Kiddies' Menus featuring low-grade food such as hot-dogs, chicken nuggets, mac & cheese, and fries with ketchup. Avoid all restaurants who advertise "Kids Eat Free"—it's not going to be high-quality food. When eating out, it's best to order small portions of adult food rather than feed children the sub-standard fare offered for kids. And remember it's best not to let kids have ice cream every day—they need to have treats to look forward to.

Children and Soft Drinks

Sodas and sweetened fruit drinks are so dangerous for kids that they deserve to be banned from homes and schools. The health implications of drinking soda are enormous, but fructose-containing beverages such as fruit juice and fruit drinks can be just as dangerous to youngsters, and that includes orange juice.

Soft drinks are almost universally sweetened with high fructose corn syrup (HFCS), which has been found to be a chronic toxin that causes liver damage. Refined sugar is half dextrose (or glucose) and half fructose, while HFCS has a higher level of fructose. Glucose is metabolized directly into the blood stream, while fructose is metabolized solely by the liver, and the excess fructose is stored in the blood stream as triglycerides. Any excess fructose that cannot be stored in the blood is stored in fat tissue in the body, around the abdomen and thighs, for instance, creating an obese individual.

One out of three kids in the U.S. is now considered overweight or obese. Until recently, children were rarely diagnosed with high blood pressure, but a new study has shown that hypertension among children is four times higher than predicted, with five percent of American children are now estimated to have high blood pressure, and among overweight children, the rate is ten percent. Even more startling is that 90 percent of adolescents who have high blood pressure have elevated uric acid levels due to fructose consumption, which leads to gout.

Kids are prime targets for soft drink advertising and marketing. The Sugary Drink FACTS report revealed some shocking statistics and covert ways that beverage companies are trying to get kids hooked on sugary drinks through TV, the Web, YouTube and Facebook:

• Children's exposure to TV ads for sugary drinks from Coca-Cola and Dr. Pepper Snapple Group nearly doubled from 2008 to 2010.

• MyCokeRewards.com was the most-visited sugary drink company website with 170,000 unique youth visitors per month (42,000 of whom were young children and 129,000 were teens); Capri Sun's website was the second-most viewed site, attracting 35,000 young children and 35,000 teens per month.

• Twenty-one sugary drink brands had YouTube channels in 2010 with more than 229 million views by June 2011, including 158 million views for the Red Bull channel alone.

• Coca-Cola was the most popular of all brands on Facebook, with more than 30 million fans; Red Bull and Monster ranked 5th and 15th, with more than 20 million and 11 million fans, respectively.

The Disaster that is School Lunch

Children cannot learn at school unless they are nourished with quality food. Starting the day with Coco Pops and having a slice of pizza and a Coke for lunch is no way for children to flourish. In schools where healthy lunch programs have been introduced, many started and inspired by celebrity chefs Alice Waters and Jamie Oliver, dramatic changes have been observed in the behavior and learning abilities of children being nourished with healthy foods low in refined carbohydrates.

The National School Lunch Program was launched in 1946 as a public safety net and many feel it should be redesigned to make our children healthier. Under the program, the United States Department of Agriculture gives public schools cash for every meal they serve—currently those amounts are $2.77 for a free lunch, $2.37 for a reduced-price lunch and 26 cents for a paid lunch, but many feel this is inadequate to cover the cost of healthy food. Much of the food consists of low-grade meat and cheese, and processed foods such as chicken nuggets and pizza. Many of the items are frozen, and then heated or just unwrapped since many schools do not have kitchens. Schools also get periodic, additional "bonus" commodities from the USDA, which pays good money for what are essentially leftovers from big American food producers.

But some parents are demanding better food for their children. Advocacy groups like Better School Food have rejected the National School Lunch Program and have turned instead to local farmers for freshly-grown food. Many schools continue to use USDA commodities, but cook food from scratch and have added organic fruits and vegetables from local farms. They have managed to cut costs by working with farmers to identify crops that they can grow in volume and sell for reasonable prices.

Many nutritional experts believe that the National School Lunch Program just needs more money spent on it, but without healthy food—and cooks to prepare it—that money will only create a larger junk-food distribution system. Others feel that the current system needs to be scrapped and the Government should give schools enough money so they can cook and serve healthy, unprocessed foods that are locally grown when possible. Many believe it would cost about $5 per child to serve them a healthy midday meal, and that it would be money well spent.

The Corruption at School Cafeterias

But the real reason the quality of school lunches is so poor may have nothing to do with value for money. According to an article in *La Vida Locavore,* manufacturers of processed foods pay "rebates," or kickbacks, to food service companies that serve school districts across the United States. More than 100 companies apparently paid rebates to Chartwells, a food service management company hired by D.C. Public Schools, said Ed Bruske, who obtained documents under the Freedom of Information Act to uncover this alleged corruption. According to Bruske: "Manufacturers pay rebates based on large volume purchases—literally, cash for placing an order. Rebates are said to be worth billions of dollars to the nation's food industry, although manufacturers as well as the food service companies who feed millions of the nation's school children every day—Chartwells, Sodexo and Aramark—treat them as a closely-guarded secret." Obviously this "rebate" system represents a conflict of interest that could prompt a food service management company to order food for school lunches based on the amount of rebate it will receive, rather than the food's nutritional value. The result is that school lunches are made up of highly processed foods such as pizza, hot-dogs, frozen meals, and flavored milk rather than fresh, nutritious food.

Chartwells is part of a huge international food services conglomerate that provides the food each day for 2.5 million children in more than 500 school districts across the U.S. Other affiliated companies in the group are Bon Appetit, Restaurant Associates, Thompson Hospitality, Morrison Management, and Wolfgang Puck Catering.

An article in *In These Times* magazine in March 2009 suggested that the giant service companies were taking in hundreds of millions of dollars in rebates by focusing on purchasing national brands that can afford to give hefty discounts, rather than smaller, local companies that sell their goods more cheaply. The article reported, "The money involved is massive. Charles C. Kirby, former USDA regional director for child nutrition in Atlanta, says he ran a Mississippi Education Department cooperative buying program from 1992 to 2001. He dealt directly with companies such as Heinz and Kellogg's and received rebates ranging from 10 percent to 50 percent. In the last year, his rebates were $15 million out of $90 million in purchasing."

A 2002 audit by the U.S. Department of Agriculture found that in a sample of Midwestern school districts, food service companies routinely ignored the rule that requires them to pass any rebates they receive on to the schools. They were just pocketing the money. A Homeland Security sub-committee in the U.S. Senate is investigating possible rebate fraud in contracts across the entire federal government. This news should encourage many parents to lobby for a healthy school lunch program at their children's schools.

Domino's Pizza for School Lunch?

Yes, the fast food chain is doing all it can to make sure your kid can eat Domino's Pizza for lunch. Their website tells us: "A revolution in school pizza! This line of delicious, nutritious pizzas created specifically for schools is delivered hot and fresh from your local Domino's Pizza store. Domino's Pizza Smart Slice is the nutritious food that kids will actually EAT and LOVE!"

Domino's pizza calibrates low on the nutritional scale—it is almost pure junk food. On their website they offer a "rich loyalty program" for those schools who sign up to serve pizza for school lunch, which sounds very much like a kick-back.

The Danger of Soy in Children's Food

Soy products are now being served in school lunches, and soy protein isolate is touted as being a healthful alternative to meat and dairy. But the latest research has shown that unfermented soy depletes the necessary nutrients needed for healthy growth and has been linked to learning disabilities. Furthermore, there are growing concerns about the potential for GM soy to create sterility in future generations.

Though *fermented* soy can be a healthy food, *unfermented* soy can cause serious health problems and may even have a disastrous impact on future generations, according to Jeffrey Smith, author of *Seeds of Deception* and *Genetic Roulette*. There are three basic problems with consuming unfermented soy: the soy itself, the genetic modification of soy beans, and the increased pesticide load from the herbicide Roundup (glyphosate) used on GM crops. These are good reasons not to let your children eat it, but soy is in just about everything, so get used to scrutinizing labels.

Soy isoflavones mimic estrogen so effectively that they are able to bind to estrogen receptors. According to one study, young female hamsters fed the soy isoflavone genistein showed physical signs of sexual maturity and interest in mating much more quickly than female hamsters that matured naturally. For boys, soy isoflavones appear to have the opposite effect; delaying or retarding sexual development. Premature development of girls has been linked to the use of soy formula and exposure to environmental estrogen-mimickers such as PCBs and DDE. Almost 15 percent of white girls and 50 percent of African-American girls now show signs of puberty before the age of eight, and some girls are showing sexual development at the age of three. Precocious puberty is worrisome, as girls who go through puberty early in life are at increased risk of developing breast and uterine cancer, both of which are strongly influenced by estrogen.

GM Foods Cause Allergies in Children

> "Swapping genes between organisms can produce unknown toxic effects and allergies that are most likely to affect children."
>
> —*Vyvyan Howard, Toxico-Pathologst, Liverpool University Hospital, England*

GM foods can have a greater impact on the structure and functioning of the fast-growing bodies of children than on adults. Children are three to four times more prone to allergies than adults and have the highest risk of death from severe food allergy, while infants under the age of two have the highest incidence of reactions, especially to new allergens encountered in the diet. Even tiny amounts of allergens can cause reactions. The EPA believes one reason for this high sensitivity is due to the fact that an immature gut is more likely to allow allergenic particles to permeate the gut and enter the blood stream and so irritate the immune system.

These new allergens from gene modification are now found in just about all the soy consumed in the U.S., as well as corn used as animal feed. According to the Royal Society of Canada, "The potentially widespread use of GM food products as food additives and staple foods, including use in baby foods, may lead to earlier introduction of these novel proteins to susceptible infants either directly or via the presence of the maternally ingested proteins in breast milk."

Scientists at the Royal Society of England have stated that genetic modification "could lead to unpredicted harmful changes in the nutritional state of foods" and recommend that "potential health effects of GM foods be rigorously researched before being fed to pregnant or breast-feeding women and babies." And biologist David Schubert warns: "Since children are the most likely to be adversely effected by toxins and other dietary problems, if the GM food is given to them without proper testing, they will be the experimental animals. If there are problems, we will probably never know because the cause will not be traceable and many diseases take a very long time to develop."

Jeffrey Smith reported on an FAO/WHO task force on GM food that said, "Attention should be paid to the particular physiological characteristics and metabolic requirements of specific population subgroups, such as infants [and] children." But in practice, he said, GM safety assessments ignore them. In fact, industry-funded studies often use mature animals instead of the more sensitive young ones in order to mask results.

The Hall of Shame

PediaSure, made by Abbott Nutrition
Truth in Advertising? Let's see if we think so:

The Pitch: "PediaSure: #1 Pediatrician Recommended Brand. The complete, balanced nutrition of PediaSure is clinically proven to help kids grow. Each delicious shake provides a source of protein, vitamins, and minerals needed for healthy child growth and development. And PediaSure is gluten-free, kosher, and halal, as well as suitable for children with lactose intolerance. PediaSure is WIC®† eligible in all 50 states and widely available in stores and pharmacies."

The Truth: PediaSure calibrates at 1,000 on the Bovis Scale of Life Force Energy, close to the level of pure sugar. Its main ingredients are corn starch, milk protein, sugar and vegetable oils, including soy oil—all guaranteed to cause inflammation and high blood sugar levels, leading to obesity and degenerative diseases over time. How is this drink considered to be better than milk? While highly processed milk isn't the greatest food for a child, it calibrates far higher than this manufactured garbage. PediaSure costs $38 for 24 eight-ounce cans ($1^1/_2$ gallons) while the same amount of supermarket milk costs about $9 or $10, with organic milk costing just a little more. Why anyone would buy this for their children is a complete mystery. Must be something do to with people actually believing the advertising.

Children's Food

The Bottom Line

THE GOOD: Organically grown and naturally-raised meat, fish, dairy, vegetables, fruits, and whole grain brown rice

THE BAD: Refined and sweetened foods such as breakfast cereals • highly-processed milk and dairy products • conventionally-raised poultry and meat • foods prepared with refined flours such as bread, baked goods, pizza, and pasta • conventionally-prepared meals served at schools and restaurants geared towards children

THE DOWNRIGHT DANGEROUS: All food containing GM ingredients, chiefly soy and corn • all food containing HFCS • bakery items made with conventional refined wheat products combined with sugar, such as cookies, cakes, pastries and pies • children's meals at fast-food restaurants

CHAPTER 29

Infant Formula and Baby Food

MOST CHILDREN ARE BORN IN A PERFECT STATE OF HEALTH. That is their birthright, and we can make sure that our children maintain that level of health by feeding them quality food from the very start. If we don't, then their health will deteriorate until they join the majority of kids in this country whose level of health is around 6,000, usually by their seventh birthday. This is the state of health of the average American, the level where inflammation develops and sets the stage for chronic disease.

There are many challenges in providing pure, healthy food for ourselves and our family, but none is more worthwhile than providing high-quality food for the very young. Because they are growing rapidly, babies and toddlers consume large amounts of food daily relative to their size and are therefore more vulnerable to toxins and other contaminants in their food than adults. Their immune systems and central nervous system are immature and still developing, so their bodies are less capable of eliminating toxins.

Without a doubt, the best food for babies is breast milk, and when they are weaned, they can eat mashed or sieved adult food until they are old enough to tackle real food on their own—and have the teeth to do so. But when you peruse the baby food isle of a supermarket, you realize that parents must feel there is something special about baby foods that confers super-good health to justify the high prices. And in fact, makers of baby food encourage a mystique about their products. But there is nothing magical about baby foods at all, in fact, quite the opposite—baby formula and jarred foods represent just about the lowest quality foods in the supermarket. And they are much more expensive, sometimes twice as much, than comparable foods marketed to adults, such as apple sauce and fruit juice.

Judging by the chart on the right, feeding your baby organic food is the best investment you can make in your child's health. A recent University of Washington study found that pre-school children aged two to four years who ate organic fruits and vegetables had six times less pesticide residues in their bodies than children who ate conventional produce.

Experts advise starting a baby on vegetables and then adding fruit to the diet later so that the child is less likely to reject vegetables in favor of the sweeter foods. And it's only common sense to delay introducing anything sweetened with sugar or high fructose corn syrup for as long as possible to avoid the chance of your baby developing a sugar addiction. It is easy enough to make a purée of most foods with a blender or food processor, while some, such as cooked sweet potatoes and bananas, can be mashed with a fork. Food for babies should always be stored in glass jars, as plastic can leach hazardous chemicals like phthalates into food.

"Our unusually large brains require large amounts of omega-3 fats, and breast milk concentrates these fats from mothers' bodily resources. Unfortunately, the omega-6 laden American diet, based on corn and soybean oil and animals fed on these crops, deprives infants of the omega-3 fats needed for healthy brain development."

—Dr. William D. Lassek, Former Assistant Surgeon General

Comparative Vibrational Levels of Health and Disease States		Comparative Nutritional Levels of Infant Formula & Baby Food
10,000 = Level of Optimal Health e.g. a healthy newborn baby / hunter/gatherer tribes	10,000	Breast milk • Similac Advance Organic baby formula • Organic unpasteurized cow/goat's milk • Organic vegetables and fruit • Sprout Organic Whole Grain Brown Rice
	9,500	
B E T T E R	9,000	Gerber Smart Nourish Organic Oatmeal
	8,500	
	8,000	
H E A L T H	7,500	
	7,000	
	6,500	
AVERAGE LEVEL OF HEALTH IN USA Inflammation	6,000	
W O R S E N I N G Arthritis starts to manifest	5,500	
Heart Disease starts to manifest	5,000	
Cancer cells form: Breast, Prostate, Lung, Colon, Pancreas	4,500	Beech Nut Oatmeal & Multigrain baby cereals
Diabetes • Osteoporosis	4,000	
H E A L T H Lymphoma • Leukemia • Dementia	3,500	Beech Nut Rice baby cereal • Gerber GHA & Probiotic Rice, Oatmeal, and Whole Wheat Cereal
Congestive heart disease Brain cancer • Multiple sclerosis	3,000	
Breast cancer metastasizes	2,500	Similac baby formula: Sensitive, Advance, Soy Isomil, Expert Care Neosure • Gerber Good Start baby formula: Protect, Gentle, Soy • Gerber Smart Nourish
Prostate cancer metastasizes • Common cold/ flu	2,000	Enfamil Enfacare, Nutramigen Lipil, A.R., Gentlease, Newborn, Infant • Gerber Nature Select Apple Juice, Carrot Juice
Melanoma	1,500	Gerber Nature Select fruit juices: white grape, pear, mixed fruit
Metastatic bone and lung cancer	1,000	Pedialyte Mainenance Solution
	500	
	50	
Decay and Death	0	

Measured in Bovis Units of Life Force Energy

Breast Milk

Human breast milk is designed especially for human babies, and there really is no suitable substitute, as breast milk provides important antibodies which bolster the immune system and bestows many health benefits on the baby. Breast-fed babies have a lower incidence of allergies and conditions such as asthma and eczema, and, according to La Leche League, breast feeding has been shown to be protective against many illnesses including ear infections, respiratory ailments, intestinal disorders, colds, viruses, staph, strep and e-coli infections, diabetes, juvenile rheumatoid arthritis, many childhood cancers, meningitis, pneumonia, urinary tract infections, salmonella, Sudden Infant Death Syndrome (SIDS), as well as lifetime protection from Crohn's Disease, ulcerative colitis, some lymphomas, insulin dependent diabetes, and for girls, breast and ovarian cancer.

Breast feeding also provides a source of beneficial bacteria for the gut. Establishing normal gut flora in the first few weeks of life plays a crucial role in the maturation of a baby's immune system. Dr. Natasha Campbell-McBride, a neurologist and nutritionist from Cambridge, England, who specializes in nutrition for children and adults with digestive and immune system disorders, says that babies who develop abnormal gut flora are left with compromised immune systems, putting them at higher risk for suffering vaccine reactions. In her research, Dr. Campbell-McBride discovered that nearly all mothers of autistic children have abnormally low levels of *bifidum infantis* gut flora, which is significant because newborns inherit their gut flora from their mothers at the time of birth. If a baby has suboptimal gut flora, vaccines can become a trigger for the development of chronic heath problems in the future.

A mother has to watch what she eats while breast feeding, however, since her baby may be allergic to something in her diet, which is passed on in her breast milk.

Baby Formula

Baby formula is supposed to simulate human breast milk, but the life force energy level of prepared formula is so low it's shocking.

Most infant formula is milk-based, but studies show that one in ten babies is allergic to cow's milk. A milk allergy occurs when the immune system mistakenly sees the milk protein as something the body should fight off. This starts an allergic reaction, which can cause excessive fussiness, colic, upset stomach, and other symptoms. But these estimates for allergies are based on *pasteurized* milk, and in fact raw cow's milk is often better tolerated by those babies who show allergic symptoms.

"The ideal milk for baby, if he cannot be breast fed, is clean, whole raw milk from old-fashioned cows, certified free of disease, that feed on green pasture," says the information on the Weston A. Price Foundation website. Studies have shown that calves fed pasteurized cow's milk instead of raw cow's milk sicken and die. Some infants who are allergic to cow's milk do better on raw goat's milk. Babies who cannot tolerate cow's milk-based formula at all are often given soy-based formula instead, but soy has issues of its own.

One of the problems with baby formula is that the baby is eating the same protein-based food day after day which can lead to food sensitivities and even full-blown allergies, and also might lead to malnutrition if the formula is substandard or contaminated. As researchers at the Royal Society of England wrote: "Infant formulas, in particular, are consumed as a single food over extended periods of time by those who are especially vulnerable and should be investigated most rigorously."

Similac Advance Organic baby formula, made from cow's milk, calibrates at the highest level and would be a safe choice for infants who can tolerate pasteurized cow's milk, but most of the others on the market offer substandard nutrition. Many commercial baby formulas are sweetened with high fructose corn syrup. Lipil, for instance, is comprised of 10 percent "corn syrup solids." The FDA website states: "Substances used in food, including infant formula, must be safe and lawful. Substances that may be used in infant formulas are food ingredients that are generally recognized as safe (GRAS) for use in infant formula and those that are used in accordance with the FDA's food additive regulations (FFDCA 201(s) and 409)." But the fact is, high fructose corn syrup has never been proven to be safe, it has just been *assumed* to be safe, and evidence is now emerging that it is in fact a chronic toxin that causes liver disease, according to the research of Dr. Robert Lustig.

Content of Some Popular Baby Formula:

- Similac Sensitive: corn syrup solids, sucrose, milk protein isolate, safflower oil, soy oil, coconut oil, and added vitamins and minerals
- Gerber Good Start: whey protein, vegetable oils, and corn maltodextrin, and added vitamins and minerals
- Nutromigan Lipil: water, corn syrup solids, vegetable oils (palm, soy, coconut, sunflower), casein hydrolysate (milk proteins), and corn starch

Soy Infant Formula

Many nutritional experts believe that soy formula is one of the most dangerous foods you can feed a baby. Feeding an infant soy-based formula can lead to many health problems including asthma, behavioral problems, thyroid disease, cancer, food allergies and digestive distress, and hormonal problems including early puberty, gynecomastia (man boobs) for boys, and fertility problems. Babies fed soy-based formula have 13,000 to 22,000 times more estrogen compounds in their blood than babies fed milk-based formula. Experts are telling us that infants exclusively fed soy formula are receiving the estrogenic equivalent of at least four birth control pills per day. In animals, studies have shown that the phytoestrogens in soy are powerful endocrine disrupters and feeding an infant soy floods the bloodstream with female hormones that inhibit testosterone. Male children exposed to DES, a synthetic estrogen, had testes smaller than normal on maturation, and infant marmoset monkeys fed soy isoflavones had a reduction in testosterone levels up to 70 percent compared to milk-fed controls.

Soy formula is also laden with toxic chemicals such as aluminum and manganese, which can cause both physical and mental health problems, learning disabilities, brain damage and behavioral problems. If a mother is unable to breast feed her baby or has adopted a baby, another option is to research recipes for homemade infant formula, such as those recommended by the Weston A. Price Foundation.

Toxins in Baby Formula and Baby Food

• Perchlorate has been found in all brands and types of infant formula tested

Concern about perchlorate pollution has intensified since a series of studies reported finding perchlorate in the urine of every American tested by the U.S. Centers for Disease Control and Prevention (CDC) and in breast milk. Perchlorate is a rocket fuel component that has been found in drinking water in more than half of U.S. states and is a potent thyroid toxin that can interfere with fetal and infant brain development.

Researchers from the CDC have reported that they found 15 brands of powdered infant formula contaminated with perchlorate. The new CDC study is the first to examine perchlorate exposure in infants fed powdered formula reconstituted with drinking water. The scientists did not identify the brands they tested, but said that the two most contaminated brands, made from cow's milk, accounted for 87 percent of the U.S. powdered formula market in 2000. "Perchlorate was found in all brands and types of infant formula tested," said the scientists.

CDC researchers warned that mixing perchlorate-contaminated powdered infant formula with tap water containing "even minimal amounts" of the chemical could result in a toxin level the EPA considers "safe," but many scientists are arguing that the level the EPA considers safe is too high to protect public health and needs to be lowered.

• Rice in baby food has been found to be contaminated with arsenic

There is concern that rice used in baby foods is often contaminated with arsenic and other heavy metals. While arsenic is known as a poison, it is also associated with the development of certain cancers. Crops can be contaminated with arsenic because of previous pesticide use in the soil in which they are grown, and also when metals and toxins produced by heavy industry find their way into the soil and food. Rice is among those plants that are efficient in taking up arsenic from the soil, regardless of whether the resulting products are considered organic. These toxins are ending up in the ingredients used in top-selling baby foods, but manufacturers insist the levels are so low they do not pose a health risk. However, scientists and food campaigners are calling for efforts to eliminate the chemicals from mass-produced products eaten by millions of youngsters.

Writing in the *Journal of Food Chemistry,* scientists from the Unit of Metals and Health at Karolinska Institute in Stockholm said: "Alarmingly, these foods may also introduce high amounts of toxic elements such as arsenic, cadmium, lead and uranium, mainly from their raw materials. These elements have to be kept at an absolute minimum in food products intended for infant consumption. The high concentrations of arsenic in the rice-based foods are of particular concern."

Professor Andrew Meharg, a biogeochemist at Aberdeen University in Scotland, is particularly concerned about the presence of arsenic in the rice used in baby food. "Baby rice is a very popular choice for parents weaning their babies onto solids, but there is a concern of arsenic contamination," he said. "Baby companies should be sourcing baby rice from regions of the world where levels of inorganic arsenic are as low as possible."

Two years ago, Britain's Food Standards Agency issued an official warning that young children should not drink rice milk because of arsenic contamination when two types of the poison were found in rice milk, including the most harmful form, inorganic arsenic. And organic brown rice syrup containing arsenic was found in infant formula by researchers at Dartmouth College, prompting them to say that there is an "urgent need" for stricter regulatory limits on the carcinogen in food. One brand of infant formula containing organic brown rice syrup had a total arsenic concentration level of as much as six times the U.S. federal limit of 10 parts per billion for drinking water, according to a study published in the journal *Environmental Health Perspectives.* Both the European Food Safety Authority and the USDA Farm Service Agency are carrying out a review to set new lower limits for arsenic in food, particularly those for babies and toddlers.

• The fungus mycoestrogen has been found in baby food

Baby food has also been found to be contaminated with mycoestrogens, or fungal hormones. Scientists at the University of Pisa in Italy found as many as 28 percent of samples of milk-based baby formulas they tested were contaminated. The substances detected in the baby products included zearalenone and its derivatives, which comes from Fusarium, a large family of fungi common in farm settings. Previous research has shown that the body rapidly breaks down zearalenone into by-products that pose no health threat, but the Italian scientists discovered that zearalenone and similar chemicals can make their way into infant foods. They believe their findings should be followed-up and ought to prompt closer scrutiny of baby formula and baby foods for toxins.

According to Reuters Health, the leader of the study, Francesco Massart, said, "Our study shows the presence of mycoestrogens in infant food. This is likely to have greater implications for infants and young children than for adults having a more varied diet." He acknowledged that many questions remain about the possible link between mycoestrogens and harm to humans, and he said the findings should give pause to parents who use baby formula. "Children, and in particular pre-term newborns, are potentially exposed to higher doses of mycotoxins during their early phases of life, but no one knows the long-term effects," he said.

Mycoestrogens such as zearalenone are a fact of life for commercial agriculture and are found in crops such as corn, wheat and soy. Cattle yards in the United States regularly use one such substance, alpha-zeralanol, as a growth stimulant for the animals, although the European Union banned this practice in the mid-1980s.

• Advanced Glycation End Products have been found in baby formula

High levels of food toxins called advanced glycation end products (AGEs) have been found in infants by researchers from Mount Sinai School of Medicine. AGES are sugar molecules that attach to and damage proteins in the body and are found in deep-fried, overcooked and charred foods and, unfortunately, in commercial infant formulas. They are also introduced to the infants through maternal blood transmission.

Infant formulas are typically processed under high heat, and this leads to the formation of these toxic substances. There is evidence that these toxins could significantly increase a child's risk for diseases, such as diabetes, from a very young age. Formulas that are processed under high heat can contain 100 times more AGEs than human breast milk.

ACEs build up in the body over time, leading to oxidation and accelerating the aging process. They also lead to inflammation, which is linked to a number of chronic diseases, including heart disease and diabetes. AGEs can be elevated as early as at birth, according to a report in *Diabetes Care* in December 2010, and researchers have found that newborn infants, expected to be practically AGE-free, had levels of AGEs in their blood as high as their adult mothers. After switching from breast milk to formula, AGEs in infants doubled during their first year of life to levels seen in diabetics, and many had elevated insulin levels.

Helen Vlassara, MD, director of the Division of Experimental Diabetes and Aging at Mount Sinai Hospital, says, "Modern food AGEs can overwhelm the body's defenses, a worrisome fact especially for young children. More research is certainly needed, but the findings confirm our studies in genetic animal models of diabetes. Given the rise in the incidence of diabetes in children, safe and low cost AGE-less approaches to children's diet should be considered by clinicians and families."

Prepared Baby Food: Junk Food for Babies and Toddlers

Gerber, formerly an American company and now a subsidiary of Nestlé, a Swiss company, makes more than 190 products which are sold in 80 countries. In the U.S., Gerber controls 83 percent of the baby food market; its main competitors are Beech-Nut and Del Monte Foods. Through public relations and advertising, Gerber has cultivated an almost sacred image in people's minds of their products, but their food is hardly better than junk food for youngsters.

Makers of baby food want parents to think that their products have special properties that make them particularly appropriate for infants and meet their nutritional needs. But those perceptions are clearly untrue. Jarred baby food is highly processed and sterilized at high temperatures for up to an hour, killing off most of the nutritional value. Parents armed with a food processor, blender, or mashing fork can prepare nutritious food for their infants at home for far less money. However, on occasion parents do need the convenience of prepared baby foods, in which case it's best to buy organic.

Babies and Food Allergies

The most common food allergies in infants are milk, eggs and soy; other common allergies in children include wheat, peanuts, tree nuts, fish and shellfish, corn, and citrus fruit. Infants under the age of two have the highest incidence of reactions, especially to new allergens encountered in the diet, and even tiny amounts of allergens can cause reactions. Babies may also experience a food intolerance, which is not an allergic reaction but any other undesirable effect experienced as a result of eating a particular food.

It's important to introduce new foods gradually to a baby, one at a time, to test for possible food allergies. Experts suggest trying a new food and then waiting for three to five days before trying another food and to be on the lookout for allergic reactions in the meantime. Food allergy symptoms usually appear very soon after the food is eaten—within a few minutes to a couple of hours. Symptoms include flushed skin or rash, swelling on face, tongue, or lip, vomiting and/or diarrhea, coughing or wheezing, difficulty breathing, and loss of consciousness. Severe allergies are to be taken seriously and can be fatal.

Many nutritional experts recommend keeping infants with any food allergies away from peanut products until the age of three. Peanuts and peanut butter can also be choking hazards, and cashew and peanut allergies commonly occur together.

Babies can have a reaction to a food even if they've eaten it before without any problem. So a baby who inherited a tendency for an allergy to eggs might not have a reaction the first few times he or she eats them— but eventually they might show symptoms.

An elimination diet is key to tracking down a child's food allergies. By eliminating certain foods from the diet systematically, you will be able to see if the symptoms clear up.

The least allergenic foods are: apples, apricots, asparagus, avocados, beets, broccoli, carrots, cauliflower, chicken, dates, grapes, lamb, lettuce, mangoes, papayas, peaches, pears, raisins, brown rice, olive oil, salmon, squash, sweet potatoes, turkey, and veal.

Infant Formula and Baby Food

The Bottom Line

THE GOOD: Breast milk • raw milk from pasture-fed cows and goats • organically-grown food • some brands of organic commercially-prepared baby formula and baby foods

THE BAD: Refined cereals, especially wheat (for allergies and pesticides), corn (for GMOs and pesticides), and rice (for toxins)

THE DOWNRIGHT DANGEROUS: Just about all baby formulas and commercially-prepared foods for infants • all baby and infant foods made with soy products

CHAPTER 30

Food for Domestic Dogs & Cats

PET FOOD INDUSTRY ADS WOULD HAVE US BELIEVE that their pet food is made from choice cuts of beef, juicy chicken and fresh vegetables—wholesome nutrition for our pets who are so dear to us they are like members of our family. But the pet food they manufacture is nothing less than junk food—processed, packaged and mass produced, made from questionable raw materials laced with rendered fat, additives, flavorings and colorings.

The pet food industry is an extension of the processed food industry, an unregulated operation that utilizes the garbage left over from the processing of food for humans. The main ingredients are often no more than rejects from the slaughterhouse floor, processed and sterilized to a such a degree that virtually no nutritional value is left. The product is then enriched with artificial vitamins and minerals and sent out into the world in cans and bags bearing slogans such as: "Every dog deserves leading nutrition" (Pedigree).

The idea that one pet food provides all the nutrition a domesticated animal will need for its entire life is just not true—in fact, it's a recipe for chronic illness and early death. It is estimated that more than 95 percent of domestic dogs and cats are now fed processed food every day of their lives, but these processed foods are very different from the meat-based diets their ancestors ate, and they have have been linked to the poor health of the animals consuming them. Research by the Pet Food Manufacturers Association shows that one in three household pets is now overweight, and Born Free, an animal advocacy organization (BornFreeUSA.org), reports that the health problems associated with inadequate diet in dogs and cats include urinary tract disease, kidney disease, dental disease, obesity, diabetes, chronic digestive problems, hyperthyroidism, and heart disease, which is now known to be caused by a deficiency of the amino acid taurine. It is tragic that so many pets fall ill and die because of substandard food, and that the pet food industry is making a huge profit at their expense, especially when pet owners believe that they are doing the best thing for their beloved animals by feeding them this food.

Anyone who has gone through the heartbreak of losing a pet to one of these degenerative diseases and has paid the vet bills that accompany them would never go that route again. The only way to raise a healthy companion animal is to feed it human grade food. I have never forgotten the advice that our veterinarian gave my mother back in the 1960s regarding our spaniel puppy: "Never feed your dog food you wouldn't eat yourself." It's the best advice anyone can give an animal owner.

> "Pet food scientists have learned that it's possible to take a mixture of inedible garbage, fortify it with artificial vitamins and minerals, preserve it so it can sit on the grocery shelf for more than a year, add dyes to make it attractive and then extrude it into whimsical shapes, making it appealing to us humans so we will purchase it."
>
> —*Michael Torchia in an article on NewsBlaze.com: "The Sickening Truth About Pet Food"*

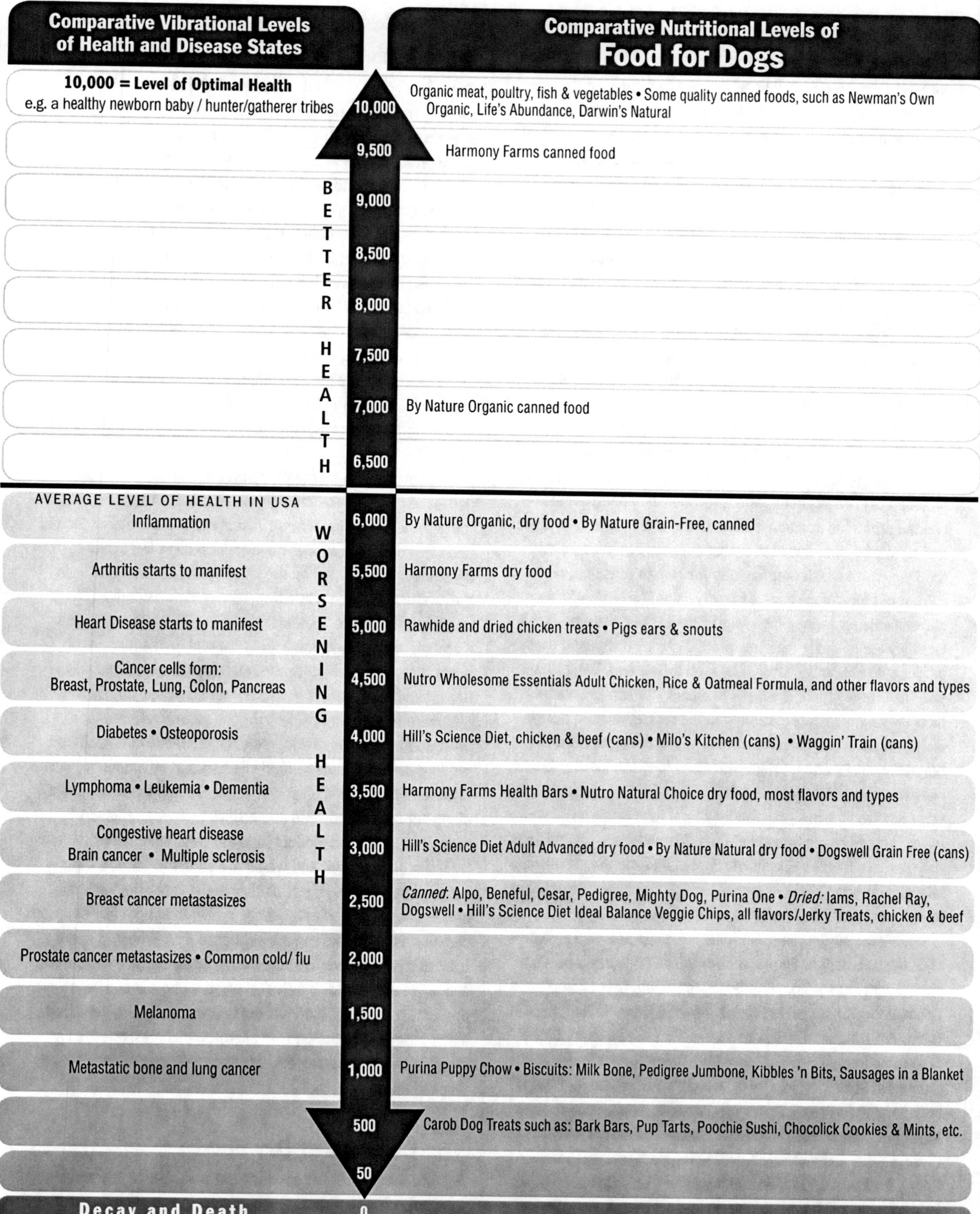
Comparative Vibrational Levels of Health and Disease States
Comparative Nutritional Levels of Food for Dogs
10,000 = Level of Optimal Health
e.g. a healthy newborn baby / hunter/gatherer tribes
10,000
Organic meat, poultry, fish & vegetables • Some quality canned foods, such as Newman's Own Organic, Life's Abundance, Darwin's Natural
9,500
Harmony Farms canned food
BETTER HEALTH
9,000
8,500
8,000
7,500
7,000
By Nature Organic canned food
6,500
AVERAGE LEVEL OF HEALTH IN USA
Inflammation
6,000
By Nature Organic, dry food • By Nature Grain-Free, canned
WORSENING HEALTH
Arthritis starts to manifest
5,500
Harmony Farms dry food
Heart Disease starts to manifest
5,000
Rawhide and dried chicken treats • Pigs ears & snouts
Cancer cells form: Breast, Prostate, Lung, Colon, Pancreas
4,500
Nutro Wholesome Essentials Adult Chicken, Rice & Oatmeal Formula, and other flavors and types
Diabetes • Osteoporosis
4,000
Hill's Science Diet, chicken & beef (cans) • Milo's Kitchen (cans) • Waggin' Train (cans)
Lymphoma • Leukemia • Dementia
3,500
Harmony Farms Health Bars • Nutro Natural Choice dry food, most flavors and types
Congestive heart disease
Brain cancer • Multiple sclerosis
3,000
Hill's Science Diet Adult Advanced dry food • By Nature Natural dry food • Dogswell Grain Free (cans)
Breast cancer metastasizes
2,500
Canned: Alpo, Beneful, Cesar, Pedigree, Mighty Dog, Purina One • Dried: Iams, Rachel Ray, Dogswell • Hill's Science Diet Ideal Balance Veggie Chips, all flavors/Jerky Treats, chicken & beef
Prostate cancer metastasizes • Common cold/ flu
2,000
Melanoma
1,500
Metastatic bone and lung cancer
1,000
Purina Puppy Chow • Biscuits: Milk Bone, Pedigree Jumbone, Kibbles 'n Bits, Sausages in a Blanket
500
Carob Dog Treats such as: Bark Bars, Pup Tarts, Poochie Sushi, Chocolick Cookies & Mints, etc.
50
Decay and Death
0
Measured in Bovis Units of Life Force Energy

The Pet Food Industry

Pet food sales have soared by 85 percent over the past decade and with rapidly expanding foreign markets, the U.S. market is now worth $15 billion a year. According to Born Free, a national animal advocacy organization, the pet food market is now dominated by large companies who have gobbled up smaller companies leaving only a few players in the field, mostly gigantic multinational corporations. These multinationals are basically recycling by-products from the human processed food industry into ingredients for pet food, which provides a convenient way for slaughterhouse offal, grains unfit for human consumption, and similar waste products to be not only utilized, but turned into a profit. From a business standpoint, this makes a lot of sense, but it's hardly a healthy choice for the pets who eat these products.

The Pet Food Institute, the trade association of pet food manufacturers, has acknowledged that the use of by-products in pet foods accounts for important additional income for food processors and farmers: "The growth of the pet food industry not only provided pet owners with better foods for their pets, but also created profitable additional markets for American farm products and for the by-products of the meat packing, poultry, and other food industries which prepare food for human consumption."

Your pet food many have a friendly name like Friskies, a refined name like Pedigree, or a high-falutin' name like Eukanuba, but in fact they are basically the same product. Many companies that sell pet food do not actually make the food themselves, but instead give their formulation, or recipe, to manufacturers. The manufacturer mixes ingredients according to the recipes to make a wide variety of pet foods for companies to sell under many different brand names. Private labelers who make food for "house" brands like Kroger and Wal-Mart, and "co-packers" who produce food for other pet food makers, are also major pet food producers. Three major companies are Doane Pet Care, Diamond, and Menu Foods; they produce food for dozens of private label and brand names, and, significantly, all three of these companies have been involved in pet food recalls that sickened or killed many pets.

Here is the current multi-national line-up in pet food companies: Nestlé's bought Purina to form Nestlé Purina Petcare Company (Fancy Feast, Alpo, Friskies, Mighty Dog, Dog Chow, Cat Chow, Puppy Chow, Kitten Chow, Beneful, One, ProPlan, DeliCat, HiPro, Kit 'n' Kaboodle, Tender Vittles, Purina Veterinary Diets). Del Monte bought Heinz (Meow Mix, Gravy Train, Kibbles 'n Bits, Wagwells, 9Lives, Cycle, Skippy, Nature's Recipe, and pet treats Milk Bone, Pup-Peroni, Snausages, Pounce). MasterFoods owns Mars, Inc., which consumed Royal Canin (Pedigree, Waltham's, Cesar, Sheba, Temptations, Goodlife Recipe, Sensible Choice, Excel). Procter and Gamble purchased The Iams Company (Iams, Eukanuba) in 1999, and Colgate-Palmolive bought Hill's Science Diet in 1976 (Hill's Science Diet, Prescription Diets, Nature's Best).

What Exactly is in Commercial Pet Food, or Are We Afraid to Ask?

The protein used in pet food comes from a variety of sources. When cattle, swine, chickens, lambs, or other animals are slaughtered, the lean muscle tissue is reserved for human consumption, along with select organs such as tongues and tripe. Whatever remains of the carcass is used to make pet food—this includes heads, feet, bones, blood, intestines, lungs, spleens, livers, ligaments, fat trimmings and other parts not generally consumed by humans. This waste also can include intestines, udders, heads, hooves, and possibly diseased and cancerous animal parts, and are known as "by-products." These are also used in feed for poultry and livestock as well as in fertilizer, industrial lubricants, soap, rubber, and other products. So-called "4D" animals (dead, dying, diseased, disabled), which were recently banned for human consumption, are still legitimate ingredients for pet food.

Meat meals, poultry meals, by-product meals, and meat-and-bone meal are common ingredients in pet foods because they cost less than fresh meat. Just about all varieties of canned and dried dog and cat food have an ingredient like "chicken by-product meal" listed on the label. The term "meal" means the product has been made from rendered parts derived from slaughtered animals. To render this material into meal, the raw materials are dumped into a large vat and boiled for several hours. Rendering separates the fat, removes water, and kills bacteria, viruses, parasites, and other organisms. But the high temperature pretty much destroys the natural enzymes and proteins found in the raw ingredients and the resulting altered proteins can contribute to food allergies and inflammatory bowel disease. Vitamins and preservatives are added to the food, and many pet food brands also add artificial colors and flavors in an attempt to make the product food look and taste better.

Grains such as corn and wheat are added to canned and dry pet food as a bulking agent as they are cheaper than animal protein, but dogs and cats did not evolve to eat grains—they are carnivores and do best on a meat-based diet. Wheat gluten is used to create shapes like slices, cuts, bites, chunks, and shreds, and as a thickener for gravy. The amount of grain and vegetable products used in pet food has risen dramatically over time, but a diet based on grains leads to allergies, diabetes, obesity and other disorders in these pets, and especially in cats, which really do need an all-meat diet.

The Dangers of Dry Food

Because the ingredients for dried pet foods are highly processed and cooked twice—first during rendering and again in the extruder—they are far more unhealthy than canned pet foods.

Comparative Vibrational Levels of Health and Disease States	Bovis Units	Comparative Nutritional Levels of Food for Cats
10,000 = Level of Optimal Health e.g. a healthy newborn baby / hunter/gatherer tribes	10,000	Organic meat, poultry, fish & vegetables • Quality organic canned food such as Newman's Own, Life's Abundance, Darwin's Natural
	9,500	Harmony Farms canned, all flavors
	9,000	
	8,500	
	8,000	
	7,500	
	7,000	By Nature Organics canned food
	6,500	Harmony Farms Chicken and Brown Rice dry food
AVERAGE LEVEL OF HEALTH IN USA		
Inflammation	6,000	Harmony Farms Indoor Cat Formula dry food
Arthritis starts to manifest	5,500	
Heart Disease starts to manifest	5,000	Hill's Science Diet Liver & Chicken, canned
Cancer cells form: Breast, Prostate, Lung, Colon, Pancreas	4,500	Hill's Science Diet Savory Seafood Entree, canned
Diabetes • Osteoporosis	4,000	By Nature Grain Free, canned • By Nature Organics dry food, chicken
Lymphoma • Leukemia • Dementia	3,500	By Nature Weight Control dry food
Congestive heart disease Brain cancer • Multiple sclerosis	3,000	Dry food: The Good Life • Hill's Science Diet, and Optimal Care Ocean Fish & Rice
Breast cancer metastasizes	2,500	
Prostate cancer metastasizes • Common cold/ flu	2,000	*Cans:* Authority, AvoDerm, Blue Buffalo, Eukanuba, Fancy Feast, Iams, Innova, Meow Mix, Nutro Max, Nutro Natural Choice, Purina Friskies/ONE, Royal Canin, Science Diet, SophistaCat, Wellness, Whiskas
Melanoma	1,500	Nutro Max dry food
Metastatic bone and lung cancer	1,000	*Dry:* Authority, AvoDerm, Blue Buffalo, Eukanuba, Fancy Feast, Iams, Innova, Meow Mix, Nutro Max, Nutro Natural Choice, Purina Friskies/ONE, Royal Canin, Science Diet, SophistaCat, Wellness, Whiskas
	500	Dry: AvoDerm, Blue Buffalo, Iams, Max Cat, Wellness Indoor, Friskies Party Mix
	50	
Decay and Death	0	

Arrow labels: BETTER HEALTH (upward) / WORSENING HEALTH (downward)

Measured in Bovis Units of Life Force Energy

Most dry pet foods contain large amounts of cereal grain or starchy vegetables to provide texture. Corn and wheat gluten meals are high-protein extracts from which most of the carbohydrate has been removed and are often used to boost protein percentages without using expensive animal-source ingredients. The vast majority of dry food is made with a machine called an extruder. Materials such as corn meal, wheat flour, rendered meat-and-bone-meal, poultry by-product meal, grains and flours are blended together to make a dough. This dough is then subjected to steam and high pressure as it is pushed through differently shaped dies. The food is allowed dry, and is then sprayed with rendered fats to make it more palatable. The fat also acts as a binding agent to which manufacturers add other flavor enhancers such as "animal digests," which are made from rendered animal or vegetable fats and oils deemed inedible for humans, such as used restaurant grease. Pet food manufacturers are skilled at enticing dogs and cats to eat something they would normally turn up their noses at, and these sprayed fats are engineered to be appealing to animals.

Animals may find that these foods taste appealing, but they are not good for their health, especially for cats. Research has linked dry cat food with urinary problems, and it is now considered to be the cause of feline diabetes. Vet and pet nutritionist Lisa Pierson says: "Chronic kidney disease is one of the main causes of death in cats and is often caused because they are chronically dehydrated by just eating dried food. Even if they drink water, often it is not enough to ensure optimum urinary health. For example, it is for hard for cats to digest the carbohydrate. Most importantly, processed food also sits like a sludge on their teeth."

Toxins in Pet Foods

Problems with processed pet foods have occurred from reactions to additives and as a result of contamination with bacteria, mold, drugs, and other toxins. In March 2007, the most lethal pet food that has ever found its way onto the market was the subject of a huge pet-food recall. Menu Foods recalled more than 100 brands, including Iams, Eukanuba, Hill's Science Diet, Purina Mighty Dog, and many store brands including Walmart's. Thousands of pets were sickened (the FDA received more than 17,000 reports) and an estimated 20 percent of affected pets died from acute renal failure caused by the food. Cats were more frequently and more severely affected than dogs. The toxin was initially believed to be a pesticide, the rat poison "aminopterin" in one of the ingredients, but shortly afterwards, scientists discovered high levels of melamine, a chemical used in plastics and fertilizers, in wheat gluten and rice protein concentrate imported from China. The melamine had been purposely added to the ingredients to falsely boost their protein content. Subsequent tests revealed that the melamine-tainted ingredients had also been used in feed for cows, pigs, and chickens and thousands of animals were quarantined and destroyed. Scientists identified the cause of the rapid onset kidney disease that had appeared in dogs and cats as a reaction caused by the combination of melamine and cyanuric acid, both unauthorized chemicals.

Pentobarbital, a drug frequently used to euthanize pets, has also allegedly been found in pet food. In an article on AlterNet entitled "Why is the pet food industry killing our pets?" the author, Ann Martin, writes that she was able to trace euthanized pets to a rendering plant, but the FDA reports that no dog or cat DNA was found there. Instead, they say that "the pentobarbital residues are entering pet food from euthanized, rendered cattle and even horses."

She writes, "As our veterinary bills mount, we have been brainwashed by the industry to think that if we feed our pets human food, we will be causing them great harm. While it is not recommended to include your pets in your junk food habits, there is no harm in sharing a well-balanced diet with your pet. You wouldn't want to eat food from the same bag every day, so don't force your pets to do just that."

When you love your pet, it makes no sense to expose him or her to these kinds of risks, so the best choice for your pet is to purchase organic pet food, or make your own at home.

Conflicts of Interest in the Veterinary Profession

With the processed pet food they often recommend so obviously unhealthy for animals, you wonder if veterinarians learn anything about nutrition at college. And in fact they do, but it appears that the veterinary industry is inextricably linked to the pet-food manufacturers. At veterinary colleges, lectures on nutrition are often paid for, and even taught, by representatives from these huge corporations, giving them a captive audience for the "benefits" of their products, and the training of veterinarians at some colleges is also funded by pet-food manufacturers. Most often when you visit an animal doctor's office you will see advertising placards for pet foods which they will prescribe for your pet and sell to you then and there. So it's hardly in these veterinarian's financial interest to promote a more natural diet for pets. And, if we want to be really cynical, we can consider the fact that poor quality food makes for an unhealthy animal, and a healthy pet doesn't make much money for the veterinarian's office.

The Best Food for your Dogs and Cats

Dogs and cats are carnivores and need a meat-based diet. Cats in their wild state will catch and kill their own prey, eating the entire animal or bird—meat, bones, intestinal tract and offal. Dogs by nature are scavengers and so are more adaptable when it comes to diet. While dogs and cats have been domesticated for thousands of years, a dog is still 99 percent related to the wolf, and a pet cat's digestive system is basically no different from a wild lion's.

As scavenging carnivores, dogs are more omnivorous than cats, but grains are not a part of their natural diet. Corn, wheat and soy have been shown to cause allergies in dogs. Meat is the most important nutrient for a dog, but only if the meat source is free of hormones, antibiotics and steroids. Dogs can survive on a plant-based diet, but cannot THRIVE on one. Dogs have no flat molars because nature didn't intend for them to eat plants, and they have an expandable stomach that enables them to hold large quantities of meat and bone. Dr. Karen Becker, an integrative wellness veterinarian, strongly believes that dogs need to be fed a meat-based diet and has expressed concern about a new brand of vegetarian dog food on the market. She writes, "If you can't tolerate the thought of feeding meat to a pet who is a carnivore, I strongly encourage you to acquire a pet that will thrive on a plant-based diet instead."

Consumption of processed foods has also been linked to poor behavior in dogs, and there are studies showing improvements in health and behavior following a change from a processed food diet to a raw food diet in both dogs and cats. It is simple to make nutritious food at home for pets using quality meats and vegetables. There are recipes on the Internet, but many recommend a diet of 30 percent grain, while most pet-care experts say that 15 percent is healthier. The only grains that are safe to feed a dog are small quantities of cooked organic oats and brown rice.

Hall of Shame

Pedigree products

On the home page of the Pedigree website is blazoned:

"At Pedigree we believe in putting dogs and their needs first." But in fact we all know that as a multinational corporation, they put profits first. "Every dog deserves leading nutrition," says Pedigree.

That is true, but they are not going to get it in a can of Pedigree. It's all marketing propaganda. A can of PEDIGREE® Healthy Longevity Food for Dogs contains a mixture of corn, chicken by-products, wheat, corn gluten, and rendered animal fat, laced with preservatives, chemical vitamins and added colorings. It's neither healthy nor going to give your dog longevity, quite the opposite in fact.

Contents of PEDIGREE® Healthy Longevity Food for Dogs: Ground Yellow Corn, Chicken By-Product Meal, Brewers Rice, Ground Whole Wheat, Corn Gluten Meal, Animal Fat (Preserved with BHA and Citric Acid), Lamb, Plain Dried Beet Pulp, Vegetable Oil (Source of Linoleic Acid), Natural Flavor, Salt, Potassium Chloride, Calcium Carbonate, Monocalcium Phosphate, Fish Oil (Preserved with Mixed Tocopherols, a Source of Vitamin E), Vitamins (dl-Alpha Tocopherol Acetate [Source of Vitamin E], Choline Chloride, L-Ascorbyl-2-Polyphosphate [Source of Vitamin C*], Vitamin A Acetate, Thiamine Mononitrate [Vitamin B1], Biotin, d-Calcium Pantothenate, Riboflavin Supplement [Vitamin B2], Vitamin D3 Supplement, Vitamin B12 Supplement), Dried Vegetables (Peas, Carrots), Minerals (Zinc, Sulfate, Zinc Proteinate, Copper Sulfate, Copper Proteinate, Manganese Proteinate, Potassium Iodide), Added FD&C Colors (Yellow 6, Yellow 5, Blue 2). Pedigree is made by Master Foods/Mars. Inc.

Pedigree has recently announced they have designed a new specially-shaped kibble biscuit that removes plaque from teeth. Plaque on the teeth of animals gets there in the first place by eating processed pet food! Contrary to the myth propagated by pet food companies, dry food is not good for animals' teeth, and given that the vast majority of pets eat dry food, yet the most common health problem in pets is dental disease, this should be obvious.

Food for Domestic Dogs & Cats

The Bottom Line

THE GOOD: Fresh meat, poultry, fish, eggs and vegetables, organic if possible • Small wild animals, such as mice • Some organic and high-quality canned foods, such as Newman's Own Organic, Life's Abundance, Darwin's Natural, Harmony

THE NOT-SO-BAD: Small amounts of organic oats and brown rice

THE DOWNRIGHT DANGEROUS: Most processed animal foods, canned and dried, and treats/biscuits

Never feed your pets: alcohol, apple pips, avocado, caffeine, chocolate, dough, garlic, grapes, milk, mushrooms, onions, potato peels, raisins, sugar, or white bread.

Appreciation goes to www.BornFreeUSA.org and Dr. Michael W. Fox for some of the information used in this chapter.

CHAPTER 31

How Our Emotions Affect our Health

"Emotional health is absolutely essential to your physical health and healing—no matter how devoted you are to the proper diet and lifestyle, you will not achieve your body's ideal healing and preventative powers if emotional barriers stand in your way."

—*Dr. Joseph Mercola, founder of the World's No. 1 Natural Health Website www.mercola.com*

AS THE CHART OPPOSITE DEMONSTRATES, our thoughts and emotions have a powerful effect on our health, both positively and negatively. We all are aware of how elated we can feel when things are going well in our life, and how down we can feel when they aren't going so well. But beyond these reactions to life's events, we also have feelings about ourselves—about our self-worth, whether people like us, whether we feel we are making a positive contribution to the world, or the feeling that we lack a sense of purpose or direction in life—and sometimes these feelings can be very deep-seated.

Our feelings represent our reactions to who we are and what we choose to do in life, and give us clues to what's working and what's not. In a sense, our feelings are our compass, guiding us in making the right choices so we can be sure we are heading in the right direction. If we ignore or suppress our feelings, we will not be able to access this crucial information, and the level of un-ease we feel will quickly turn into dis-ease.

Conscious Feelings

Sometimes our negative feelings will be *conscious,* but we choose to ignore them. Negative feelings can be frightening; many of us are not taught how to handle them when we are young. And we may feel "bad" that we have them in the first place. But we will also find that when we ignore our feelings, they become repressed and then reappear in the most unexpected ways and places; we find ourselves suddenly bursting into tears at a board meeting, or exploding in anger when our four-year-old asks a simple question. But a more significant way that repressed emotions can appear is through disease. Most of us will have had friends or relatives who've faced a life-threatening disease and heard them say that it was a "wake-up call" and because of it, they were inspired to change their life, to finally make those changes that seemed so impossible *before* the health crisis.

Unconscious Feelings

Some people are completely unaware of how they feel. They find it more convenient that way, so not only do they not have to *feel* the feelings, they also don't feel bad about having them in the first place—they just don't exist! This is the most dangerous emotional condition since the more out of touch we are from our feelings, the more our feelings and emotions will run our lives unconsciously. We may find ourselves in life situations where we are desperately unhappy without really understanding why and feel powerless to do anything about it, such as being in the wrong career, married to the wrong person, or living in a partnership with a person of the "wrong" gender, which, sadly, is more common than you can possibly imagine.

Suppressed Truths

One psychological cause of disease, especially cancer, is what I call the Repressed Inconvenient Truth (RIT). This is a truth so huge that to accept it would turn someone's life upside down. In fact, some people would rather die than face

Comparative Vibrational Levels of Health and Disease States		How Our Emotions Affect Our Health
10,000 = Level of Optimal Health e.g. a healthy newborn baby / hunter/gatherer tribes	10,000	Bliss • Compassion • Contentment • Ecstasy • Empathy • Enthusiasm • Gratitude • Meditation • Prayer
	9,500	Reverence
BETTER HEALTH	9,000	Affection • Altruism • Caring for others • Forgiveness • Joy • Laughter • Love • Optimism • Serenity
	8,500	
	8,000	Happiness • Hopefulness • Satisfaction
	7,500	
	7,000	Trust
	6,500	Conscientiousness • Responsibility
AVERAGE LEVEL OF HEALTH IN USA Inflammation	6,000	Gossip • Infatuation
Arthritis starts to manifest	5,500	Anger
Heart Disease starts to manifest	5,000	Complaining • Dependence
Cancer cells form: Breast, Prostate, Lung, Colon, Pancreas	4,500	Irritation
Diabetes • Osteoporosis	4,000	Criticism • Feelings of impotence • Grief • Judgmentalism • Regret • Worry
Lymphoma • Leukemia • Dementia	3,500	Boredom • Disappointment • Envy • Guilt • Humiliation • Pride
Congestive heart disease Brain cancer • Multiple sclerosis	3,000	Blame • Bullying • Fear • Hostility • Regret • Negativity
Breast cancer metastasizes	2,500	Hatred • Scorn
Prostate cancer metastasizes • Common cold/ flu	2,000	Apathy • Anxiety • Betrayal • Bitterness • Contempt • Pessimism • Repressed Inconvenient Truth
Melanoma	1,500	Depression • Jealousy • Rage
Metastatic bone and lung cancer	1,000	Despair • Hopelessness • Loathing • Obsession • Shame
	500	Cravings • Revulsion
	50	Evil thoughts • Planning evil deeds • Fury
Decay and Death	0	

(Arrow labels: BETTER HEALTH upward; WORSENING HEALTH downward)

Measured in Bovis Units of Life Force Energy

their truth. I have seen this so many times—a person who has a RIT they cannot accept about themselves will get sick and very often cannot be cured, no matter what treatment they have. The main RITs I have come across have to do with work and relationships. Karl was a surgeon but hated his profession; for financial reasons he did not feel he could change his career. Eventually, he contracted pancreatic cancer, which claimed his life. Tim didn't love his wife, but they were pillars of the community and church; he felt trapped, but just couldn't admit that he had "failed" in his marriage. He died of prostate cancer. George was married to a wonderful woman but perplexed his family and friends by trying to seduce everything on his radar screen wearing a skirt. He could not accept that fact that, in his heart, he realized he was homosexual; he died of colon cancer. Mary was very much involved with her family, raising her two sons, and insisted she loved her husband, even though deep in her heart she realized she would be happier living with a woman. She eventually died after a long battle with breast cancer

This is the incredible power that suppressing the truth has on our psyche. Each one of us has a crucial role to play in this complex drama we call Life. We need to be free to be who we are, otherwise we are not contributing all that we can and should be. Truly being who we are and being the best that we can be are good not just for ourselves and our community, but also for society at large and for the multi-celled organism that is the human race. When an individual is deprived of this opportunity to blossom into who they *really are* because they feel they cannot express themselves fully, often because someone close to them is prejudiced, then we all lose.

Feeling Our Feelings

Another problem with suppressing our negative feelings is that we run the risk of suppressing ALL our feelings, the positive ones too. And these are life-affirming. Laughter calibrates at 9,000. You cannot get sick if you laugh! But you will most assuredly get sick if you get stuck in a negative emotion. The idea is to FEEL our feelings, experience them, and then let them move out of our bodies. An e-motion is energy in motion. We sob when we are sad, laugh when we are happy, shake when we are angry, shiver when we are frightened, tense up when we are startled.

We all need to learn to experience a negative emotion, observing it work its way through our body, and then *letting it go.* Learning to do this, consciously observing the process, will give us confidence that next time we have a negative emotion, we can open ourselves up to experiencing it, letting it work its way through our body, and know that our sunny disposition will eventually return. Remaining "stuck" in anger or fear or guilt will only cause illness in the long-run. Many people learned to suppress their emotions during childhood, a time in our lives when we feel so vulnerable. But this little exercise, of observing the emotions as they move through us, helps break that pattern. Remember the story of the Velveteen Rabbit? That's how he became "real"—by shedding a tear of sorrow and thereby learning how to experience emotions.

Conversely, consciously focusing on nurturing emotions that are "above the line" means we will stay healthy. In Norman Cousins' book, *Anatomy of an Illness*, he describes how he cured himself of ankylosing spondylitis by checking himself out of hospital and into a hotel room and spending the next couple of weeks watching comedies and literally laughing himself back to health. Since then—that was in 1964—a large amount of research has been done on the effects of emotions on our health.

But this method will only work with people who WANT to get well. We have to accept that everyone is on their own personal journey and there are some people, especially those with Repressed Inconvenient Truths, who, at the soul level, may not want to get well—they may subconsciously want to "check out" of life. They may not be able to accept their own personal truth at the deepest level, and although they will fight valiantly to "cure" their illness, in their hearts it's not what they want.

Encouraging Positive Emotions

So how can we encourage more positive emotions, such as reverence, compassion, gratitude and joy, in our lives? Most people agree that helping others is a sure way to feel positive emotions. We feel good about ourselves because we are focusing more on others and doing something they are grateful for. "Giving is better than receiving," we are told, and it is so true. Another saying is that having "an attitude of gratitude" is bound to lift you higher. The reverence that we experience at the wonders of nature or in a place of worship, or at some group event that stirs our heart, has the same effect. It would make sense, then, to encourage these moments in our lives and try to limit the experiences that cause stress and the more negative emotions, such as irritation, frustration, fear, and anger. If we are unhappy at work, or the morning commute drives us nuts, or we just can't stand our spouse, be aware that these unaddressed emotions act as powerful irritants to the psyche and can cause serious disease. So don't wait until after the wake-up call to re-arrange your life so it works *for you,* do it now before serious illness sets in.

It was when my closest friend contracted breast cancer in the mid 1980s and I witnessed all that she went through that I decided I would learn the life-lessons, the wake-up call, she was being given—but without, hopefully, ever having to have cancer myself, or like her, losing my life to that disease.

One method that helps release and control emotions is the Emotional Freedom Technique, or EFT, a psychological acupressure technique which is often recommended by physicians to optimize emotional health. EFT is a form of psychological acupressure, based on the same energy meridians used in traditional acupuncture, but without the use of needles. A combination of tapping the energy meridian points on the body while saying positive affirmations helps to clear emotional blocks from the body's bioenergy system. This system is now used around the world.

Our Thoughts Affect our Health

Our thoughts, too, have been found to dramatically affect our health. In fact, recent research shows that our mind basically cannot tell the difference between what we tell it and what is reality. Imagine that—our thoughts are so powerful that we literally create our own reality. This is a phenomenon that quantum mechanics has demonstrated with Max Planck's particle-wave duality. So we must remember to use our thoughts wisely. Sending peace and love out into the world is a very productive thing to do; complaining about how violent and depressing the world is right now, with the "we've all gone to hell in a handbasket" type of thought, is sending out a negative message.

It's good to aim whenever possible to have positive thoughts: "I am so blessed. This is such a beautiful world. So many people are doing good things to make the world a better place. I am so grateful to live in a free country, to have a roof over my head and food on the table. I have everything I need. I am in perfect health. I attract abundance into my life." My favorite is, "Everything is as it should be; everything is in Divine order." Having these kinds of thoughts will attract health and abundance into our lives and resonate out into the world.

CHAPTER 32

How Our Surroundings Affect our Health

OUR ENVIRONMENT AFFECTS US MUCH MORE than most people realize. All things vibrate with energy, and this includes the earth and the things we surround ourselves with, from buildings to furniture to clothing. They all have an impact on the delicate electrical workings of the body, so any interference in the electrical field around us can influence us in different ways, affecting our mood, our physical body, and even our thinking process.

As can be seen in the chart on the opposite page, the quality of our environment can vary greatly depending upon where we are—being surrounded by nature is much healthier for us than being in public buildings, such as schools, hospitals and airports, for instance. We can simply be sensitive to the different kinds of energy given off by some places, such as the hushed atmosphere of an ancient church or the hustle and bustle of a busy department store, or we might be affected by other energies that are echoes from the past, as in old houses, antique shops, and places of worship. But whatever the cause, places with a powerful energy field can affect us all. Sensitive people are often more aware of this phenomenon and can pick up energy vibrations in any place or situation, from the chaos of a railway station at rush-hour to the peace of the countryside; many cannot live in cities because of this extreme sensitivity, and prefer to live and work in places where they are surrounded by nature. At the other end of the spectrum are people who live and/or work in a high-rise building and daily walk city streets on asphalt pavement, which is just about as unnatural a life as you can get. People who live and work in this kind of environment can benefit from being out in nature as much as they are able.

According to Clinton Ober, Stephen T. Sinatra, M.D., and Martin Zucker, authors of the book *Earthing*, we humans evolved having a continuous connection to the earth. They describe the earth as an "electrical planet that pulsates with primordial natural energies," making it in essence a vast battery that is charged by various sources, such as lightning, solar radiation, and heat from its molten core. The energy that emanates from the earth nourishes us and heals us, but only if we are in direct contact with it. As early human beings, we evolved walking barefoot on the ground and slept close to the earth on natural materials like straw, heather, moss, or animal skins—materials that allowed the earth's energy to pass through them. When we began to wear leather shoes, we were still connected to the earth since leather is a natural substance, but the adoption of rubber and composite soles meant that this connection was severed and we became cut off from this vital energy due to our insulated shoes.

"Exposure to the ground provides an electrical 'nutrient' in the form of electrons," write the authors in their book. They believe that "earthing" protects the body's delicate bio-electrical circuitry against static electrical charges and interferences, and facilitates the reception of free electrons and stabilizing electrical signals from the earth. Since there is more electromagnetic activity around us now than ever before, it's been found to be beneficial for us to connect directly to the earth whenever possible—work in your garden with bare hands, lie on the grass, go barefoot when you can, walk on the beach, hug a tree or a pet. More suggestions about how we can connect to the earth can be found in the book.

Just becoming aware of the positive and negative effects that the environment has on your mood is a step in the right direction. If you find you are becoming irritable in a department store, depressed in a municipal building, or airport, or under fluorescent lighting at work, it may be because you are being affected by the energy around you. An environment that affects you negatively can cause physical ills and depression, and when combined with a poor diet can lead to serious illness.

Comparative Vibrational Levels of Health and Disease States	Bovis Units	How Our Surroundings Affect Our Health
10,000 = Level of Optimal Health e.g. a healthy newborn baby / hunter/gatherer tribes	10,000	Lying on the beach or grass • walking barefoot • gardening with bare hands • swimming or paddling in salt water, fresh pond water, or river water • being in direct sunshine
	9,500	
BETTER HEALTH	9,000	Walking in the woods in sneakers • gardening with gloves on • living in a stone or brick house
	8,500	Interior of the average health food store • Swimming in a chlorinated pool, outdoors
	8,000	Living in an uninsulated wooden house
	7,500	Walking on a city sidewalk • Living in an insulated wooden house
	7,000	Being in a Whole Foods Market grocery store
	6,500	Checking in at the average international airport • Being in a Trader Joe's grocery store • Living in a wooden house with vinyl siding
AVERAGE LEVEL OF HEALTH IN USA		
WORSENING HEALTH		
Inflammation	6,000	Swimming in a chlorinated pool, indoors • average Starbucks cafe • 42nd Street, New York City
Arthritis starts to manifest	5,500	Being in an office in a high-rise building in a major US city • average high school
Heart Disease starts to manifest	5,000	Being in the average supermarket, or average "big box" store: Home Depot, Macy's, Bed & Bath
Cancer cells form: Breast, Prostate, Lung, Colon, Pancreas	4,500	Being in a K-Mart store, or a McDonald's, Burger King, KFC or Wendy's fast-food outlet
Diabetes • Osteoporosis	4,000	Going through airport security at Logan Airport • being in an average city hospital
Lymphoma • Leukemia • Dementia	3,500	Average rural courthouse
Congestive heart disease Brain cancer • Multiple sclerosis	3,000	Average dry cleaning store/carpet store • average city courthouse/hospital emergency room
Breast cancer metastasizes	2,500	
Prostate cancer metastasizes • Common cold/ flu	2,000	Average county jail
Melanoma	1,500	Maximum security prison
Metastatic bone and lung cancer	1,000	
	500	
	50	
Decay and Death	0	

Measured in Bovis Units of Life Force Energy

A Final Word

BY NOW IT SHOULD BE CLEAR THAT BY CHOOSING FOOD of the highest vibrational level, we will resonate with good health. Imagine not having to worry about being ill! No more visits to the doctor or painful medical tests! Likewise, we can choose a healthy environment for ourselves at home and at work, surrounded by supportive, sane people so we are living and working in a safe and calm atmosphere.

There are four important factors that I measure on the same scale as the charts in this book when I see clients for nutritional consulting or a medical intuitive reading:

1. Level of general physical health
2. Quality of nutritional intake
3. Level of emotional health
4. Quality of environment at home and at work

Just like food and diseases, these can calibrate anywhere from a high of 10,000 to a low of 0, but for a person to be healthy and happy, all four need to be "above the line," and as close to 10,000 as possible for optimal health and happiness. Anyone can learn to calibrate these levels for themselves—the method is clearly described by Dr. David Hawkins in his amazing book *Power vs. Force*.

Our physical health can be affected by our emotions and by our surroundings, but it is what we eat that has the most impact on our general health. It is important that we learn to pay attention to what we eat—we are all different, and we each need to find out what kind of food and what kind of eating schedule suits us best. Food is meant to make us *feel good*, so we feel full of energy—"bright-eyed and bushy-tailed," eager to get out there and start the day—not groggy from a donut and a cup of sweetened coffee or from overdoing it the night before. If a particular food doesn't make us feel good, then we can cut it out of our diet for a while and try something else. Food is like high octane fuel for our body, and if we feed our body high quality fuel, it will run perfectly and won't break down. Illness is not inevitable—in most cases, it is the result of a choice, and the choice is ours.

Sources of Life Force Energy

These are the major sources of Life Force Energy available to us to nourish the body:

1. Food: Make sure the food you eat calibrates high on the nutrition chart.

2. Sunshine: Spend time outside every day, even in winter. Sunlight needs to reach your brain through your eyes to stimulate your endocrine system, so if you wear glasses or contact lenses, remove them for at least 20 minutes while you are outside (but of course do not look directly at the sun).

3. Water: Drink plenty of fresh spring water daily.

4. Earth: Be connected to the Earth whenever possible: lie on the beach or the grass, swim or paddle in salt or fresh water, garden with your hands in the dirt, hug a tree or an animal—or another person.

5. Air: It's important to breathe deeply and with awareness at some point during the day, preferably during a period of meditation or quiet sitting.

6. Energy Healing Modalities: Chiropractic, massage, homeopathy, hands-on healing, energy healing/Reiki, sound and color therapy, crystals, and flower essences can all increase vibrational levels in the body.

Recommended Reading

Books

"Ageless Body, Timeless Mind" by Deepak Chopra, MD

"Anti Cancer: A New Way of Life" by David Servan-Schreiber, MD, PhD

"The Basic Code of the Universe: The Science of the Invisible in Physics, Medicine, and Spirituality" by Massimo Citro, MD

"The Biology of Belief" by Bruce H. Lipton, PhD

"The Divining Hand" by Christopher Bird

"Colloidal Minerals and Trace Elements: How to Restore the Body's Natural Vitality" by Marie-France Muller MD, ND PhD

"Cross Currents: The Perils of Electropollution, The Promise of Electromedicine" by Dr. Robert O. Becker

"Earthing" by Clinton Ober, Stephen T. Sinatra, MD, and Martin Zucker

"Eat Right For Your Type" by Dr. Peter J. D'Adamo

"Energy Medicine: The Scientific Basis" by James L. Oschman, PhD

"Good Calories, Bad Calories: Challenging the Conventional Wisdom on Diet, Weight Control, and Disease" by Gary Taubes

"The Field: The Quest for the Secret Force of the Universe" by Lynne McTaggart

"Healing is Voltage: The Handbook" by Jerry Tennant, MD

"Light: Medicine of the Future" by Jacob Liberman, OD, PhD

"Morphic Resonance: The Nature of Formative Causation" by Rupert Sheldrake

"Nutrition and Physical Degeneration" by Weston A. Price, DDS

"The Omnivore's Dilemma" by Michael Pollan

"Optimal Digestive Health" edited by Trent W. Nichols, MD, and Nancy Faass, MSW, MPH

"The Perricone Prescription" by Nicholas Perricone, MD

"Points of Cosmic Energy" by Blanche Merz

"Power vs. Force: The Hidden Determinants of Human Behavior" by David Hawkins, MD, PhD

"A Practical Guide to Vibrational Medicine: Energy Healing and Spiritual Transformation" by Richard Gerber, MD

"Science and the Akashic Field: An Integral Theory of Everything" by Ervin Laszlo

"Science and Psychic Phenomena: The Fall of the House of Skeptics" by Chris Carter

"Science Set Free: 10 Paths to New Discovery" by Rupert Sheldrake

"The Seat of the Soul" by Gary Zukav

"The Secret Life of Plants" by Peter Tompkins and Christopher Bird

"Seeds of Deception: Exposing Industry and Government Lies About the Safety of the Genetically Engineered Foods You're Eating" by Jeffrey M. Smith

"Spontaneous Evolution" by Bruce H. Lipton, PhD, and Steve Bhaerman

"Sugar Blues" by William Dufty

"Sugar: The Bitter Truth" by Samantha Quinn

"Survival of the Sickest" by Dr. Sharon Moalem

"The True Power of Water" by Masaru Emoto

"Vibrational Medicine" by Richard Gerber, MD

"The Way of the Explorer" by Edgar Mitchell, PhD

"You Are What You Eat" by Victor Lindlahr

Newsletters and Websites

"Alternatives" newsletter by David Williams, PhD
www.drdavidwilliams.com

"Health Alert" newsletter by Dr. Bruce West
www.healthalert.com

"Real Cures" newsletter by Frank Schallenberger, MD
www.realcuresletter.com

"Nutrition & Healing" newsletter by Jonathan V. Wright, MD
www.wrightnewsletter.com

Dr. Joseph Mercola on-line newsletter
www.mercola.com